DSM-IV-TR Case Studies

A Clinical Guide to Differential Diagnosis

DSM-IV-TR Case Studies

A Clinical Guide to Differential Diagnosis

Allen Frances, M.D.
Chair, Task Force on DSM-IV
Professor of Psychiatry,
Duke University, Durham, North Carolina

Ruth Ross, M.A.
Science Editor, DSM-IV
Managing Editor,
Journal of Psychiatric Practice
Independence, Virginia

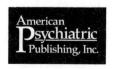

American Psychiatric Publishing, Inc.

Washington, DC
London, England

American Psychiatric Publishing, Inc.
1000 Wilson Boulevard
Arlington, VA 22209-3901
www.appi.org

Library of Congress Cataloging-in-Publication Data
Frances, Allen, 1942–
     DSM-IV-TR case studies : a clinical guide to differential diagnosis /
Allen Frances, Ruth Ross.
        p.   cm.
     Includes bibliographical references and index.
     ISBN 1-58562-049-1 (casebound). — ISBN 1-58562-055-6 (alk. paper)
     1. Diagnostic and statistical manual of mental disorders. 2. Mental
illness—Diagnosis—Case studies. 3. Diagnosis, Differential—
Case studies. I. Ross, Ruth 1952–   .   II. Diagnostic and statistical
manual of mental disorders, 4th ed., text revision. III. Title.
     [DNLM: 1. Mental Disorders—diagnosis—Case Report.
2. Diagnosis, Differential—Case Report. 3. Mental Disorders—
therapy—Case Report.   WM 40 F815d 2001]
     RC473.D54 F73   2001
     616.89'075—dc21
                                                          2001041368
British Library Cataloguing in Publication Data
A CIP record is available from the British Library.

To Vera, Craig, Stacey, and Bobby,
and to David, Emma, and Fred

Contents

Acknowledgments

We first want to acknowledge all those who made DSM-IV possible. Over a thousand people (and numerous professional organizations) worked on this project, including the DSM-IV Task Force, Work Groups, advisers and consultants, and the DSM-IV staff. We also want to acknowledge all those at the American Psychiatric Association and the American Psychiatric Press who worked so tirelessly on DSM-IV. Our special thanks go to Michael First, Harold Pincus, Thomas Widiger, Claire Reinberg, Pam Harley, Cindy Jones, Betty Collins, and Tammy Gentry.

Some of the case descriptions in this book are based on a series of columns in *Hospital and Community Psychiatry* edited by Allen Frances in the 1980s. These cases have been revised to more accurately illustrate the DSM-IV-TR diagnostic categories. We gratefully acknowledge the opportunity to use these columns and the contributions of the many clinicians who helped with them. We are also grateful to a number of experts who have shared their clinical experience with us specifically for this book: Daniel Buysse, M.D., C. Keith Conners, Ph.D., Richard Frances, M.D., Tana A. Grady, M.D., Harold Koenig, M.D., Ronald L. Martin, M.D., Katherine A. Phillips, M.D., Richard Rosenthal, M.D., Mary Soderstrom, M.D., Suzanne M. Sutherland, M.D., Fred Volkmar, M.D., and B. Timothy Walsh, M.D.

Finally, and most important, we would like to acknowledge the contribution of our patients to this endeavor. Without the life experience shared with them, this book would not have been possible.

Introduction

All clinicians quickly come to realize that we learn much more from our patients than from our teachers or from books. Although DSM-IV-TR, the text revision of DSM-IV, published in 2000, is very useful and informative, it is necessarily a dry book that cannot begin to capture the complexity of dealing with human lives and problems. The DSM-IV-TR diagnostic criteria are attempts to codify the great diversity of human emotional and behavioral problems. These criteria can help clinicians establish diagnoses, choose appropriate treatments, and communicate clearly with one another. But the wise clinician will never lose sight of the importance of clinical insight in evaluating actual people with all their symptoms and behaviors, talents and weaknesses, and loves and hates. It is the richness of human experience that makes therapeutic relationships so rewarding and endlessly diverse, and so impossible to capture within the construct of bloodless diagnostic criteria.

In this casebook, we hope to make DSM-IV-TR human—to bring to life dry diagnostic descriptions and criteria by using three-dimensional examples. We use the terms *case* and *casebook* reluctantly and only because they are the traditional way of describing this sort of undertaking. People are never merely "cases," and we dislike the implication that something as complex as human behavior can be adequately captured by a few pages of written description. We do hope these case descriptions will illustrate both the usefulness and the limitations of the DSM-IV-TR diagnostic criteria in a clinical setting. Although a necessary and important tool, DSM-IV-TR is not a substitute for the expert judgment that can be acquired only by experience on the front lines of clinical practice. We will stress the essential role of clinical judgment in diagnostic evaluation over and over again as we take you through the examples in this book.

Throughout this book we focus on the process of differential diagnosis—how to distinguish one disorder from another. On paper this seems deceptively easy to do—simply follow algorithms, decision trees, arrows, and little boxes. But, fortunately or unfortunately, depending on how you look at it, people don't fit so neatly into little boxes and diagnostic algorithms. Nobody's presentation is as cut-and-dried as the DSM-IV-TR criteria would lead one to believe. In clinical practice, boundary situations and multiple diagnoses are very common. The value of the case study method is that it provides an opportunity to see how clinical judgment can be applied to the complexity of the individual clinical situation. Please remember that the DSM-IV-TR criteria are no more than guidelines. You should not apply them in a rigid or "cookbook" fashion. For example, if a person's symptoms meet only four criteria for a disorder that by DSM-IV-TR definition requires the presence of five items, but those four items are present to a degree that is severely impairing, such a presentation would very likely warrant a diagnosis. In contrast, a presentation in which an individual's symptoms meet six criteria items, but only in a very mild way that does not appear to be causing any serious distress or impairment, would likely not require a diagnosis. Never forget to use your common sense. We hope that this book will help the reader gain an understanding of how we use DSM-IV-TR in actual clinical situations.

In revising *DSM-IV Case Studies* to reflect DSM-IV-TR, published in 2000, we have made some changes in criteria sets and case discussions to reflect relevant changes in criteria sets and text discussions in DSM-IV-TR. We also have updated some of the treatment discussions to reflect up-to-date information concerning medications and psychosocial interventions.

How to Use This Book

We wondered how best to structure this casebook and experimented with several different formats before arriving at the one that you will soon encounter. Because we hope to illustrate the use of DSM-IV-TR, we decided to follow its organizational pattern and the order of its chapters. We tried to be fairly comprehensive and provide case samples for most of the commonly encountered disorders discussed in DSM-IV-TR. The book ends with a final chapter titled "Test Yourself" in which we provide a number of fairly complex cases for you to consider, each accompanied by a brief discussion.

For the sake of convenience as a teaching tool, we have listed each example under a specific diagnostic category in the first 16 chapters of the book. The disadvantage of this organizational structure is that the reader may feel tipped off about the diagnosis by the location. A similar situation often occurs in clinical practice. Patients may come in with diagnostic labels, but these are often incorrect or misleading. Moreover, there are studies that show that clinicians tend to come to their first diagnostic conclusions within 3 or 4 minutes from the beginning of their interview with the patient. Although this can be helpful in generating a set of useful questions to confirm or disprove an initial impression, some clinicians reach premature closure and become too fixed on their first impressions. Always remember that your initial intuition can be wrong and that the diagnoses we propose here are only tentative—other possibilities must always be considered and may be correct. Even though a case is listed under Schizophrenia, this does not mean that Schizophrenia is the only possible diagnosis. We hope that you will read each case with a critical eye and an open mind and consider all of the alternatives.

In using this casebook, study the DSM-IV-TR and its criteria sets and try to figure out why we chose our diagnosis based on the criteria set. By doing this, you will gain greater familiarity with the symptoms that constitute each diagnosis. A good understanding of, and memory for, the symptoms that define the most commonly encountered diagnoses will help you to be a more empathic interviewer and a better diagnostician. For example, if you remember most of the symptoms of depression, you will be able to ask the appropriate questions that indicate to patients that you have extensive experience and keen insight into their problems. We hope that these case studies will add to your clinical experience and serve as easily remembered examples to help you recall the criteria sets and increase your ability to be a comprehensive and accurate interviewer.

To use this book most effectively, we recommend that you follow this procedure: Read the case, try to visualize the person, and decide what diagnosis you would initially consider and what alternatives are possible. Then read our suggested diagnosis, but do not accept it as necessarily correct. Review the criteria set that we think supports the diagnosis, and read our "Guidelines for Differential Diagnosis" to see whether our reasoning agrees with yours or how they differ. We have also included a few words on treatment for each diagnosis, because it is not much fun for us or useful for the patient to discuss diagnosis in isolation. Indeed the real importance of accurate diagnosis is the role it plays as a tool in treatment planning. Finally, we usually provide a "Summary" section at the end of each case or series of cases to highlight particularly pertinent points that merit special attention.

As an additional aid to understanding how clinical judgment can be applied to the DSM diagnoses, in Chapter 17, "Test Yourself," we provide more complicated cases that present intriguing diagnostic problems and are somewhat less clear-cut than the illustrative examples included in the first 16 chapters. Again, the best way to use this section of the book is to form your own conclusions about each of the presentations and read the pertinent DSM-IV-TR criteria sets before reviewing our diagnostic choices and supporting discussion.

Steps in Differential Diagnosis

The clinician should use six basic steps in evaluating symptoms and arriving at a differential diagnosis. Throughout this book, we discuss different aspects of these steps in more detail as they apply to specific presentations. Here we briefly outline the steps so that the reader can keep them in mind while reviewing all the cases in the book. To remind clinicians to include these considerations in their diagnostic evaluations, the DSM-IV-TR criteria often contain exclusion criteria that list diagnoses that need to be ruled out (e.g., when the symptoms are not caused by the direct physiological effects of a substance or a general medical condition).

Six Steps to Differential Diagnosis

1. **Rule out a substance-related etiology (e.g., a drug of abuse, a medication, or toxin exposure).**   Substance and medication use are ubiquitous in our society, and their role in causing psychopathology is frequently missed. This step involves taking a careful history and perhaps performing a physical examination and/or laboratory tests to discover whether a substance has been used. If so, the clinician must then ascertain whether an etiological relationship exists between the Substance Use and the psychiatric symptoms and what type of relationship it is. This involves evaluating temporal sequences by determining whether the psychiatric symptoms preceded Substance Use or developed soon after and whether the psychiatric symptoms persist or remit when Substance Use and Withdrawal effects cease. The clinician must also consider whether the nature, amount, and duration of the Substance Use are consistent with the type of psychiatric symptoms present.

2. **Rule out an etiology related to a general medical condition.**   This can be a difficult and complicated determination because the symptoms of some psychiatric disorders and general medical conditions can be identical, and some medical conditions (e.g., Parkinson's disease) can first present with psychiatric symptoms. General medical conditions can cause psychiatric symptoms through a direct physiological effect on the central nervous system (Mental Disorder Due to a General Medical Condition) or can cause symptoms such as depression or anxiety that are psychological reactions (Adjustment Disorder). Clinicians evaluating patients in a mental health setting need to be careful to consider etiologies related to general medical conditions, especially in patients with atypical presentations.

3. Determine the specific primary disorder that is present.   After ruling out etiologies related to Substance Use or a general medical condition, the clinician must determine which primary mental disorder best describes the presenting symptoms. DSM-IV-TR is organized by presenting symptoms (e.g., mood, anxiety, dissociative), and you should first review the diagnoses in the section that seems most applicable to ascertain which disorder best fits the presentation. DSM-IV-TR provides three types of assistance in this process:

1. The criteria sets for many of the disorders in the manual provide exclusion criteria that list other disorders with similar symptoms that need to be considered in the differential diagnosis (e.g., the G criterion for Social Phobia rules out fear or avoidance that is due to Panic Disorder With or Without Agoraphobia, Separation Anxiety Disorder, Body Dysmorphic Disorder, Pervasive Developmental Disorder, or Schizoid Personality Disorder).
2. The differential diagnosis section in the text for each disorder gives a detailed discussion of which other disorders should be considered and how to distinguish them.
3. Appendix A gives Decision Trees for Differential Diagnosis that alert the clinician to consider disorders in all pertinent sections when evaluating a certain type of symptom.

4. Differentiate Adjustment Disorder from Not Otherwise Specified.
If the symptoms do not meet criteria for a specific DSM-IV-TR diagnosis but the clinician judges that a mental disorder is present, either a diagnosis of Adjustment Disorder or the appropriate Not Otherwise Specified category should be considered. Adjustment Disorder is diagnosed if it is judged that the symptoms are a maladaptive response to a psychosocial stressor. If no stressor appears to be responsible for the symptoms, then the appropriate Not Otherwise Specified category can be diagnosed (e.g., impairing depressive symptoms that do not meet criteria for a specific Mood Disorder and do not appear to be the result of the effects of a stressor would be diagnosed as 311 Depressive Disorder Not Otherwise Specified).

5. Establish the boundary with no mental disorder.   Current psychiatric diagnosis includes many conditions that are close to the boundary with normality. For the clinician to decide that a mental disorder is present, the symptoms must be judged to cause clinically significant problems. For this reason, most criteria sets in DSM-IV-TR include the following criterion: "The disturbance causes clinically significant distress or impairment in social, occupational, or other important areas of functioning." The determination of what is "clinically significant" must be based on the clinician's own judgment and should take into account the individual's environment and cultural background. For example, a person with a specific phobia of snakes who lives in a city where snakes are almost nonexistent would not be considered to have clinically significant impairment because of the phobia. If the same person moves to an environment where snakes are common and finds it hard to function normally because of excessive fear of encountering a snake, the problem would be considered clinically significant and would warrant treatment as a mental disorder.

6.   Rule out Factitious Disorder or Malingering.   Unfortunately, clinicians are not particularly good at determining when patients are feigning or intentionally producing symptoms. To be productive, the therapeutic relationship between clinician and patient must be based on collaboration and trust. Nevertheless, clinicians must not be overly gullible, especially in settings in which patients might intentionally produce or feign symptoms (e.g.,prisons, courtrooms, disability hearings, and emergency rooms). When a patient produces or feigns symptoms to achieve an external goal (e.g., compensation from insurance companies, evading legal or military duties, or obtaining drugs), it is considered Malingering. When a patient produces or feigns symptoms not for external gain but to assume the sick role, the clinician should consider a diagnosis of Factitious Disorder.

The Multiaxial System

Each case presentation in this book is followed by our assessment of the DSM-IV-TR multiaxial diagnosis. To make the best possible treatment plan for a particular patient, the clinician needs to know not only what mental disorder(s) are present, but also whether general medical conditions exist that may influence the course of the mental disorder or its management, whether psychosocial or environmental stressors are affecting the patient, and the level at which the patient is currently functioning. The multiaxial diagnostic system, with its five axes, was developed to allow the clinician to record all these types of information in a concise format. The system prompts the clinician to evaluate for mental disorders, including Personality Disorders or maladaptive personality features, general medical conditions, psychosocial and environmental problems, and the level of functioning.

All mental disorders, including those problems listed in the DSM-IV-TR chapter for Other Conditions That May Be a Focus of Clinical Attention, are recorded on Axis I, with the exception of the Personality Disorders, Mental

Retardation, and Borderline Intellectual Functioning, which are coded on Axis II. Comorbid general medical conditions are specified on Axis III, and DSM-IV-TR includes a list of commonly used Axis III codes in Appendix G. Psychosocial and environmental problems that may affect the diagnosis, treatment, and prognosis of a mental disorder are noted on Axis IV (see box below).

☐   **Axis IV**   ☐
Psychosocial and Environmental Problems

Problems with primary support group
Problems related to the social environment
Educational problems
Occupational problems
Housing problems
Economic problems
Problems with access to health care services
Problems related to interaction with the legal system/crime
Other psychosocial and environmental problems

The Axis V Global Assessment of Functioning (GAF) Scale (see next page) provides a method for numerically rating the patient's level of psychological, social, and occupational functioning. This can help the clinician plan treatment and evaluate its effectiveness, as well as predict outcome. The scale is usually used to rate the patient's current level of functioning; however, in many cases, evaluating the highest level of functioning achieved over a longer period (e.g., over the past year) may also be useful. For most cases in this book, we provide a GAF rating for the patient's current level of functioning as well as the highest rating achieved during the past year.

Readers who would like more detail on how to use the GAF Scale are referred to DSM-IV-TR, which provides greatly expanded instructions for using the scale and outlines a 4-step method to ensure that no elements of the scale are overlooked when making a GAF rating.

Global Assessment of Functioning (GAF) Scale

Consider psychological, social, and occupational functioning on a hypothetical continuum of mental health–illness. Do not include impairment in functioning due to physical (or environmental) limitations.

Code   (**Note:**   Use intermediate codes when appropriate, e.g., 45, 68, 72.)

100 **Superior functioning in a wide range of activities, life's problems never seem | to get out of hand, is sought out by others because of his or her many positive** 91 **qualities. No symptoms.**

90 Absent or minimal symptoms (e.g., mild anxiety before an exam), **good function-** | **ing in all areas, interested and involved in a wide range of activities, socially effec-** | **tive, generally satisfied with life, no more than everyday problems or concerns** 81 (e.g., an occasional argument with family members).

80 **If symptoms are present, they are transient and expectable reactions to** | **psychosocial stressors** (e.g., difficulty concentrating after family argument); **no** | **more than slight impairment in social, occupational, or school functioning** (e.g., 71 temporarily falling behind in schoolwork).

70 Some mild symptoms (e.g., depressed mood and mild insomnia) **OR some diffi-** | **culty in social, occupational, or school functioning** (e.g., occasional truancy or | theft within the household), **but generally functioning pretty well; has some** 61 **meaningful interpersonal relationships.**

60 Moderate symptoms (e.g., flat affect and circumstantial speech, occasional panic | attacks) **OR moderate difficulty in social, occupational, or school functioning** 51 (e.g., few friends, conflicts with peers or co-workers).

50 Serious symptoms (e.g., suicidal ideation, severe obsessional rituals, frequent | shoplifting) **OR any serious impairment in social, occupational, or school func-** 41 **tioning** (e.g., no friends, unable to keep a job).

40 Some impairment in reality testing or communication (e.g., speech is at times illog- | ical, obscure, or irrelevant) **OR major impairment in several areas, such as work or** | **school, family relations, judgment, thinking, or mood** (e.g., depressed man avoids | friends, neglects family, and is unable to work; child frequently beats up younger 31 children, is defiant at home, and is failing at school).

30 Behavior is considerably influenced by delusions or hallucinations OR serious im- | pairment in communication or judgment (e.g., sometimes incoherent, acts grossly | inappropriately, suicidal preoccupation) **OR inability to function in almost all** 21 **areas** (e.g., stays in bed all day; no job, home, or friends).

20 Some danger of hurting self or others (e.g., suicide attempts without clear expecta- | tion of death; frequently violent; manic excitement) **OR occasionally fails to** | **maintain minimal personal hygiene** (e.g., smears feces) **OR gross impairment in** 11 **communication** (e.g., largely incoherent or mute).

10 Persistent danger of severely hurting self or others (e.g., recurrent violence) **OR** | **persistent inability to maintain minimal personal hygiene OR serious suicidal act** 1   **with clear expectation of death.**

0   Inadequate information.

We have tried to indicate how a wide variety of factors influence diagnostic evaluation and treatment planning in our discussions of the cases and in the multiaxial diagnoses we provide.

Final Thoughts

The DSM-IV-TR criteria sets are necessarily generic and are meant to capture what is common among patients. They apply across the developmental cycles (from children to the elderly), to males and females, and across different cultures. The fact that the criteria sets work as well as they do shows that people are in many ways more alike than they are different. However, all of us are unique, and the clinician must never lose sight of that individuality by trying to apply the diagnostic criteria in a rigid and mechanistic fashion. A strong reliance on clinical judgment and respect for the tremendous variations in human nature must form the foundation for any interpretation of the generic DSM-IV-TR criteria.

We hope that you enjoy learning from the patients described here and share our wonder at the privilege of clinical practice.

Chapter 1

Disorders Usually First Diagnosed in Infancy, Childhood, or Adolescence

DSM-IV-TR (American Psychiatric Association 2000) includes a section for disorders that are usually first diagnosed in infancy, childhood, or adolescence merely as a convenient method for organizing the manual. This can be misleading, however. The clinician should remember that many of the disorders listed in this section are often diagnosed in adulthood and that many disorders included in other sections of the manual (e.g., Major Depressive Disorder) may have their onset in childhood or adolescence. Therefore, every adult psychiatrist must be familiar with this section and every child psychiatrist must know the rest of the manual.

The following main categories of disorders are included in this section:

❖ Mental Retardation
❖ Learning Disorders
❖ Motor Skills Disorder
❖ Communication Disorders
❖ Pervasive Developmental Disorders
❖ Attention-Deficit and Disruptive Behavior Disorders
❖ Feeding and Eating Disorders of Infancy or Early Childhood
❖ Tic Disorders
❖ Elimination Disorders

❖ Other Disorders of Infancy, Childhood, or Adolescence (which include Separation Anxiety Disorder, Selective Mutism, Reactive Attachment Disorder of Infancy or Early Childhood, and Stereotypic Movement Disorder)

❖ Disorders of Infancy, Childhood, or Adolescence Not Otherwise Specified

We will present specific cases illustrating the following disorders: Autistic Disorder, Attention-Deficit/Hyperactivity Disorder, Disorder of Written Expression, Conduct Disorder, Tourette's Disorder, and Separation Anxiety Disorder. We will also discuss a number of the other disorders in the differential diagnostic sections of these case studies.

Pervasive Developmental Disorders

Pervasive Developmental Disorders

299.00   Autistic Disorder
299.80   Rett's Disorder
299.10   Childhood Disintegrative Disorder
299.80   Asperger's Disorder
299.80   Pervasive Developmental Disorder Not Otherwise Specified

Autistic Disorder

❖ Case Study: Strange Behaviors in a
Teenager With Developmental Disorder[1]

James is a 15-year-old boy, the second of three children, with a long history of unusual and delayed development. His parents bring him for evaluation because of a worsening in his behavioral functioning. Over the 2 years before this evaluation, James has become progressively more rigid and inflexible, and his insistence on elaborate routines causes much difficulty. He has no real friends and displays a number of idiosyncrasies. He repeats certain phrases from television over and over and displays a fascination with bits of

---

1. Thanks to Fred Volkmar, M.D., of the Child Study Center at Yale University for supplying this case.

string and lint. He has collected considerable quantities of these items, which he insists on carrying with him. Any attempt to divert him from this unusual interest leads to agitation with periods of body rocking or head banging.

Upon examination, James exhibits an unusual pattern of social related-ness—making eye contact infrequently and seeming relatively uninterested in social interaction. He does not use facial expressions, gestures, or body posture to regulate the interaction and lacks emotional reciprocity. His parents report that he has great trouble sustaining a conversation and is interested in discussing only certain television programs and his string collection. His language is stereotyped and repetitive with a monotonic quality. His parents also report that he exhibits some stereotyped behaviors when excited and tends to adhere to various nonfunctional routines (e.g., he always walks around a chair three times before sitting in it, a practice observed by the clinician during the evaluation). His affective range is highly constricted, and his insight and judgment are poor. No evidence of delusions, hallucinations, or other psychotic phenomena are observed.

James was born to a working-class family after a normal pregnancy, labor, and delivery. According to his mother, as an infant he was undemanding and relatively placid and seemed "different" from the first weeks of life. In contrast to his two siblings, James seemed much less interested in social interaction. Motor milestones occurred at the expected times, but language development was significantly delayed. There was some concern that James might be deaf, but a hearing test indicated apparently normal hearing. Although initially reassured by their pediatrician that James was a "late talker," his parents continued to be concerned and, when he was 36 months old, they sought additional evaluations. On examination, James exhibited scattered developmental skills with severe delay in language and language-mediated cognitive skills, but with some motor and nonverbal cognitive abilities close to age level. James said only a few single words that were used for requests for food rather than for social contact. He was unable to follow simple requests and had marked difficulties with tasks that involved imitation. James was particularly intolerant of change. For example, he insisted that his parents follow exactly the same complicated routine at bedtime each night and became extremely agitated if any change in the usual pattern occurred. He was also very sensitive to the inanimate environment so that, although he often seemed almost completely oblivious to his mother's voice, he would panic when he heard the vacuum cleaner. His play involved simple object manipulation with considerable perseveration. A comprehensive medical evaluation revealed a normal electroencephalogram and computed tomography scan. Genetic screening and chromosome analysis were normal as well. Family history consisted of a much less severe speech-language delay in his older brother.

As a result of this evaluation, a diagnosis of Infantile Autism was made when James was 3 years old. He was enrolled in an intensive early intervention program where he made gains, particularly in terms of expressive vocabulary. However, his speech was characterized by echolalia, extreme literalness, and a monotonic voice quality. James had particular difficulties with using language in social situations.

By school age, James developed more differentiated social skills, but he also developed various self-stimulatory behaviors, especially body rocking and head banging, and a fascination with collecting string. Although he remained extremely sensitive and resistant to change in his environment, uneven but steady progress was observed. Formal psychological assessment at age 10 revealed a full-scale IQ in the mildly retarded range, with considerable scatter in subtest results. By the time James was 12, his unusual interests and his difficulty dealing with change had diminished somewhat, and he was mainstreamed for a few class periods a day in public school.

With the onset of adolescence, however, James's behavior deteriorated, particularly after the onset of seizure disorder at age 14. He became more behaviorally rigid, his childhood interest in collecting unusual materials returned, and it was difficult for him to focus on educational or vocational activities.

DSM-IV-TR Diagnosis

Axis I: 299.00   Autistic Disorder
             317   Mild Mental Retardation
Axis II: V71.09   No diagnosis
Axis III: 345.9   Seizure disorder
Axis IV: Onset of adolescence, seizure disorder
Axis V: GAF = 35 (current); 40 (highest level past year)

DSM-IV-TR diagnostic criteria for 299.00 Autistic Disorder

A. A total of six (or more) items from (1), (2), and (3), with at least two from (1), and one each from (2) and (3):
    (1) qualitative impairment in social interaction, as manifested by at least two of the following:
        (a) marked impairment in the use of multiple nonverbal behaviors such as eye-to-eye gaze, facial expression, body postures, and gestures to regulate social interaction

(continued)

DSM-IV-TR diagnostic criteria for
299.00 Autistic Disorder *(continued)*

       (b) failure to develop peer relationships appropriate to developmental level

       (c) a lack of spontaneous seeking to share enjoyment, interests, or achievements with other people (e.g., by a lack of showing, bringing, or pointing out objects of interest)

       (d) lack of social or emotional reciprocity

  (2) qualitative impairments in communication as manifested by at least one of the following:

       (a) delay in, or total lack of, the development of spoken language (not accompanied by an attempt to compensate through alternative modes of communication such as gesture or mime)

       (b) in individuals with adequate speech, marked impairment in the ability to initiate or sustain a conversation with others

       (c) stereotyped and repetitive use of language or idiosyncratic language

       (d) lack of varied, spontaneous make-believe play or social imitative play appropriate to developmental level

  (3) restricted repetitive and stereotyped patterns of behavior, interests, and activities, as manifested by at least one of the following:

       (a) encompassing preoccupation with one or more stereotyped and restricted patterns of interest that is abnormal either in intensity or focus

       (b) apparently inflexible adherence to specific, nonfunctional routines or rituals

       (c) stereotyped and repetitive motor mannerisms (e.g., hand or finger flapping or twisting, or complex whole-body movements)

       (d) persistent preoccupation with parts of objects

B. Delays or abnormal functioning in at least one of the following areas, with onset prior to age 3 years: (1) social interaction, (2) language as used in social communication, or (3) symbolic or imaginative play.

C. The disturbance is not better accounted for by Rett's Disorder or Childhood Disintegrative Disorder.

Guidelines for Differential
Diagnosis of Autistic Disorder

The recent exacerbation of James's behavioral difficulties has occurred in the context of a long history of markedly impaired development and deficits in social interaction; delayed and distorted communication; and restricted, repetitive, and stereotyped patterns of behavior that are consistent with a diagnosis of Autistic Disorder.

At the time of his most recent examination, James exhibited "qualitative impairment in social interaction": He was unable to use nonverbal cues to regulate social interaction, had failed to develop peer relationships appropriate to his developmental level, and lacked the skill of social reciprocity. Similarly, "qualitative impairments in communication" were present and included James's marked difficulties in sustaining a conversation and his stereotyped use of language. Finally, James exhibited "restricted, repetitive, and stereotyped patterns of behavior, interests, and activities" as seen in his compulsive adherence to nonfunctional routines, his stereotyped motor mannerisms, and his preoccupation with his string collection. His social and language deficits were apparent well before he was 3 years old. Therefore a DSM-IV-TR diagnosis of Autistic Disorder would be consistent with both his current presentation and the initial diagnosis of DSM-III (American Psychiatric Association 1980) Infantile Autism made when he was 3 years old.

The differential diagnosis of Autistic Disorder includes other disorders in the category of Pervasive Developmental Disorders. This category was expanded in DSM-IV by the addition of Rett's Disorder, Childhood Disintegrative Disorder, and Asperger's Disorder. These diagnoses were included to improve differential diagnosis and allow clinicians to more accurately and specifically describe symptoms that would have been diagnosed as Autistic Disorder or Pervasive Developmental Disorder Not Otherwise Specified in DSM-III-R (American Psychiatric Association 1987).

Rett's Disorder has been observed only in females and is characterized by a typical pattern of head growth deceleration, loss of motor skills, and the development of severe psychomotor retardation. In Childhood Disintegrative Disorder, development is normal until at least 2 years of age, after which a severe regression occurs with the development of features suggestive of autism. In Asperger's Disorder, marked language delay is not observed; Asperger's is not diagnosed if criteria for Autistic Disorder are met.

The diagnosis of Pervasive Developmental Disorder Not Otherwise Specified is used to describe presentations in which the criteria for Autistic Disorder or one of the other specifically defined Pervasive Developmental Disorders are not met but there is a severe and pervasive impairment in the development of reciprocal social interaction associated with impairment in either verbal or nonverbal communication skills or with the presence of stereotyped behavior, interests, and activities. For example, a child who displays communicative features typical of Autistic Disorder along with stereotyped movements, but who does not exhibit qualitatively impaired social skills, would appropriately be diagnosed as having Pervasive Developmental Disorder Not Otherwise Specified. Pervasive Developmental Disorder Not Otherwise Specified is also not diagnosed if criteria are met for Schizophrenia or Schizotypal or Avoidant Personality Disorder.

The differential diagnosis of Autistic Disorder also includes certain disorders outside the class of Pervasive Developmental Disorders. Schizophrenia occasionally has its origins in childhood, although usually after a period of some years of normal or near normal development. This is unlike Autistic Disorder in which certain delays or abnormal functioning must be present before 3 years of age. An additional diagnosis of Schizophrenia is made in individuals with Autistic Disorder only if they go on to develop prominent delusions or hallucinations that meet criteria for Schizophrenia.

The Communication Disorders, Expressive Language Disorder and Mixed Receptive-Expressive Language Disorder, are characterized by marked language problems but, unlike Pervasive Developmental Disorders, Communication Disorders are not associated with qualitative abnormalities of social interaction or with a pattern of restricted, repetitive, and stereotyped interests. Because stereotypic movements form part of the definition of Pervasive Developmental Disorders, they do not warrant a separate diagnosis of Stereotypic Movement Disorder. When, as is often the case, Mental Retardation coexists with autism, both diagnoses may be given.

Treatment Planning for Autistic Disorder

The symptoms of Autistic Disorder may vary with developmental level. Particularly during adolescence, some degree of behavioral deterioration (as in James's case) or, somewhat less frequently, of improved adjustment may be observed. Although the cause or causes of autism remain unknown, there is considerable evidence that sustained educational and behavioral intervention is associated with improved long-term outcome. It is important to focus on helping the individual acquire the basic adaptive skills necessary for the highest possible level of adult self-sufficiency. Behavioral interventions that positively reinforce desired behaviors and discourage inappropriate behaviors are also important. A number of medications may be helpful in facilitating behavioral adjustment and learning. In James's case, an evaluation of his current educational and behavioral program and consultation with the neurologist who manages the seizure disorder are indicated. Approximately 25% of individuals with Autistic Disorder also exhibit seizures of various types.

Summary

Many children and adolescents present with odd behavior but do not meet the threshold for a diagnosis of Autistic Disorder. Depending on the specifics of the presentation, these individuals might be diagnosed with Asperger's Disorder; Pervasive Developmental Disorder Not Otherwise Specified; or Schizoid, Schizotypal, or Avoidant Personality Disorder. Frequently, adults with continuing symptoms of Autistic Disorder are misdiagnosed as having Schizophrenia. A thorough developmental history indicating an early onset of symptoms will help the clinician to make this distinction. If the individual had an onset and symptoms consistent with Autistic Disorder and prominent hallucinations or delusions are also present, then both diagnoses are appropriate.

Attention-Deficit and Disruptive Behavior Disorders

Attention-Deficit and Disruptive Behavior Disorders

314.xx	Attention-Deficit/Hyperactivity Disorder
.01	Combined Type
.00	Predominantly Inattentive Type
.01	Predominantly Hyperactive-Impulsive Type
314.9	Attention-Deficit/Hyperactivity Disorder Not Otherwise Specified
312.xx	Conduct Disorder
.81	Childhood-Onset Type
.82	Adolescent-Onset Type
.89	Unspecified Onset
313.81	Oppositional Defiant Disorder
312.9	Disruptive Behavior Disorder Not Otherwise Specified

Attention-Deficit/Hyperactivity Disorder

We present two cases of Attention-Deficit/Hyperactivity Disorder to illustrate the varying subtypes of this disorder. The issues related to differential diagnosis and treatment will be discussed for both cases together.

❖ Case Study: A Hyperactive
Boy Who Is Failing in School[2]

Kevin is a cheerful 9-year-old third grader who is brought to the outpatient clinic after the teacher at the private school he attends repeatedly called his

---

2. Thanks for supplying these cases go to C. Keith Conners, Ph.D., of the Psychiatry Department of Duke University Medical Center.

mother about his worsening classroom behavior. His teacher described him as a likable and friendly youngster who always obeyed when spoken to but also repeatedly disrupted the class by his antics and could no longer be tolerated in the classroom. The teacher reported that he hummed and made noises under his breath, blurted out answers without raising his hand, and always tried to be first when the teacher asked a question, even though he often did not have the answer when called upon. The teacher had to remind him constantly to stay in his seat. On the playground, Kevin was a whirlwind of energy. Although he often elicited guffaws from his classmates by his antics and daredevil behavior, he seemed to have few playmates who spent any time with him because of his tendency to disrupt games and invent his own rules. He was often the last to be chosen for playground teams; in games such as softball he was totally unreliable in the outfield, usually concentrating on vapor trails in the sky or interesting pebbles underfoot.

Although Kevin seemed very bright, he seldom managed to complete his assignments in class. As a result, papers were often sent home but rarely returned. When Kevin's mother was informed of this at a teacher conference, she was very surprised because she spent a good deal of time helping Kevin complete his homework. In fact, daily homework had become a gruesome hour-long exercise during which Kevin needed frequent reminders to stop running into the living room to see what was on television or to stop interrupting the conversations of people around him. He investigated any sounds or movement in the kitchen where he did his daily homework. His mother noted that he constantly forgot to take his materials to school and that he often had crumpled papers left inside his book bag.

During an interview at the clinic, Kevin's mother describes him as "the sweetest boy imaginable," with a winning smile and happy-go-lucky style that most people find endearing. On the other hand, she does admit that he is "all boy" and "a real handful." His kindergarten teacher had told her that he was "immature" and should spend another year in kindergarten before entering the first grade. He seemed to like school at first but began complaining about his teachers in the second grade, saying they were mean and unfair and "always on his case."

At home, Kevin was always on the go, usually leaving a trail of toys in his wake as he sped through the house looking for things to do. Despite a roomful of toys and games, he usually complained that "Everything here is boring." His mother could always locate him in the house by the loud sounds that accompanied his play. He was usually unwilling to play any of the quiet games his sister adored, such as puzzles or board games. He went full tilt until mid-evening when he would suddenly wind down, in his mother's words, "like a motor that ran out of gas."

On the weekends, Kevin had a number of minor chores to accomplish, such as taking out the garbage and cleaning his room. He would almost invariably get distracted along the way and leave his chores partially completed or not done at all. He was never unwilling or defiant when asked to do these tasks but could be derailed by the simplest distractions. At other times, he would become highly engrossed in a video game or movie, and his mother found she had to place her hands on his face and look him in the eye before any request was attended to.

In contrast to the vivid descriptions of his overactive behavior, when Kevin is observed in the waiting room on his first visit, he is playing quietly on the floor with a number of small robots and transformers he brought with him. He comes with the examiner calmly and willingly, his eyes lighting up when told that he will be playing some computer games. Upon examination, Kevin is found to be a healthy, well-nourished boy in good physical condition except for several scrapes and bruises and several healed lacerations on the scalp and forearm. There is no significant medical history except for a fractured wrist at age 3, sustained when Kevin fell from a high wall he had somehow managed to climb. Kevin's birth and early development were unremarkable, with language and motor milestones always normal or slightly early. His early activity level was high, and he had a short duration of attention for toys as a toddler. Although he was a friendly, affectionate baby who liked to be cuddled, his mother noticed very early that when she was holding him he would struggle to turn around to see what was going on if there was any movement or activity in the vicinity. Kevin always woke up early, and as young as age 2 would get out of bed in the morning and explore the household. Kevin's mother admitted that she had been worried about the early difficulty she had in managing him, especially because he seemed not to learn to stop doing dangerous or innocently destructive acts despite constant reminders.

Kevin's father berated her, saying that Kevin was just a boy and that he had been no different when he was a boy. Kevin's mother began to cry when it was suggested that she had been spending a great deal of her waking life dealing with Kevin. She described Kevin's father, who did not attend the first clinic visit, as a moderately successful sales manager for a medical supply firm. He was frequently away on sales trips and, when working in town, usually did not arrive home until 7 P.M. She reported that he was a restless and somewhat disorganized man who nevertheless was fairly successful because of his drive and energy. She said he would have been even more successful if he could have tolerated doing office work. He was hopeless at keeping his checkbook and tended to procrastinate at anything requiring paperwork. He had finished high school and was frequently told he was an underachiever. He would often complain about the messy state of the household, saying that if she were firmer with Kevin, the house wouldn't be such a mess. Although his father enjoyed playing outdoor games with Kevin, he frequently ended up yelling at him and was usually impatient with his antics.

DSM-IV-TR Diagnosis

Axis I: 314.01   Attention-Deficit/Hyperactivity Disorder,
Combined Type

              V62.3   Academic Problem

Axis II: V71.09   No diagnosis

Axis III: None

Axis IV: Impending school expulsion

Axis V: GAF = 50 (serious impairment in schoolwork moderate
impairment in social relationships)

❖   Case Study: Daddy's Little Space Cadet

Darlene is a 12-year-old sixth grader whose parents bring her in for evaluation following a psychoeducational evaluation by the school psychologist
who found that she had a superior IQ and "a mild visually based reading disorder." Darlene did not qualify as having a learning disorder by school standards, however. The psychologist noted that compared with other parts of
her IQ test Darlene's performance on recalling digits, mental arithmetic,
and symbol coding was much lower, which he attributed to anxiety. He recommended an evaluation for a possible Anxiety Disorder. Darlene has had
failing or near-failing grades since the third grade but, because of high IQ
and model behavior, she was passed on to the next grade. She received numerous admonishments because of her apparent "laziness." She appeared
to be uninterested, bored, and more concerned about her busy social life
than about her studies. She complained that the middle school environment was too noisy for her to concentrate.

At home, Darlene was generally cooperative except for a growing resistance to homework. Her school papers were sloppy and disorganized. Her
handwriting was notably immature and she printed rather than using cursive
whenever possible. Further examination with the Test of Written Language
revealed a 2-year delay in writing skills, particularly involving expressive
writing as opposed to writing from dictation. Her spelling had been a problem since the second grade but was only moderately delayed. Darlene
tended to rush through her work and had to be reminded to check it. Even
so, she would often make many careless errors, even in areas where she had
demonstrated previous competence. Although generally willing to do everything she was asked by her parents, she was unreliable and frequently
had to be reminded about chores that were well established and should
have been routine.

Darlene often appeared to be in a fog at home. When asked a question,
she frequently failed to answer or would appear as if startled out of a rev-
erie. She was considered a daydreamer. Since at least the first grade, her father's favorite nickname for her had been "my little space cadet." Darlene

was usually bored around the house and often importuned her mother to do something with her. Her mother taught her needlepoint, macramé, and drawing, but, despite her obvious pleasure at doing these things with her mother, she could seldom stick with them long enough to finish a project. She had even more trouble completing difficult homework. She said that when she was studying, she couldn't remember what was at the top of a page by the time she got to the bottom. She complained that she couldn't concentrate on her homework because there was so much "racket" in the house, but nevertheless would play rock music while doing homework if allowed to. According to her mother, Darlene had a fantastic memory for details that other family members had forgotten, yet she was forgetful about appointments, calendar events, or even meetings with friends that she had planned. She was known among her peers as an unreliable person who was usually late or missing altogether. Her favorite activity was browsing in the mall.

DSM-IV-TR Diagnosis

Axis I: 314.00   Attention-Deficit/Hyperactivity Disorder,
                         Predominantly Inattentive Type
             315.2   Disorder of Written Expression
Axis II: V71.09   No diagnosis
Axis III: None
Axis IV: Educational problems (noisy school and home study
             environment)
Axis V: GAF = 50 (current; serious impairment in school
             performance)

DSM-IV-TR diagnostic criteria for
Attention-Deficit/Hyperactivity Disorder

A.   Either (1) or (2):
     (1)   six (or more) of the following symptoms of **inattention** have persisted for at least 6 months to a degree that is maladaptive and inconsistent with developmental level:
     Inattention
     (a)   often fails to give close attention to details or makes careless mistakes in schoolwork, work, or other activities
     (b)   often has difficulty sustaining attention in tasks or play activities
     (c)   often does not seem to listen when spoken to directly

(continued)

DSM-IV-TR diagnostic criteria for
Attention-Deficit/Hyperactivity Disorder *(continued)*

  (d) often does not follow through on instructions and fails to finish schoolwork, chores, or duties in the workplace (not due to oppositional behavior or failure to understand instructions)

  (e) often has difficulty organizing tasks and activities

  (f) often avoids, dislikes, or is reluctant to engage in tasks that require sustained mental effort (such as schoolwork or homework)

  (g) often loses things necessary for tasks or activities (e.g., toys, school assignments, pencils, books, or tools)

  (h) is often easily distracted by extraneous stimuli

  (i) is often forgetful in daily activities

 (2) six (or more) of the following symptoms of **hyperactivity-impulsivity** have persisted for at least 6 months to a degree that is maladaptive and inconsistent with developmental level:

Hyperactivity

  (a) often fidgets with hands or feet or squirms in seat

  (b) often leaves seat in classroom or in other situations in which remaining seated is expected

  (c) often runs about or climbs excessively in situations in which it is inappropriate (in adolescents or adults, may be limited to subjective feelings of restlessness)

  (d) often has difficulty playing or engaging in leisure activities quietly

  (e) is often "on the go" or often acts as if "driven by a motor"

  (f) often talks excessively

Impulsivity

  (g) often blurts out answers before questions have been completed

  (h) often has difficulty awaiting turn

  (i) often interrupts or intrudes on others (e.g., butts into conversations or games)

B. Some hyperactive-impulsive or inattentive symptoms that caused impairment were present before age 7 years.

C. Some impairment from the symptoms is present in two or more settings (e.g., at school [or work] and at home).

D. There must be clear evidence of clinically significant impairment in social, academic, or occupational functioning.

E. The symptoms do not occur exclusively during the course of a Pervasive Developmental Disorder, Schizophrenia, or other Psychotic Disorder and are not better accounted for by another mental disorder (e.g., Mood Disorder, Anxiety Disorder, Dissociative Disorder, or a Personality Disorder).

(continued)

DSM-IV-TR diagnostic criteria for
Attention-Deficit/Hyperactivity Disorder *(continued)*

Code based on type:

314.01   Attention-Deficit/Hyperactivity Disorder, Combined Type: if both Criteria A1 and A2 are met for the past 6 months

314.00   Attention-Deficit/Hyperactivity Disorder, Predominantly Inattentive Type: if Criterion A1 is met but Criterion A2 is not met for the past 6 months

314.01   Attention-Deficit/Hyperactivity Disorder, Predominantly Hyperactive-Impulsive Type: if Criterion A2 is met but Criterion A1 is not met for the past 6 months

Coding note: For individuals (especially adolescents and adults) who currently have symptoms that no longer meet full criteria, "In Partial Remission" should be specified.

Because Darlene also meets criteria for Disorder of Written Expression, we also include here the generic criteria for Learning Disorders.

Generic DSM-IV-TR diagnostic criteria for
315.00 Reading Disorder, 315.1 Mathematics
Disorder, and 315.2 Disorder of Written Expression

A.   Academic achievement (i.e., reading, mathematics, or written expression), as measured by individually administered standardized tests, is substantially below that expected given the person's chronological age, measured intelligence, and age-appropriate education.

B.   The disturbance in A significantly interferes with academic achievement or activities of daily living.

C.   If a sensory deficit is present, the difficulties are in excess of those usually associated with it.

Note: DSM-IV-TR gives separate criteria sets for Reading Disorder, Mathematics Disorder, and Disorder of Written Expression. This is a generic criteria set that summarizes the features essential to each of these disorders.

Guidelines for Differential Diagnosis of Attention-Deficit/Hyperactivity Disorder

Attention-Deficit/Hyperactivity Disorder is a diagnosis that is being made increasingly often in both children and adults. For this reason, the thresholds established by the criteria set were the subject of considerable controversy during the development of DSM-IV. There is no clear boundary between children who are normally active and those who would be considered hyperactive, just as there is no clear boundary between those who are normally distractible and those who have an attention deficit. Moreover, expectations concerning what is normal in this regard may vary greatly across different cultures and depend on the situations with which the individual is confronted. The DSM-IV (and DSM-IV-TR) definition of this disorder is fairly inclusive in an effort to encourage early case finding and treatment intervention. As a result, however, some clinicians and parents are concerned that individuals with attention or hyperactivity problems best conceived as normal variants may inappropriately receive a diagnosis of Attention-Deficit/Hyperactivity Disorder with the resulting risk of overmedication. Therefore, it is important to evaluate the behavior, especially the hyperactivity, in relation to what would be considered normal in other children of the same age and developmental level and from the same cultural background.

The DSM-IV-TR criteria set includes several requirements that are meant to reduce the risk of overdiagnosis. The behaviors must occur in multiple settings rather than representing the more or less expectable fidgeting or loss of interest that may occur in a particular unstimulating environment. The criterion requiring clinically significant impairment also serves as a check to prevent the overdiagnosis of normally active or normally distractible children. The third way to prevent overdiagnosis is the requirement that the symptoms must have caused impairment before the individual was 7 years old. In fact, in most individuals, attention-deficit/hyperactivity symptoms are first apparent in infancy or early childhood, a feature that sharply distinguishes this disorder from the many other psychiatric disorders (e.g., Substance-Related Disorders, Bipolar Disorders, and Schizophrenia and Other Psychotic Disorders) that are characterized by hyperactivity and inattention but generally have a later onset. One of the most difficult and interesting differential diagnoses is between Attention-Deficit Disorder, Hyperactive Type, and Bipolar Disorder in adolescents who are irritable, hyperactive, and distractible. To make this distinction, it is especially important to ascertain the age at onset of symptoms, which must be before age 7 in Attention-Deficit/Hyperactivity Disorder and is rarely before age 7 in Bipolar Disorder. It is also useful to inquire whether there is a family history of Bipolar Disorder. Of course, both disorders may sometimes be present. As mentioned above, Kevin's mother reported that even as an infant and young toddler Kevin seemed unusually distractible and impulsive and had a very short attention span. Darlene had been her father's "little space cadet" even before the first grade. This issue is particularly important when making the diagnosis of Attention-Deficit/Hyperactivity Disorder in adults, which should be done only after obtaining a careful history that documents the early onset of symptoms and evaluating for other psychiatric disorders that may be responsible for the symptoms.

A major issue in the diagnosis of Attention-Deficit/Hyperactivity Disorder is the relationship between the attention deficit and the hyperactivity. In DSM-III-R, the major emphasis was on those individuals who displayed both attention deficit and hyperactivity, whereas those who displayed attention deficit alone were included in what was regarded as a residual category (undifferentiated attention deficit disorder). The literature reviews, data reanalyses, and field trials for DSM-IV suggested that, although there are occasional pure cases of attention deficit and occasional pure cases of hyperactivity, aspects of attention deficit and hyperactivity very often occur together, even if the criteria thresholds for one or the other are not met. As a result, DSM-IV has created one unified category of Attention-Deficit/Hyperactivity Disorder with subtypes that allow for greater specificity. Adolescents and adults are relatively more likely to present with the Predominantly Inattentive Type because individuals tend to gain greater control over their activity level as they grow older.

The diagnosis of Attention-Deficit/Hyperactivity Disorder is less frequently missed in those individuals who have the Combined Type or who are predominantly hyperactive because they make their presence known by disruptive behavior that intrudes on the space or privacy of others, as did Kevin's. In contrast, an individual with the Primarily Inattentive Type, like Darlene, is more likely to be dismissed as lazy, unintelligent, or a "space cadet," without the realization that a specific attention deficit problem may be responsible for the individual's inability to perform. The clinician should also be careful to distinguish behaviors that are the result of inattention from other problems (e.g., oppositional behavior, depression, Learning Disorders, failure to understand instructions). The difficulty that Kevin and Darlene have in focusing on tasks does not appear to be the result of any oppositional attitude (they are both willing to do what they are asked once their attention is gained), nor do they exhibit other problems that would account for their inability to complete a task.

Attention-Deficit/Hyperactivity Disorder is often comorbid with, and may predispose to, the development of other disorders (particularly Oppositional Defiant Disorder, Conduct Disorder, Learning and Communication Disorders, Mood and Anxiety Disorders, and Substance Abuse).

As often happens, Darlene's clinical presentation combines Attention-Deficit/Hyperactivity Disorder with a Learning Disorder. Darlene was also diagnosed with Disorder of Written Expression because individualized testing demonstrated a 2-year delay in expressive writing skills, despite her high IQ. It should be noted that Learning and Communication Disorders are probably not best considered mental disorders and have been included in DSM-IV only because they are often present in children who are being evaluated in a mental health setting and may be important in differential diagnosis.

Treatment Planning for Attention-Deficit/Hyperactivity Disorder

Attention-Deficit/Hyperactivity Disorder is a widespread condition of great public health significance. It is a disorder that causes much concern for the individuals themselves and for their families and schools. There is considerable controversy about the treatment of Attention-Deficit/Hyperactivity Disorder, which has resulted in widely disparate practice habits. The stimulant medications have consistently been documented to produce significant gains in focusing attention and regulating activity levels, and they remain the major treatment modality for individuals who have severely impairing symptoms. However, these medications are accompanied by side effects, especially a risk of growth retardation, and must be prescribed judiciously and under careful supervision. A number of psychosocial interventions are very promising when employed either in addition to or instead of medication. For children and adolescents, these interventions include psychoeducation, school-based interventions, parent training, contingency management, clinical behavior therapy, and skills-based training, depending on the type of prominent symptoms and age of the patient. For adults with ADHD, psychoeducation, bibliotherapy, and skills-based training have been recommended. Children and adults with ADHD may also require treatment for comorbid psychiatric disorders, including mood or anxiety disorders, if present.

Summary

Hyperactivity and inattention are common aspects of normal, if not ideal, functioning, but they may also accompany a wide variety of mental disorders. The diagnosis of Attention-Deficit/Hyperactivity Disorder should be reserved for those who have the characteristic symptom pattern at a sufficient level of severity and pervasiveness to warrant clinical attention. To distinguish this disorder from other psychiatric causes of hyperactivity and inattention, it is necessary to establish an early onset and continuous course of symptoms and to rule out other more acute etiologies.

Conduct Disorder

❖   Case Study: A Young Boy
With Serious Behavioral Problems

Robert is a 10-year-old boy who is admitted to a child psychiatry hospital unit after he attempted to jump off the 20th-floor balcony of the apartment house where he lives. The incident occurred on a Monday morning, when he and his mother were scheduled to meet with the school principal because Robert had been caught the previous week stealing from other students in his class. Robert refused to go to school, saying he would run away if she forced him. They began to argue, and Robert got violently out of control. He threw a clock and a lamp and then suddenly ran toward the balcony. His mother raced toward him, knocked him down, and held him, while he pleaded with her: "Please let me go and jump. It will be better if I'm dead. I won't have to think. I won't have to worry. There's a better place. Maybe it's pretty there. It'll be beautiful." Robert eventually calmed down enough for his mother to stop restraining him. She called her therapist, who advised her to take Robert to the emergency room for immediate evaluation.

Robert lives with his mother and stepfather. The family has recently moved away from the town where Robert's father lives. Robert's stepfather often becomes angry with him for taking money out of his wallet, setting fires, and staying out late at night without permission. Two days before the suicide attempt, Robert talked to his father on the telephone and cried about how much he missed him and how he wished he had not moved away. He told his father that he both hated and feared his stepfather.

The child psychiatrist who was called to see Robert in the emergency room recommended that he be hospitalized because he might attempt to hurt himself again. Hearing this recommendation, Robert became agitated and attempted to throw an ashtray at the doctor. During his initial evaluation after admission to the hospital, Robert is calm but sad and anxious. He states that he "wanted to jump off the balcony because my mom and I were fighting so much and I wanted it to stop. I went too far, I guess. I was very sad for several days and angry since we moved."

During the early days of his hospitalization, additional history is obtained about Robert's early developmental period. Although Robert is physically healthy and intellectually advanced, his mother reports that he has always been a difficult child who tends to react to changes and criticism with anger. She describes a pattern of aggressive behavior going back to the time Robert was very young. For example, when he was 6 years old, he had a violent argument with his 13-year-old brother, after which he hit his sleeping brother on the head with a can of soda. Three years before this evaluation, Robert became enraged and hit a male teacher who was attempting to discipline him. This event precipitated the beginning of outpatient psychotherapy: Robert attended a nearby child psychiatry clinic twice a week for a year, until his therapist left the clinic. Robert refused to see a new therapist, saying that no one else could help him.

Robert reports that he often thinks about "killing someone, then the police will get me and take care of me. Then I can get out of the house." Robert is often truant from school, and his mother reports that he has twice run away from home after arguments with her. On one occasion he stayed out until well after dark, and the other time he was gone until the next day. Robert was first caught stealing from classmates in the second grade. Robert's mother says she also suspects that he often takes money from her purse without permission, although he always denies this even when he clearly has money she has not given him, claiming instead that he "found" it. Robert's teacher has called his mother in on many occasions to discuss his disruptive and aggressive behavior. He frequently starts fights on the playground and refuses to do any schoolwork he finds boring. On several occasions, he has taken notebooks and paperback books away from classmates with whom he was angry and torn them up.

Robert has experienced numerous environmental stresses since the time he was 4 years old. At that time, his mother was hospitalized for 4 months with a fever of unknown origin. Two years later, his parents separated after a great deal of animosity, including numerous physical altercations. Robert's father had been unemployed for approximately a year and drank excessively. Robert's parents divorced when Robert was almost 8 years old. His father remarried shortly after, began to work again, and controlled his drinking. When Robert was 9 years old, his mother remarried. Her new husband has three teenage children who spend much time in their new home with Robert, his mother, and brother. Although he wants to get along with Robert, his stepfather finds it difficult to cope with Robert's willfulness and anger. When verbal efforts at discipline fail, his stepfather resorts to harsh corporal punishment, often with a belt.

DSM-IV-TR Diagnosis

Axis I: 312.81   Conduct Disorder, Childhood-Onset Type, Mild
           309.0   Adjustment Disorder, With Depressed Mood
Axis II: V71.09   No diagnosis
Axis III: None
Axis IV: Family move, school change, loss of contact with father,
           harsh discipline by stepfather
Axis V: GAF = 45

DSM-IV-TR diagnostic criteria for Conduct Disorder

A. A repetitive and persistent pattern of behavior in which the basic rights of others or major age-appropriate societal norms or rules are violated, as manifested by the presence of three (or more) of the following criteria in the past 12 months, with at least one criterion present in the past 6 months:

Aggression to people and animals

  (1) often bullies, threatens, or intimidates others
  (2) often initiates physical fights
  (3) has used a weapon that can cause serious physical harm to others (e.g., a bat, brick, broken bottle, knife, gun)
  (4) has been physically cruel to people
  (5) has been physically cruel to animals
  (6) has stolen while confronting a victim (e.g., mugging, purse snatching, extortion, armed robbery)
  (7) has forced someone into sexual activity

Destruction of property

  (8) has deliberately engaged in fire setting with the intention of causing serious damage
  (9) has deliberately destroyed others' property (other than by fire setting)

Deceitfulness or theft

  (10) has broken into someone else's house, building, or car
  (11) often lies to obtain goods or favors or to avoid obligations (i.e., "cons" others)
  (12) has stolen items of nontrivial value without confronting a victim and without breaking and entering (e.g., shoplifting, forgery)

Serious violations of rules

  (13) often stays out at night despite parental prohibitions, beginning before age 13 years
  (14) has run away from home overnight at least twice while living in parental or parental surrogate home (or once without returning for a lengthy period)
  (15) is often truant from school, beginning before age 13 years

B. The disturbance in behavior causes clinically significant impairment in social, academic, or occupational functioning.

C. If the individual is age 18 years or older, criteria are not met for Antisocial Personality Disorder.

(continued)

DSM-IV-TR diagnostic criteria for
Conduct Disorder *(continued)*

Code based on age at onset:
312.81   Conduct Disorder, Childhood-Onset Type: onset of at least one criterion characteristic of Conduct Disorder prior to age 10 years
312.82   Conduct Disorder, Adolescent-Onset Type: absence of any criteria characteristic of Conduct Disorder prior to age 10 years
312.89   Conduct Disorder, Unspecified Onset: age at onset is not known

Specify severity:
Mild: few if any conduct problems in excess of those required to make the diagnosis **and** conduct problems cause only minor harm to others
Moderate: number of conduct problems and effect on others intermediate between "mild" and "severe"
Severe: many conduct problems in excess of those required to make the diagnosis **or** conduct problems cause considerable harm to others

---

Guidelines for Differential
Diagnosis of Conduct Disorder

There are those who believe that Conduct Disorder is really not best considered a mental disorder but instead represents either a defect in the individual's moral development or the result of a disadvantaged or violent environment. They argue that there is no effective treatment for Conduct Disorder and that providing a diagnostic label may inappropriately afford the sick role to those who should be held more responsible for their behavior. The diagnosis is particularly difficult to make in environments in which violent or illegal behaviors are common and encouraged by peer pressure or the need for self-protection. Indeed, an alarming and increasing percentage of young people carry and use weapons as part of everyday life in what they perceive to be a threatening environment. To assist in making this distinction, DSM-IV-TR states that "the Conduct Disorder diagnosis should be applied only when the behavior in question is symptomatic of an underlying dysfunction within the individual and not simply a reaction to the immediate social context" (p. 96). This was also a powerful rationale for providing a Childhood-Onset Type, in which symptoms are present before age 10. Children whose Conduct Disorder begins early are more likely to be male, to have a positive family history, to have disturbed peer relationships, to commit violent acts, and to go on to meet criteria for Antisocial Personality Disorder as adults. It is more difficult to decide whether Conduct Disorder is an appropriate diagnosis when the conduct problems begin in adolescence, are sanctioned or encouraged by peers, and do not cause severe consequences.

A second issue is the boundary between Conduct Disorder and Oppositional Defiant Disorder, a disorder that is less severe and has less prognostic significance. Because individuals with Conduct Disorder usually also meet the criteria for Oppositional Defiant Disorder (which is often a precursor to Conduct Disorder), when the full criteria for Conduct Disorder are met, only that disorder is diagnosed. Thus, although Robert's behavior would clearly meet the criteria for Oppositional Defiant Disorder (he often loses his temper; often actively defies or refuses to comply with adults' requests or rules; often deliberately annoys people; and is often angry, resentful, spiteful, and vindictive), he also shows a pattern of aggression, destructiveness, truancy, and theft that meets criteria for Conduct Disorder. Although Oppositional Defiant Disorder is a common precursor of Conduct Disorder, in many children it does not progress to Conduct Disorder.

Because children with Conduct Disorder often also meet criteria for Attention-Deficit/Hyperactivity Disorder, it is important to evaluate for the presence of hyperactive or attentional symptoms. Although Robert does have a low tolerance for frustration, is easily bored, and acts impulsively, his symptoms do not appear to meet full criteria for Attention-Deficit/Hyperactivity Disorder.

Depressive symptoms also commonly accompany Conduct Disorder. In fact, Conduct Disorder is an important predictor of suicide risk in teenagers. Robert's case describes a typical pattern in which depressive symptoms and suicidal ideation (or behavior) rapidly develop when the individual is frustrated or confronted by authorities after being caught in wrongdoing. Very often these symptoms are a reaction to changes in environmental circumstances and do not last long enough to meet criteria for Major Depressive Disorder. For example, Robert's depressive symptoms also appear to be related to his disturbed home life, recent move, and loneliness for his father, although these symptoms are not severe enough to meet criteria for a Depressive Disorder. For this reason, an additional diagnosis of Adjustment Disorder With Depressed Mood appears appropriate.

The causal relationship between Conduct Disorder and Substance Use is often difficult to tease out. Individuals with Conduct Disorder are inclined to have precociously early, persistent, and severe Substance Abuse. On the other hand, individuals who abuse substances may get into trouble as a result of either disinhibition resulting from intoxication or the need to acquire funds to support their Substance Use. Conduct Disorder should be diagnosed only when there is a repetitive and persistent pattern of behavior, not just an isolated misdeed. However, the diagnosis of Conduct Disorder remains appropriate even when the behaviors are closely associated with Substance Use if they are sufficiently repetitive and persistent.

The relationship between childhood or adolescent Conduct Disorder and adult Antisocial Personality Disorder is interesting. The definition of Antisocial Personality Disorder requires that there be evidence of Conduct Disorder beginning before age 15. However, only about one-third of those individuals who are diagnosed as having Conduct Disorder in childhood or adolescence go on to develop Antisocial Personality Disorder as adults. Rarely, an older adolescent or young adult may be diagnosed as having Conduct Disorder if the individual continues to demonstrate severe and impairing conduct problems that do not meet criteria for Antisocial Personality Disorder. In contrast, Antisocial Personality Disorder cannot be diagnosed in those under 18 years of age, in whom the symptom pattern would be considered Conduct Disorder.

One remaining area of controversy and uncertainty is the diagnosis of Conduct Disorder in females. In most studies, Conduct Disorder is diagnosed much more frequently in males than in females. Although this undoubtedly reflects real gender differences in the prevalence of delinquent behavior, it may also result in part from the definition of the disorder which, in DSM-III-R at least, tended to stress aggressive and confrontational behaviors rather than those more characteristic of female delinquency (e.g., lying, truancy, running away, substance use, and prostitution). The criteria set for Conduct Disorder was revised in DSM-IV to try to more accurately describe how this disorder may present in females as well as in males.

Treatment Planning for Conduct Disorder

Treatment of Conduct Disorder is an area of controversy. A number of clinicians believe that nothing works, despite the considerable clinical and research efforts to find a treatment or prophylaxis for this disorder. Others are much less pessimistic. Ongoing research is investigating a variety of cognitive/behavioral, parent training, teacher training, and environmental approaches—the ultimate efficacy of which remains to be seen. In treating Conduct Disorder, it is often useful to focus initial attention on the target symptoms of Substance Abuse because substance-related problems are often important in the pathogenesis of the behavioral problems and may be more amenable to change than the other features of the disorder. The diagnosis and treatment of comorbid conditions are also high priorities. Depression is commonly associated with Conduct Disorder, and there is a suicide risk of perhaps 5% with this condition.

Summary

Conduct Disorder is on the boundary between psychiatry and the legal system and at present is often poorly handled by both. Any evaluation for Conduct Disorder should focus on the degree to which the delinquent behaviors are the direct result of substance use or environmental pressures, because behaviors resulting from these causes are more amenable to intervention than the kind of delinquency that seems to be driven more by factors inherent in the individual. The latter is associated with early onset, heavy family loading, and violent behavior. It may seem like small comfort, but time is on our side with this disorder because the majority of individuals seem to outgrow it and do not go on to develop adult Antisocial Personality Disorder. Even those who do go on to develop Antisocial Personality Disorder tend to mellow somewhat with age.

Tic Disorders

Tic Disorders
307.23   Tourette's Disorder
307.22   Chronic Motor or Vocal Tic Disorder
307.21   Transient Tic Disorder
307.20   Tic Disorder Not Otherwise Specified

Tourette's Disorder

❖   Case Study: Multiple Tics
in a 9-Year-Old Boy[3]

Bob is a 9-year-old boy who is seen at the request of his pediatrician to evaluate the need for possible inpatient admission. The pediatrician is concerned that Bob may be becoming psychotic because he has begun swearing under his breath. When his parents and teacher ask him to stop, he is able to do so for a time but eventually the swearing returns. Bob and his parents are seen together and the three of them provide Bob's history.

---

3. Thanks to Fred Volkmar, M.D., of the Child Study Center at Yale University for this case.

The first of two children, Bob was born following a planned pregnancy and uncomplicated labor and delivery. Early developmental milestones were within normal limits. Bob was a sociable child who was enrolled in a preschool program at age 3. His preschool teacher noted that he had greater than usual difficulties with activities that required sustained attention. His attentional problems continued when he entered primary school but were not sufficiently severe to merit diagnosis or pharmacological intervention. Although Bob has had some difficulties learning, his academic performance is at expected levels for his grade.

Bob's father says that he noticed that Bob developed some "funny movements" (e.g., eye blinking, quick movements of the head and neck, and shoulder shrugs) after he entered school. These seemed to come and go over time and to be exacerbated by stress or anxiety. These movements were relatively infrequent, although Bob's peers sometimes made fun of him because of them. In the year before this referral, however, the movements continued and began to be accompanied by sounds that Bob makes "under his breath." When asked to stop doing this, Bob is able to do so only for a brief time. The subvocal comments have gradually become more audible and include various swear words. Over the past year, there has not been a period of more than a few days when this behavior has not been present.

By the time he was evaluated, Bob's problems had become a source of great embarrassment to him, causing him to become withdrawn and upset. His school performance has also declined and, although he has always been socially outgoing, his peer relationships have deteriorated dramatically. Bob is in good general health and has no history of any exposure to psychotropic medications. Bob's father reports that he also exhibited some unusual head movements as a child but that these seemed to diminish as he grew older.

On examination, Bob exhibits recurrent motor and vocal tics. The motor tics include eye blinking and shoulder shrugs. The vocal tics include both simple throat-clearing sounds and occasional coprolalia. Bob is clearly distressed by these behaviors, particularly the vocal tics. Although he can suppress the tics briefly, he experiences an internal and ultimately irresistible urge to perform these acts. He tries to cover up by incorporating the movements in what appear to be purposeful behaviors, like scratching his head or yawning. Although clearly upset, anxious, and suffering from some problems with poor self-esteem, he does not exhibit features of depression. His speech is well articulated and logically organized, and he does not have major difficulties with attention or concentration. No symptoms suggestive of Schizophrenia or other psychotic conditions are observed. Apart from being worried about his disorder and the possibility that he might be "going crazy," Bob is not particularly preoccupied with recurrent thoughts or worries, and compulsive behaviors are not evident. Psychological testing reveals an IQ within the normal range with commensurate achievement scores.

DSM-IV-TR Diagnosis

Axis I: 307.23   Tourette's Disorder
Axis II: V71.09   No diagnosis
Axis III: None
Axis IV: Poor peer relations
Axis V: GAF = 50 (current); 60 (highest level past year)

DSM-IV-TR diagnostic criteria for 307.23 Tourette's Disorder

A. Both multiple motor and one or more vocal tics have been present at some time during the illness, although not necessarily concurrently. (A *tic* is a sudden, rapid, recurrent, nonrhythmic, stereotyped motor movement or vocalization.)
B. The tics occur many times a day (usually in bouts) nearly every day or intermittently throughout a period of more than 1 year, and during this period there was never a tic-free period of more than 3 consecutive months.
C. The onset is before age 18 years.
D. The disturbance is not due to the direct physiological effects of a substance (e.g., stimulants) or a general medical condition (e.g., Huntington's disease or postviral encephalitis).

Guidelines for Differential
Diagnosis of Tourette's Disorder

Although Bob's symptoms do cause him distress and interfere with his social functioning, they are not, as his parents and pediatrician feared, a sign of psychosis. Note that, although Bob did experience distress, the criteria for Tourette's Disorder, as revised in DSM-IV-TR, no longer require "clinically significant distress or impairment" to make the diagnosis. This change was made because clinical experience indicates that many children with Tourette's Disorder do not experience marked distress or impairment.

Bob has a history of long-standing motor tics, with the more recent onset of vocal tics. The diagnosis of Tourette's Disorder requires both motor and vocal tics that occur intermittently for a period of more than 1 year with no more than 3 months in which tics do not occur.

The natural history of Tourette's Disorder often includes a history of attentional problems that are sometimes severe enough to merit an additional diagnosis of Attention-Deficit/Hyperactivity Disorder (although Bob's attentional problems were not severe enough to warrant an additional diagnosis). Tourette's Disorder has its onset before age 18, with motor tics usually appearing several years before vocal tics.

Distinctions between the different disorders in the Tic Disorders category are based on the duration, variety, and onset of the tics. In Transient Tic Disorder, motor and/or vocal tics last for at least 4 weeks but for no longer than 1 year. In Chronic Motor or Vocal Tic Disorder, either motor or vocal tics are present, but not both. Tic Disorder Not Otherwise Specified would be used to describe a clinically significant tic condition that does not meet criteria for any of the specifically defined Tic Disorders (e.g., a condition that has lasted for less than 4 weeks or begins after age 18 years).

The tics in Tourette's Disorder and the other Tic Disorders must be differentiated from other movement problems such as choreiform, dystonic, athetoid, myoclonic, and hemiballistic movements. In contrast to such movements, tics are sudden, rapid, stereotyped, nonrhythmic, and recurrent. Tics can be classified as simple (e.g., eye blinking or throat clearing) or complex (facial gestures or coprolalia). Tics usually diminish markedly during sleep. Although the tics can be suppressed for periods of time, they may be exacerbated by stressful situations such as the clinical interview. Abnormal movements associated with various general medical conditions (e.g., Huntington's disease, Wilson's disease, head injury, etc.) must be distinguished from Tourette's Disorder. Similarly, if tics are a direct result of the use of a medication, the appropriate diagnosis would be Medication-Induced Movement Disorder Not Otherwise Specified.

Tourette's Disorder must also be distinguished from the stereotyped movements that occur in Autistic Disorder and other Pervasive Developmental Disorders and in Stereotypic Movement Disorder. Although simple tics can usually be readily differentiated, the distinction between complex tics and stereotyped movements may be more difficult. Stereotyped movements appear to be more intentional and are rhythmic in nature.

Complex motor tics may also sometimes be difficult to distinguish from the compulsions of Obsessive-Compulsive Disorder; however, compulsions are usually very complex and are performed in response to an obsession or obsessional rule. Some individuals exhibit both Tourette's Disorder and Obsessive-Compulsive Disorder, and accumulating research suggests that these disorders may be on a spectrum with a shared family history. Occasionally, motor and vocal tics will be mistaken for the unusual behavior of Schizophrenia.

Treatment Planning for Tourette's Disorder

Tourette's Disorder is a chronic condition that often waxes and wanes over time. If tics have been misperceived as intentional behaviors on the part of the child and have led to negative experiences, educational and supportive psychotherapy interventions can have a major impact. Because children with Tourette's Disorder sometimes also have attentional and learning problems, educational interventions may be necessary. Providing parents with information about the condition is also often very helpful. Pharmacological intervention may be indicated. The relatively more selective D_2 antagonists (haloperidol and pimozide) have been proven effective in carefully controlled, double-blind studies. Symptom reduction is often striking, although side effects sometimes limit the usefulness of such agents. Clonidine, a selective α_2-adrenergic receptor agonist, may be helpful in a smaller group of patients and has the advantage of fewer side effects.

Summary

The diagnosis of Tourette's Disorder can be difficult, especially in younger children who do not yet display both motor and vocal tics. Sometimes Attention-Deficit/Hyperactivity Disorder is diagnosed before the symptoms of Tourette's Disorder develop.

Other Disorders of Infancy, Childhood, or Adolescence

309.21   Separation Anxiety Disorder
313.23   Selective Mutism
313.89   Reactive Attachment Disorder of Infancy or Early Childhood
307.3   Stereotypic Movement Disorder
313.9   Disorder of Infancy, Childhood, or Adolescence Not Otherwise Specified

Other Disorders of Infancy, Childhood, or Adolescence

Separation Anxiety Disorder

❖   Case Study: An 8-Year-Old Boy
Who Refuses to Go to School

Cal is an 8-year-old boy who is referred because of social withdrawal, overwhelming fears, multiple somatic complaints, and refusal to attend school. Cal's difficulties first began with trouble falling asleep and frequent nightmares. He is preoccupied with morbid daydreams of family members' dying or being injured and of threatening and terrifying antisuperheroes. He categorically refuses to go to bed unless his mother sits beside him and most nights will fight sleep for more than an hour so that she will not leave him.

Especially on school days, Cal complains of many headaches and stomachaches for which no physical basis could be found on a recent pediatric examination. Because of these physical complaints, he frequently stays home from school and has trouble paying attention when he does go to school. He often insists that he is sick and needs to go home. His school performance has deteriorated, and his grades have dropped from an A average to barely passing.

Cal's social relations have also become increasingly restricted because he is reluctant to play away from home at friends' houses and absolutely refuses to sleep at a friend's house overnight. Nonetheless he is glad to have friends come to play at his house. When he does go to a friend's house, he insists on writing down the phone number at which his mother can be reached and insists that his mother tell him the exact time she will be picking him up. He frequently asks to call his mother to reassure himself that she is there. He also repeatedly asks what time it is and how long it will be until his mother is supposed to come. If she is by some chance delayed by even a few minutes in picking him up, he becomes fretful and unable to focus his attention on activities with his friends.

The mental status exam shows Cal to be a worried, anxious, sad child with increased activity and difficulty attending to the examiner. He brightens up immediately, however, whenever his mother returns to the room. Cal describes his multiple problems with difficulty and says that he is afraid matters will never improve, although he does relate well to the examiner and states a desire to feel better and to attain his previous level of school achievement. There is no evidence of a thought disorder, cognitive impairment, or suicidal risk. Cal's mother reports that his development was normal, except that almost from birth he was an anxious and worried child. His symptoms became much worse, however, soon after his father retired from a desk job and began to work as a factory security officer at night and his mother was hospitalized for acute emphysema and began experiencing intermittent dysphoric episodes. Cal is the youngest of three children; two older sisters are married and live away from home.

DSM-IV-TR Diagnosis

Axis I:	309.21	Separation Anxiety Disorder
Axis II:	V71.09	No diagnosis
Axis III:	None	
Axis IV:	Mother's hospitalization and illness, father's new job	
Axis V:	GAF = 60	

DSM-IV-TR diagnostic criteria for
309.21 Separation Anxiety Disorder

A. Developmentally inappropriate and excessive anxiety concerning separation from home or from those to whom the individual is attached, as evidenced by three (or more) of the following:
    (1) recurrent excessive distress when separation from home or major attachment figures occurs or is anticipated
    (2) persistent and excessive worry about losing, or about possible harm befalling, major attachment figures
    (3) persistent and excessive worry that an untoward event will lead to separation from a major attachment figure (e.g., getting lost or being kidnapped)
    (4) persistent reluctance or refusal to go to school or elsewhere because of fear of separation
    (5) persistently and excessively fearful or reluctant to be alone or without major attachment figures at home or without significant adults in other settings
    (6) persistent reluctance or refusal to go to sleep without being near a major attachment figure or to sleep away from home
    (7) repeated nightmares involving the theme of separation
    (8) repeated complaints of physical symptoms (such as headaches, stomachaches, nausea, or vomiting) when separation from major attachment figures occurs or is anticipated
B. The duration of the disturbance is at least 4 weeks.
C. The onset is before age 18 years.
D. The disturbance causes clinically significant distress or impairment in social, academic (occupational), or other important areas of functioning.
E. The disturbance does not occur exclusively during the course of a Pervasive Developmental Disorder, Schizophrenia, or other Psychotic Disorder and, in adolescents and adults, is not better accounted for by Panic Disorder With Agoraphobia.

Specify if:
Early Onset: if onset occurs before age 6 years

Guidelines for Differential Diagnosis of Separation Anxiety Disorder

The first, and most important, differential to consider in diagnosing Separation Anxiety Disorder is that the discomfort must be beyond that which is normal and developmentally appropriate when one is separated from loved ones. The clinician must take into account the child's age and the cultural values of the family group. If Cal were 4 or 5 years old, his reluctance to stay away from home at night and his preoccupation with his mother's whereabouts would probably not be considered excessive. However, at 8 years old, in our society at least, Cal would be expected to be learning how to begin separating more readily from his mother. By bringing Cal in for evaluation, the family has clearly indicated that they too find that Cal's anxiety about separation goes beyond what they consider acceptable and is distressing to both him and them.

It is also important to rule out other disorders in which separation anxiety may be an associated feature that does not require a separate diagnosis. Based on the mental status exam, Cal clearly does not show symptoms of autism or psychosis. The diagnosis of Separation Anxiety Disorder is usually restricted to childhood and early adolescence because most individuals either outgrow it or go on to develop Panic Disorder With Agoraphobia or another Anxiety Disorder. If Panic Disorder develops in adolescence or adulthood in such individuals, only the Panic Disorder is diagnosed.

Two other disorders should be considered in diagnosing Separation Anxiety Disorder. If the child's anxieties are wide ranging and involve a number of everyday concerns beyond fear of separation, a diagnosis of Generalized Anxiety Disorder may be appropriate. In Cal's case, however, his anxiety is focused almost entirely on separation from home and family. A Major Depressive Disorder should also be considered if the child's fears are accompanied by marked depressive symptoms. Although Cal is unhappy, this is probably secondary to his separation fears and is not severe enough to meet full criteria for a depressive disorder.

Treatment Planning for Separation Anxiety Disorder

There has been little systematic research on the treatment of Separation Anxiety Disorder, but parent training, cognitive-behavioral therapy, and time all may be effective.

Summary

It is important to avoid both underdiagnosing and overdiagnosing this disorder. Underdiagnosing may result in the perpetuation of persistent patterns of intolerance to anxiety that may culminate in adult Panic Disorder and Agoraphobia. Overdiagnosis may result in the stigmatization and overtreatment of normal developmentally appropriate separation anxiety that will take care of itself in time.

Chapter 2

Delirium, Dementia, and Amnestic and Other Cognitive Disorders

The cognitive disorders section of DSM-IV-TR includes Delirium, Dementia, and Amnestic and Other Cognitive Disorders, which are coded as 294.9 Cognitive Disorder Not Otherwise Specified. All the disorders in this section are characterized by a cognitive impairment of some sort that is due to a general medical condition, to a substance or medication, or to a combination of these. These disorders were formerly referred to as "organic disorders," a misleading term that was dropped in DSM-IV because it mistakenly implied that there was some sort of mind-body dichotomy that separated the "organic" mental disorders from the other mental disorders. No one now believes that Schizophrenia, Mood Disorders, or even Personality Disorders are without biological foundation. In fact, the view in DSM-IV (and DSM-IV-TR) is that all disorders in the manual have at least some biological component and that all of them, including those in this section, are also influenced by psychological factors and environmental context. In this section, we present case examples illustrating Delirium Due to Multiple Etiologies, Dementia of the Alzheimer's Type, Vascular Dementia, and Amnestic Disorder Due to a General Medical Condition.

Delirium

Delirium may have one or more etiologies. The DSM-IV-TR classification for the types of delirium is shown below:

Delirium

293.0   Delirium Due to . . . *[Indicate the General Medical Condition]*
——.–   Substance Intoxication Delirium *(refer to Substance-Related Disorders for substance-specific codes)*
——.–   Substance Withdrawal Delirium *(refer to Substance-Related Disorders for substance-specific codes)*
——.–   Delirium Due to Multiple Etiologies *(code each of the specific etiologies)*
780.09   Delirium Not Otherwise Specified

❖   Case Study: An Elderly Woman Who
Has Suddenly Become Confused

Mrs. T is a 79-year-old retired schoolteacher who is brought to the emergency room after being found wandering around her neighborhood in a confused and disoriented state. She seemed to be in good health until a few months ago when her husband was hospitalized for 10 days for relatively minor surgery. About a month after her husband returned home, he and their two married daughters, who do not live at home, reported a noticeable change in Mrs. T's mental status. She became somewhat hyperactive and seemed to have excessive energy, was irritable and agitated, had difficulty getting to sleep at night, and became preoccupied with concerns that she was going to die. She began to prepare for death and wanted to visit relatives in the Midwest to see them for the last time.

After Mrs. T's confused and depressive symptoms had gone on for about a week, she was taken to see a psychiatrist, who made a diagnosis of depression and started her on imipramine and haloperidol. Shortly after beginning these medications, her agitation decreased slightly, but she began to have difficulty remembering recent events and seemed even more confused and disoriented. These difficulties continued, and one day Mrs. T called the police telling them she was being poisoned by the pills she was being given. She became disoriented to time and place, markedly confused, and incontinent and began wandering away from home. When she encountered anyone, she became verbally and physically abusive.

When Mrs. T was brought in for evaluation, the initial diagnostic impression was of a psychotic depression superimposed on a dementing illness. The consultant also noted that Mrs. T was experiencing a number of anticholinergic side effects, such as dry mouth, constipation, and racing heart, and suggested that she be removed from all medications. After she discontinued all medications, Mrs. T's condition improved rapidly: Her psychotic thinking and assaultiveness disappeared, and her agitation and confusion decreased.

During the next several weeks, however, Mrs. T continued to have intermittent episodes of clouding of consciousness during which she became confused and disoriented. She was found wandering around her neighborhood in a confused state and was brought to the emergency room for this evaluation.

Mrs. T's mental status examination upon admission shows her to be disoriented to time and place, agitated, and confused. During an interview with the patient's husband, an important piece of information about Mrs. T's recent history is brought to light for the first time. This information was not elicited in the early evaluations and was therefore not taken into account in the initial treatment planning. Mrs. T has for many years suffered from dizziness and light-headedness upon standing and has had occasional falls, none of which have caused any lasting damage. Shortly before her depressive and confused symptoms began, Mrs. T apparently suffered a fall during the night and was found by her husband in the morning lying next to her bed in a confused state. Because they were accustomed to such falls, neither Mr. nor Mrs. T made much of this experience, nor did they report it to any of Mrs. T's physicians until now. A computed tomography (CT) scan reveals the presence of a subdural hematoma, which is then evacuated. After this procedure Mrs. T's confusion and disorientation clear completely and she returns to her previous level of functioning.

DSM-IV-TR Diagnosis

Axis I:	Delirium Due to Multiple Etiologies:	
	293.0	Delirium Due to Head Trauma
	292.81	Anticholinergic-Induced Delirium
Axis II:	V71.09	No diagnosis
Axis III:	E941.1	Central anticholinergic syndrome
	852.2	Head trauma with subdural hematoma
	733.00	Osteoporosis
Axis IV:	Hospitalization of husband, financial worries	
Axis V:	GAF = 20 (on admission); 70 (after subdural hematoma cleared and medications discontinued)	

DSM-IV-TR diagnostic criteria for Delirium

A. Disturbance of consciousness (i.e., reduced clarity of awareness of the environment) with reduced ability to focus, sustain, or shift attention.

B. A change in cognition (such as memory deficit, disorientation, language disturbance) or the development of a perceptual disturbance that is not better accounted for by a preexisting, established, or evolving dementia.

C. The disturbance develops over a short period of time (usually hours to days) and tends to fluctuate during the course of the day.

D. [Varies based on etiology—see specific disorders for discussion.]

DSM-IV-TR diagnostic criteria for 293.0 Delirium Due to . . . *[Indicate the General Medical Condition]*

A. Disturbance of consciousness (i.e., reduced clarity of awareness of the environment) with reduced ability to focus, sustain, or shift attention.

B. A change in cognition (such as memory deficit, disorientation, language disturbance) or the development of a perceptual disturbance that is not better accounted for by a preexisting, established, or evolving dementia.

C. The disturbance develops over a short period of time (usually hours to days) and tends to fluctuate during the course of the day.

D. There is evidence from the history, physical examination, or laboratory findings that the disturbance is caused by the direct physiological consequences of a general medical condition.

Coding note: If delirium is superimposed on a preexisting Vascular Dementia, indicate the delirium by coding 290.41 Vascular Dementia, With Delirium.

Coding note: Include the name of the general medical condition on Axis I, e.g., 293.0 Delirium Due to Hepatic Encephalopathy; also code the general medical condition on Axis III (see Appendix G for codes).

> # DSM-IV-TR diagnostic criteria for
> ## Substance Intoxication Delirium
>
> A. Disturbance of consciousness (i.e., reduced clarity of awareness of the environment) with reduced ability to focus, sustain, or shift attention.
> B. A change in cognition (such as memory deficit, disorientation, language disturbance) or the development of a perceptual disturbance that is not better accounted for by a preexisting, established, or evolving dementia.
> C. The disturbance develops over a short period of time (usually hours to days) and tends to fluctuate during the course of the day.
> D. There is evidence from the history, physical examination, or laboratory findings of either (1) or (2):
>   (1) the symptoms in Criteria A and B developed during Substance Intoxication
>   (2) medication use is etiologically related to the disturbance*
>
> **Note:**   This diagnosis should be made instead of a diagnosis of Substance Intoxication only when the cognitive symptoms are in excess of those usually associated with the intoxication syndrome and when the symptoms are sufficiently severe to warrant independent clinical attention.
>
> *Note: The diagnosis should be recorded as Substance-Induced Delirium if related to medication use. Refer to Appendix G for E-codes indicating specific medications.
>
> Code [Specific Substance] Intoxication Delirium:
> (291.0 Alcohol; 292.81 Amphetamine [or Amphetamine-Like Substance]; 292.81 Cannabis; 292.81 Cocaine; 292.81 Hallucinogen; 292.81 Inhalant; 292.81 Opioid; 292.81 Phencyclidine [or Phencyclidine-Like Substance]; 292.81 Sedative, Hypnotic, or Anxiolytic; 292.81 Other [or Unknown] Substance [e.g., cimetidine, digitalis, benztropine])

Guidelines for Differential Diagnosis of Delirium

This presentation illustrates the crucial point that late-onset psychopathology is much more likely to be due to medication side effects, to a general medical condition, or to the combined effects of both than to the development of a new primary mental disorder. It is surprising how often this is missed. Patients presenting with delirium are often misdiagnosed as depressed and treated with medications that compound and exacerbate the symptoms further, thus leading to a vicious cycle. Very often "psychopathology" will improve when the medication that has in fact been its cause and not its cure is reduced or discontinued. It is thus instructive that Mrs. T improved markedly when all medications were discontinued.

This case also illustrates the importance of trying to gather as much information as possible about the patient's history, especially when there is a sudden late onset of symptoms. Incidents that may not seem at all important to the patient or family, like Mrs. T's history of falls and her recent head trauma, may be very important in proper evaluation and treatment.

To diagnose delirium, the clinician must determine whether a cognitive disturbance and attentional difficulties are responsible for the symptoms. The symptoms of delirium usually develop over a short period of time and tend to fluctuate during the course of the day. Mrs. T did present with a change in cognition (i.e., memory deficits, confusion, and disorientation) and a disturbance of consciousness, as evidenced by her confusion about time and place and her tendency to wander away from home.

Delirium may be caused by a general medical condition or a substance or medication, or, as often happens, it may have multiple causes. For this reason, a category for "Delirium Due to Multiple Etiologies" is included in DSM-IV-TR to alert clinicians to the need to consider this possibility. A very common pattern of multiple etiologies is a causative general medical condition that is being treated with a medication that is also contributing to the delirium. Mrs. T's initial symptoms appear to have been caused by a subdural hematoma resulting from a head trauma, but they were then compounded and exacerbated by the medications with which she was treated. When evaluating the symptoms of delirium, it is important to try to find and correct the specific cause if there is only one. However, it is also always useful to carefully check if additional causes may be contributing to the symptoms. The clinician should not consider the diagnostic evaluation complete until all possible causes have been ruled out. This is especially true for Alcohol Withdrawal Delirium (delirium tremens [the DTs]), which is very likely to occur with and be exacerbated by the presence of an underlying general medical condition. When more than one etiology is present, each should be coded separately. Note that Substance Intoxication Delirium should be diagnosed only when the cognitive symptoms are in excess of what would usually be seen in an individual intoxicated with that substance.

It is often difficult to evaluate whether dementia is also present until the acute symptoms of delirium have cleared. Mrs. T's symptoms arose suddenly and were of relatively short duration, a presentation that is consistent with a diagnosis of delirium. A characteristic symptom pattern involving marked confusion and attentional problems is also much more typical of delirium, as is a fluctuating pattern of symptoms and disturbances in the sleep-wake cycle.

The diagnosis of delirium is much less likely to be missed when it occurs in the agitated form, as seen in Mrs. T's case. It is more likely to be missed when the patient is quiet. In such cases, delirium may be misinterpreted as depression, dementia, or normal passivity. Many patients in a nursing home or hospital may be unobtrusively disoriented in a manner that will be picked up only with systematic clinical interviewing.

Treatment Planning for Delirium

Delirium is a medical emergency. In treating it, the focus is on quickly carrying out a medical workup and implementing treatment interventions. Delirium has serious risks and complications that can be reduced by prompt intervention once the causes are identified. The underlying cause is often correctable but, if left untreated, whatever is causing the delirium can ultimately result in serious medical complications and irreversible cognitive impairments (e.g., dementia or Amnestic Disorder). The clinician must be aware that untreated delirium is associated with a high mortality rate. Because of their poor judgment and reduced awareness, individuals in delirious states are at risk for accidents, suicide, or violent behavior. For example, Mrs. T wandered off from home in a disoriented state and was verbally and physically abusive to strangers on the street. The management of delirium usually requires the provision of a structured environment, with measures taken to ensure the patient's safety, and appropriate medical evaluation and treatment.

Summary

This diagnosis is probably one of the most likely to be missed and, when missed, to cause the most mischief. The best way to avoid this is to maintain a very high index of suspicion, particularly concerning symptoms in the elderly and among substance users. The second crucial issue is that you must not stop the workup once you have found one cause because other causes are also frequently present. Delirium is particularly likely to occur in the strange, unfamiliar hospital environment, especially at night.

Dementia

In this section, we present a case example illustrating Dementia of the Alzheimer's Type and an example illustrating Vascular Dementia. Dementia may be caused by a number of general medical conditions (e.g., 294.1 Dementia Due to HIV Disease, 294.1 Dementia Due to Head Trauma,

294.1 Dementia Due to Parkinson's Disease, etc.), by the long-term effects of substances or medications (Substance-Induced Persisting Dementia), or by a combination of these (Dementia Due to Multiple Etiologies), in which case all the causes are coded separately (e.g., Vascular Dementia and Dementia of the Alzheimer's Type). Although the etiologies vary, the descriptive features of each type of dementia are the same and involve a memory impairment accompanied by at least one of four additional cognitive disturbances: aphasia, apraxia, agnosia, or a disturbance in executive functioning. The DSM-IV-TR classification for dementia is shown below:

Dementia

294.xx   Dementia of the Alzheimer's Type, With Early Onset *(also code 331.0 Alzheimer's disease on Axis III)*
   .10   Without Behavioral Disturbance
   .11   With Behavioral Disturbance
294.xx   Dementia of the Alzheimer's Type, With Late Onset *(also code 331.0 Alzheimer's disease on Axis III)*
   .10   Without Behavioral Disturbance
   .11   With Behavioral Disturbance
290.xx   Vascular Dementia
   .40   Uncomplicated
   .41   With Delirium
   .42   With Delusions
   .43   With Depressed Mood
   Specify if: With Behavioral Disturbance
Code presence or absence of a behavioral disturbance in the fifth digit for Dementia Due to a General Medical Condition:
   0 = Without Behavioral Disturbance
   1 = With Behavioral Disturbance
294.1x   Dementia Due to HIV Disease *(also code 042 HIV on Axis III)*
294.1x   Dementia Due to Head Trauma *(also code 854.00 head injury on Axis III)*
294.1x   Dementia Due to Parkinson's Disease *(also code 331.82 Dementia with Lewy bodies on Axis III)*
294.1x   Dementia Due to Huntington's Disease *(also code 333.4 Huntington's disease on Axis III)*
294.1x   Dementia Due to Pick's Disease *(also code 331.11 Pick's disease on Axis III)*

(continued)

Dementia *(continued)*

294.1x Dementia Due to Creutzfeldt-Jakob Disease *(also code 046.1 Creutzfeldt-Jakob disease on Axis III)*

294.1x Dementia Due to . . . *[Indicate the General Medical Condition not listed above] (also code the general medical condition on Axis III)*

——.— Substance-Induced Persisting Dementia *(refer to Substance-Related Disorders for substance-specific codes)*

——.— Dementia Due to Multiple Etiologies *(code each of the specific etiologies)*

294.8 Dementia Not Otherwise Specified

Coding note: Also code 331.0 Alzheimer's disease on Axis III. Indicate other prominent clinical features related to the Alzheimer's disease on Axis I (e.g., 293.83 Mood Disorder Due to Alzheimer's Disease, With Depressive Features, and 310.1 Personality Change Due to Alzheimer's Disease, Aggressive Type).

Dementia of the Alzheimer's Type

❖ Case Study: An Elderly Man Whose
Wife Can No Longer Care for Him

Mr. E is a 68-year-old married man with two children who has been followed by a multidisciplinary team at a Department of Veterans Affairs (VA) geriatric research and clinical center for the past 6 years. The occasion for this evaluation is Mrs. E's request for residential placement for her husband.

Mr. E was first evaluated 9 years ago when his wife observed changes in his memory and behavior and suggested that they seek medical advice. At that time, Mr. E was still employed as a security guard. During the couple's initial visit to a physician, Mr. E acknowledged that he had been aware of increasing memory problems for at least the past 2 years. He said that he frequently forgot his keys or would go into the house to get something and then forget what he wanted. Mrs. E noted that he had changed from an outgoing, pleasant person to one who avoided conversation. She said that he also seemed hostile at times for no apparent reason. Mr. E was in good general health and was not taking any medications. His alcohol consumption was limited to two to three beers a day. He had no significant medical or psychiatric history and no significant family history for either cognitive or psychiatric disorders.

Three years later, Mrs. E contacted the VA center for treatment of her husband's cognitive and behavioral symptoms. The general physical examination conducted during this visit was unremarkable. The neurological examination demonstrated an absence of focal abnormalities, but glabellar, snout, and palmomental responses were present. Mr. E was hesitant and had difficulty with sustained attention, which made determination of visual fields difficult. There was no evidence of any disturbance of mood. On examination of his sensorium, Mr. E was disoriented about place and date: He missed the actual date by 2 years and 1 month. However, he seemed to comprehend most of the questions and was aware that he was experiencing cognitive difficulties.

On neuropsychological testing, Mr. E showed moderate to severe impairment in memory, attention, visual spatial reasoning, set shifting, and judgment and planning abilities. Results of laboratory screening tests were unremarkable. An electroencephalogram (EEG) was mildly abnormal, showing nonspecific theta waves and sharp discharges bilaterally. A CT head scan showed slight enlargement of the lateral ventricles and the third ventricle, which was consistent with mild atrophy.

Mrs. E reported that her husband had begun exposing himself to neighbors, especially children who walked by their windows. She said that he had become sexually aggressive toward her and at times would chase her around the house and try to remove her clothing. When told of these activities, he claimed to have no recollection of them.

Mr. E was started on 1 mg of haloperidol at bedtime. Shortly after this, his wife became concerned that the medication was actually increasing his agitated behavior because he had begun to lock himself in the bedroom and would not allow her to clean him up after he was incontinent of stool in his clothing. The haloperidol was then reduced to .5 mg/day. Mr. E's behavior did not improve after 4 months of medication, so the drug was discontinued at Mrs. E's request.

A year and a half after Mr. E's initial visit to the geriatric center (and 6 years after he began experiencing cognitive and behavioral symptoms), Mrs. E first began discussing long-term placement for Mr. E with the treatment team. By this time, the dementia was severe: Mr. E paced most of the night, experienced frequent crying spells, and had become physically threatening to his wife. On one occasion, Mrs. E had gotten up during the night to find that her husband had turned up the thermostat to the maximum temperature, turned on all the burners on the stove, and turned the oven on at 500 degrees.

However, after exploring family support options with the team, Mrs. E decided to continue to care for her husband in their home. A selective serotonin reuptake inhibitor was prescribed for him, after which Mrs. E noted an initial decrease in Mr. E's crying, an improvement in his sleep, and an increased willingness to help with some of the household chores. However,

Mrs. E soon felt the medication was making Mr. E more confused and unmanageable and after 4 months it was discontinued.

About 7 months later, Mrs. E brings her husband in for this evaluation to seriously investigate residential placement for him. She says she is at the end of her rope because Mr. E constantly wanders off when she isn't watching him and has nearly been run over on several occasions. Although she describes feeling terribly guilty about "abandoning" him, she does not think she can cope any longer with the responsibility of ensuring his safety. She doesn't see any alternative but to arrange for his placement in a residential facility. Mr. E is therefore transferred from the geriatric center to a VA long-term-care center 120 miles away.

DSM-IV-TR Diagnosis

Axis I: 294.11   Dementia of the Alzheimer's Type,
                     With Early Onset, With Behavioral Disturbance
Axis II: V71.09   No diagnosis
Axis III: 331.0   Alzheimer's disease
Axis IV: Financial difficulties
Axis V: GAF = 15 (current); 20 (highest level in the past year)

DSM-IV-TR diagnostic criteria for 294.1x Dementia of the Alzheimer's Type

A. The development of multiple cognitive deficits manifested by both
   (1) memory impairment (impaired ability to learn new information or to recall previously learned information)
   (2) one (or more) of the following cognitive disturbances:
       (a) aphasia (language disturbance)
       (b) apraxia (impaired ability to carry out motor activities despite intact motor function)
       (c) agnosia (failure to recognize or identify objects despite intact sensory function)
       (d) disturbance in executive functioning (i.e., planning, organizing, sequencing, abstracting)
B. The cognitive deficits in Criteria A1 and A2 each cause significant impairment in social or occupational functioning and represent a significant decline from a previous level of functioning.
C. The course is characterized by gradual onset and continuing cognitive decline.

(continued)

DSM-IV-TR diagnostic criteria for
294.1x Dementia of the Alzheimer's Type *(continued)*

D. The cognitive deficits in Criteria A1 and A2 are not due to any of the following:

   (1) other central nervous system conditions that cause progressive deficits in memory and cognition (e.g., cerebrovascular disease, Parkinson's disease, Huntington's disease, subdural hematoma, normal-pressure hydrocephalus, brain tumor)

   (2) systemic conditions that are known to cause dementia (e.g., hypothyroidism, vitamin B_{12} or folic acid deficiency, niacin deficiency, hypercalcemia, neurosyphilis, HIV infection)

   (3) substance-induced conditions

E. The deficits do not occur exclusively during the course of a delirium.

F. The disturbance is not better accounted for by another Axis I disorder (e.g., Major Depressive Disorder, Schizophrenia).

Code based on presence or absence of a clinically significant behavioral disturbance:

294.10 Without Behavioral Disturbance: if the cognitive disturbance is not accompanied by any clinically significant behavioral disturbance.

294.11 With Behavioral Disturbance: if the cognitive disturbance is accompanied by a clinically significant behavioral disturbance (e.g., wandering, agitation).

Specify subtype:

  With Early Onset: if onset is at age 65 years or below

  With Late Onset: if onset is after age 65 years

Coding note: Also code 331.0 Alzheimer's disease on Axis III. Indicate other prominent clinical features related to the Alzheimer's disease on Axis I (e.g., 293.83 Mood Disorder Due to Alzheimer's Disease, With Depressive Features, and 310.1 Personality Change Due to Alzheimer's Disease, Aggressive Type).

Vascular Dementia

❖   Case Study: A Late Onset
of Depression and Memory Loss

Mr. A is a 67-year-old retired factory worker who is referred from another hospital for inpatient evaluation after he "failed to respond" to therapy for a depressive episode. Before transfer, Mr. A had a 2-month history of depressed mood, decreased interest in his usual activities, withdrawal from family and friends, a 10-pound weight loss, and difficulty falling and staying asleep. He also had problems with memory and with making decisions, suicidal ideation, and a growing belief that the government was out to get him for presumed misdeeds, which Mr. A's wife insisted was without any foundation.

During his stay in the other hospital, Mr. A underwent a 3-week trial of doxepin (with 2 weeks at a maximum dose of 150 mg/day) and haloperidol 2 mg bid. He developed urinary retention, constipation, orthostatic effects, and pseudoparkinsonian symptomatology on this psychopharmacological regimen, and his depressive symptoms worsened, leading to his referral to our facility. Mr. A was tapered off the doxepin and haloperidol during the week before transfer.

Although Mr. A has no history of previous depressive episodes, his wife reports that his memory has been "getting bad" for at least several years and that he began acting "suspicious" about the government as long as a year ago. There is no evidence of mental illness in Mr. A's family except that his father was placed in a nursing home at age 70 because "his mind couldn't work right."

When evaluated on transfer, Mr. A appears to be a sad and hopeless-looking elderly man who is quite difficult to engage in conversation. Initially, he shows clear evidence of motor retardation, although he becomes somewhat agitated later in the interview when discussing his condition. Mr. A is oriented except to day and month. He is unable to remember any of three items after 5 minutes.

The physical examination is essentially within normal limits except for a blood pressure of 190/110 and neurological findings that include the presence of snout and bilateral grasp reflexes. Both plantar reflexes are flexor, however.

The neurological consultant concludes that the data support a possible diagnosis of dementia and suggests further laboratory studies, including magnetic resonance imaging (MRI) of the brain, an EEG, and lumbar puncture. The MRI shows diffuse mild cerebral atrophy and a slight enlargement of the lateral ventricles. The neuroradiologist reports that both changes are abnormal for Mr. A's age. Also noted in the T2-weighted MRI are several patchy and diffuse hyperintense foci in the periventricular and deep white matter. The EEG reveals mild generalized slowing, again more than would be expected for a patient of Mr. A's age. Analysis of cerebrospinal fluid is normal.

Results of other laboratory studies, including a thyroid function test and vitamin B_{12} and folate levels, are all normal except for the electrocardiogram (ECG), which demonstrates a bifascicular block. The cardiology consultant cautions against the further use of antidepressant medication for Mr. A and suggests that electroconvulsive therapy (ECT) be considered instead.

A psychological examination is done to further assess the level of Mr. A's cognitive dysfunction. The results of a Minnesota Multiphasic Personality Inventory (MMPI) are compatible with the presence of a depressive episode with psychotic ideation. A Wechsler Adult Intelligence Scale—Revised (WAIS-R) reveals a marked discrepancy between verbal IQ (95) and performance IQ (70). This evidence for cerebral dysfunction is further supported by the results of a Halstead-Reitan Battery, which is interpreted as compatible with a moderate diffuse cognitive impairment that is affecting memory function and other cognitive areas.

After this evaluation, Mr. A is referred for a consultation with the chief of the ECT service, who agrees with the clinical team that a recommendation for ECT is appropriate. A subsequent pre-ECT workup is unremarkable. Mr. A agrees to receive ECT and provides signed consent.

Mr. A receives a total of eight brief-pulse unilateral nondominant ECT treatments three times a week. (The right side is stimulated because Mr. A is right-body dominant.) Initial improvement in sleep and appetite is noted after the second treatment. By the sixth treatment, both affective and vegetative symptoms have all but disappeared. What is particularly remarkable to Mr. A's wife, as well as to many of the ward staff, is that Mr. A's problem with memory also seems to be diminished, as opposed to the worsening they expected to see over the ECT course.

By the time Mr. A is discharged from the hospital, 4 days after completion of the course of ECT, he is verbal, outgoing, and able to focus on plans to use the time available to him in his retirement more constructively. Because of the cardiac findings, it is decided to begin maintenance ECT on an outpatient basis.

DSM-IV-TR Diagnosis

Axis I: 290.43   Vascular Dementia, With Depressed Mood
Axis II: V71.09   No diagnosis
Axis III: 426.2   Bifascicular block
Axis IV: Recent retirement
Axis V: GAF = 40 (on admission); 65 (on discharge)

DSM-IV-TR diagnostic criteria for 290.4x Vascular Dementia

A. The development of multiple cognitive deficits manifested by both
    (1) memory impairment (impaired ability to learn new information or to recall previously learned information)
    (2) one (or more) of the following cognitive disturbances:
        (a) aphasia (language disturbance)
        (b) apraxia (impaired ability to carry out motor activities despite intact motor function)
        (c) agnosia (failure to recognize or identify objects despite intact sensory function)
        (d) disturbance in executive functioning (i.e., planning, organizing, sequencing, abstracting)

B. The cognitive deficits in Criteria A1 and A2 each cause significant impairment in social or occupational functioning and represent a significant decline from a previous level of functioning.

C. Focal neurological signs and symptoms (e.g., exaggeration of deep tendon reflexes, extensor plantar response, pseudobulbar palsy, gait abnormalities, weakness of an extremity) or laboratory evidence indicative of cerebrovascular disease (e.g., multiple infarctions involving cortex and underlying white matter) that are judged to be etiologically related to the disturbance.

D. The deficits do not occur exclusively during the course of a delirium.

Code based on predominant features:

290.41 With Delirium: if delirium is superimposed on the dementia
290.42 With Delusions: if delusions are the predominant feature
290.43 With Depressed Mood: if depressed mood (including presentations that meet full symptom criteria for a Major Depressive Episode) is the predominant feature. A separate diagnosis of Mood Disorder Due to a General Medical Condition is not given.
290.40 Uncomplicated: if none of the above predominates in the current clinical presentation

Specify if:
With Behavioral Disturbance
Coding note: Also code cerebrovascular condition on Axis III.

Guidelines for Differential Diagnosis of Dementia

Although ongoing research into Alzheimer's disease is very promising and is likely to supply us with more accurate and accessible means of diagnosis in the not too distant future, Dementia of the Alzheimer's Type currently remains a residual and descriptive diagnosis that cannot be proven except by autopsy or brain biopsy findings. The diagnosis is made based on the inability to find other causes for the dementia and its characteristic course, which is usually slowly progressive and insidious.

It is therefore important to consider and evaluate for all other possible causes of the dementia, especially because some of these can be effectively treated so that the progression of the dementia may be stopped or even reversed (e.g., subdural hematoma, vitamin deficiency, hypertension, or vascular disease). History, physical examination, laboratory testing, and information from family members are all helpful in making this determination.

Elderly patients are at risk for both cerebrovascular and Alzheimer's disease; therefore, it may be difficult to distinguish Vascular Dementia from Dementia of the Alzheimer's Type, and the two types may co-occur, in which case the diagnosis would be Dementia Due to Multiple Etiologies and both types would be coded separately. No other general medical condition could be found that accounted for Mr. E's dementia, however, and therefore his diagnosis would be Dementia of the Alzheimer's Type. Of course, it would be important to corroborate his alcohol use to ensure that it was limited to only a few beers a day and that the appropriate diagnosis was not Substance-Induced Persisting Dementia.

Although the most prominent symptom of dementia is cognitive impairment, the differential diagnosis is complicated because dementia may often be accompanied by delirium, psychotic symptoms, depressive symptoms, personality changes, and behavioral disturbances. When these symptoms are part of the presentation of the Dementia of the Alzheimer's Type or Vascular Dementia, they would not be separately diagnosed, but rather a subtype would be used to indicate which symptoms are predominant (e.g., With Delirium, With Delusions, With Depressed Mood). For the other types of dementia (i.e., those due to other general medical conditions or to substances), if a delirium or clinically significant mood or psychotic symptoms are present, two separate diagnoses are made (e.g., 294.1 Dementia Due to Parkinson's Disease and 293.83 Mood Disorder Due to Parkinson's Disease).

Individuals who have dementia are particularly vulnerable to developing delirium. This is partly because their central nervous system functioning is impaired and vulnerable to physical and environmental changes. They also often have a number of other general medical conditions that may directly cause the delirium, or they may require medications that contribute to the delirium. Although individuals with dementia with superimposed delirium may also present with dysphoria, the subtype With Delirium takes precedence. In addition, when individuals with dementia require hospitalization, the unfamiliar setting may serve as a stressor to provoke confusion, which should be distinguished from delirium.

The first symptoms of Alzheimer's disease in some individuals may be depression, and this can be confused with Major Depressive Disorder. It is also not unusual for individuals with Major Depressive Disorder to present with some cognitive impairment (often referred to somewhat misleadingly as pseudodementia), which often improves as the depressive symptoms improve. To distinguish between dementia and Major Depressive Disorder, the clinician should make a careful clinical evaluation and take into account the results of neuropsychological testing, brain imaging, and the patient's response to antidepressant treatment. This situation is further complicated because individuals with late-onset depression have been found to have subtle lesions on sophisticated MRI testing.

It is important to distinguish the cognitive impairment associated with dementia from the "nonpathological" memory impairment of old age, which is listed in the DSM-IV system as 780.93 Age-Related Cognitive Decline, a new category included in the section for Other Conditions That May Be a Focus of Clinical Attention. To help sharpen this boundary, DSM-IV-TR requires that for a diagnosis of dementia to be made, the memory loss must cause significant impairment in functioning and must be accompanied by at least one of four other types of cognitive disturbance that itself also causes significant impairment in functioning. Aphasia (language disturbance) may be receptive or expressive or both. The problems with language must be severe enough to cause impairment. Occasional difficulty finding the right word is fairly common, especially among older individuals, and would not meet this criterion. Apraxia (impaired ability to carry out motor abilities despite intact motor function) will be apparent when the individual is asked to perform tasks such as brushing teeth, combing hair, tying shoes, and buttoning a shirt. The patient's problem is not with motor function but with the inability to organize the set of relatively complex actions required to carry out the task. Again, occasional clumsiness would not meet this criterion, which requires that the apraxia cause significant impairment in a person's ability to function. Agnosia (failure to recognize or identify objects despite intact sensory function) might be revealed by a person's inability to identify a quarter by touch with eyes closed. Just as apraxia does not result from a problem with peripheral motor function, agnosia is not the result of a peripheral sensory deficit but rather is a failure of an individual's ability to correctly integrate sensory input. The disturbance in executive functioning (i.e., planning, organizing, sequencing, and abstracting) must be evaluated in relation to a person's previous level of functioning. For example, someone who had a very high level of baseline functioning may still be able to perform adequately on standard tests of sequencing and abstracting, despite being impaired by a significant loss of functional ability.

Mr. A clearly has both memory impairment and other severe cognitive impairments, especially in executive functioning, that severely restrict his ability to function. If a memory impairment is present that is severe enough to interfere significantly with functioning but is not accompanied by other significant cognitive deficits, the appropriate diagnosis is Amnestic Disorder. Presentations involving clinically significant cognitive impairments that do not meet the full criteria for dementia or Amnestic Disorder may fit the criteria for a proposed new category, mild neurocognitive disorder, that is included in an appendix to DSM-IV-TR for diagnoses needing further study. Such presentations would currently be coded as 294.9 Cognitive Disorder Not Otherwise Specified.

Mr. E's case illustrates a very common and confounding clinical situation. Late-onset depression (i.e., the first episode of depression occurring at an advanced age) should always alert the clinician to the possibility of an underlying general medical condition or medication side effect. What makes this situation particularly confusing is that Major Depressive Disorder can present with cognitive symptoms, especially in elderly patients, and that dementia can often present with depressive symptoms even before other cognitive symptoms emerge. Recent evidence from MRI suggests that late-onset depression is often associated with central nervous system lesions that would not have been detected with less sophisticated testing. Moreover, both depression and cognitive symptoms can be caused or made worse by many of the medications taken for mental disorders or general medical conditions. A thorough neurological workup is indicated when patients present with a late-onset first episode of depression, especially when accompanied by cognitive problems.

Treatment Planning for Dementia

Several medications to prevent memory loss are currently available, and others are being evaluated. However, there is no specific cure or prevention for Alzheimer's disease at present. Treatments are often directed toward the symptoms (i.e., depression, psychosis, agitation, and behavioral disturbance) that may be associated with Alzheimer's disease.

In managing patients with Alzheimer's disease, it is very important for the clinician to evaluate the extent to which the person can function in the home environment and to help family members learn how to manage the patient and locate sources of help in the home. Those who are trying to care for Alzheimer's patients at home are often under a good deal of stress and experience extremely high rates of depression. They may benefit by referrals to a number of community agencies. Adult day-care programs and nurse and aide services from local home health agencies can be very helpful in assisting the family to care for the patient at home. Family support groups can also help to provide moral support for the caretakers and reduce their sense of isolation. Finally, the patient's situation and functional level should be regularly reevaluated with input from caretakers to determine at what point treatment in a facility may be needed, either on a long-term basis or as a means of reevaluating the patient's status and providing a respite for family members.

Patients with dementia often display "sundowning"—an increase in confusion and disorientation at night— and they have special difficulty dealing with unstructured and unfamiliar situations. The confusion associated with dementia can often be improved by providing a predictable, structured, and orienting environment. It may be helpful to place calendars, clocks, familiar pictures and objects, and night-lights in the room to help orient the individual.

When delirium occurs in someone with dementia, it is very important to search for and try to correct the underlying cause. This may be a general medical condition (perhaps the one that is also causing the dementia or perhaps another condition accompanying the clinical presentation) or a medication side effect, particularly in elderly individuals who are likely to be receiving multiple medications and are less able to metabolize or eliminate them.

Summary

Dementia is not just a cognitive disorder but involves a complex combination of symptomatology that may include delirium, psychotic symptoms, depressive symptoms, personality changes, and behavioral disturbances. Because dementia can present with such a wide range of symptoms, each type of symptom must be considered in the differential diagnosis of the dementia. Furthermore, the possibility of a dementia must also be considered in the differential diagnosis of other disorders that present with these symptoms (e.g., Major Depressive Disorder). Note that if the symptoms occur only during the course of a delirium, a diagnosis of dementia would not be made.

Amnestic Disorders

The DSM-IV-TR classification for Amnestic Disorders is shown below:

DSM-IV-TR diagnostic criteria for 294.0 Amnestic Disorder Due to . . . [Indicate the General Medical Condition]

A. The development of memory impairment as manifested by impairment in the ability to learn new information or the inability to recall previously learned information.
B. The memory disturbance causes significant impairment in social or occupational functioning and represents a significant decline from a previous level of functioning.
C. The memory disturbance does not occur exclusively during the course of a delirium or a dementia.
D. There is evidence from the history, physical examination, or laboratory findings that the disturbance is the direct physiological consequence of a general medical condition (including physical trauma).

Specify if:
Transient: if memory impairment lasts for 1 month or less
Chronic: if memory impairment lasts for more than 1 month

Coding note: Include the name of the general medical condition on Axis I, e.g., 294.0 Amnestic Disorder Due to Head Trauma; also code the general medical condition on Axis III.

❖   Case Study: A Woman Who Can't Remember

Ms. R is a 48-year-old woman who is divorced and has three teenage children. Until 3 years earlier, Ms. R worked as a buyer for a department store. At that time, she experienced fatigue, forgetfulness, a sense of apathy, and headaches, which she attributed to a preexisting migraine condition. She visited a psychiatrist who prescribed an antidepressant to which she did not respond. The headaches worsened, and Ms. R visited a neurologist who found nothing on neurological examination but recommended a CT scan as a precautionary measure. The CT scan revealed a large, Grade II out of IV right frontal glioma. This was resected surgically followed by 7,500 rads of radiotherapy focused on the right frontal quadrant. Ms. R recovered well from the surgery and radiation, with no focal neurological deficits. She had a surprisingly benign course and was able to return to work. The only medication she was taking was carbamazepine as a prophylactic against seizures, which she has never had.

Three years after her surgery, the patient and her family began to notice a problem in her short-term memory, which began with forgetting appointments and losing objects. On one occasion, she was unable to find her car in the airport parking lot because she forgot its make and where she had parked it. With time, this forgetfulness progressed and became severe enough to interfere with her work. For example, she would forget she had placed orders and would repeat them. At first, Ms. R became irritable about these incidents and often blamed others for her problems (e.g., her secretary for losing her papers, her children for misplacing things at home). Ms. R's memory problems were especially distressing to her because she had always prided herself on her memory and had been the one to find things for others in the household. With time, however, she developed insight and accepted that this memory problem was a result of the radiation she had received. Her long-term memory is intact as are her other cognitive abilities, except for some reduced ability to plan ahead, but, because this had been very well developed before, the patient can still function better than average. Ms. R eventually began to make so many mistakes at work that it was obvious she could no longer continue in her job. She is able to function reasonably well at home, however, with the assistance of "things to do" lists and cuing bulletin boards in many rooms of the house.

DSM-IV-TR Diagnosis

Axis I: 294.0   Amnestic Disorder Due to Central Nervous System
                    Radiation, Chronic
Axis II: V71.09   No diagnosis
Axis III: 990   Postradiation for brain tumor
Axis IV: Inability to work causing financial stress
Axis V: GAF = 55

Guidelines for Differential Diagnosis of Amnestic Disorder

In diagnosing Amnestic Disorder, the clinician must focus on the differential diagnosis, keeping in mind the normal forgetting of everyday life. Memory, in particular short-term memory, tends to decline with age, especially after age 50, in a fashion analogous to the deterioration of vision that usually causes people to become farsighted sometime after reaching the age of 40. Unfortunately, no mental equivalent to reading glasses has yet been developed. Amnestic Disorder differs from Age-Related Cognitive Decline in the severity of the memory loss and the presence of clinically significant impairment. For example, when Ms. R first began forgetting things but was still able to continue working, her presentation did not warrant a diagnosis of Amnestic Disorder. Because it is not considered a mental disorder, 780.93 Age-Related Cognitive Decline is included in DSM-IV-TR in the category for Other Conditions That May Be a Focus of Clinical Attention (p. 731).

The other boundary that should be considered in the differential diagnosis of Amnestic Disorder is with dementia, which is also characterized by memory impairment but requires the presence of at least one additional cognitive impairment item from a list that includes aphasia, apraxia, agnosia, and disturbance in executive functioning. This differential is much more difficult than meets the eye because it is not uncommon for individuals, particularly as they age, to have mild degrees of aphasia, apraxia, agnosia, and reduced planning abilities. DSM-IV-TR does not provide any definite guidelines except to require that the additional cognitive impairments be severe enough to be impairing in and of themselves in order to count toward the diagnosis of dementia. Occasional inability to remember a word is completely compatible with the normal, expectable, and nonimpairing loss of cognitive efficiency that goes with aging and would not result in a change of diagnosis from Amnestic Disorder to dementia. In Ms. R's case, there do not appear to be any additional cognitive impairments of sufficient severity to cause impairment, and, therefore, the appropriate diagnosis in this case would be Amnestic Disorder.

Although it is not an issue in this case, a third disorder, Dissociative Amnesia, should be considered in the differential diagnosis of Amnestic Disorder. This determination is most difficult in situations in which the amnesia follows a traumatic incident such as an auto accident. In these cases, the clinician must judge whether the memory impairment is the direct physical result of a head trauma, a psychological phenomenon following the shock of an accident, or both. In such circumstances, a thorough neurological examination should always be performed to rule out brain injury as a causal factor in the amnesia before assuming that it results from dissociation. One differentiating point is that memory loss due to direct physiological effects on the brain tends to be less reversible, whereas memory loss associated with Dissociative Disorders is more likely to be spotty, to be related to emotionally charged events, and to yield to hypnosis or suggestions that the memory can be recovered.

In diagnosing Amnestic Disorder Due to a General Medical Condition, the clinician must determine that the memory loss is not due to the immediate or persisting effects of substance or medication use. If blackouts occur during intoxication but do not represent a persisting memory loss, only Substance Intoxication would be diagnosed, and it would not be considered Substance-Induced Persisting Amnestic Disorder. A diagnosis of Substance-Induced Persisting Amnestic Disorder would be warranted when long-term memory loss caused by a substance occurs. Although Ms. R has been taking carbamazepine as a prophylactic against seizures, the amnesia does not appear to be related to the medication because it is more severe than what would be expected with carbamazepine and because a reduction in the dosage did not produce any improvement.

Clinicians should be alert to the possibility that individuals may pretend to have Amnestic Disorder to escape responsibility for their actions, especially in forensic settings. In general, clinicians tend to be poor in spotting malingering but should be mindful of the possibility in situations in which memory loss produces an obvious gain.

Treatment Planning for Amnestic Disorder

There is currently no specific treatment for Amnestic Disorder. Treatment strategies must be targeted toward the underlying etiology of the disturbance, whether it is a general medical condition, Substance Use, or a medication side effect. It may be helpful to teach the patient strategies for enhancing memory or working around memory gaps. These might include such techniques as keeping a daily calendar and reminder board.

Summary

This is a disorder that must be distinguished from ordinary forgetting and dementia. It is probably underdiagnosed because many clinicians are not as familiar with it as they are with other types of cognitive impairment. Nevertheless, Amnestic Disorder can be severe and impairing in its own right. The most common and preventable cause of this disorder is Wernicke's encephalopathy. This condition results from thiamine deficiency related to chronic alcoholism and can lead to the development of 291.1 Alcohol-Induced Persisting Amnestic Disorder, or Korsakoff's syndrome, if not treated with large doses of thiamine.

Chapter 3

Substance-Related Disorders

The Substance-Related Disorders in DSM-IV-TR include disorders that are related to drugs of abuse, medications, and toxins. Text and criteria are given for disorders related to 11 classes of drugs of abuse:

- ❖ Alcohol
- ❖ Amphetamine (or Amphetamine-Like Substances)
- ❖ Caffeine
- ❖ Cannabis
- ❖ Cocaine
- ❖ Hallucinogens
- ❖ Inhalants
- ❖ Nicotine
- ❖ Opioids
- ❖ Phencyclidine (or Phencyclidine-Like Substances)
- ❖ Sedatives, Hypnotics, and Anxiolytics

The category Other (or Unknown) Substance-Related Disorders is included to allow clinicians to classify 1) presentations involving other types of drugs of abuse; 2) presentations in which it is clear that a substance is etiological, but it is not possible to determine specifically what substance is involved; and 3) presentations in which the symptoms are related to a medication or toxin exposure.

The Substance-Related Disorders are divided into the Substance Use Disorders—Dependence and Abuse—and the Substance-Induced Disorders—Intoxication, Withdrawal, Substance-Induced Delirium, Substance-

Induced Persisting Dementia, Substance-Induced Persisting Amnestic Disorder, Substance-Induced Psychotic Disorder, Substance-Induced Mood Disorder, Substance-Induced Anxiety Disorder, Substance-Induced Sexual Dysfunction, Substance-Induced Sleep Disorder, and Hallucinogen Persisting Perception Disorder (Flashbacks). Note that not all diagnoses apply to every class of drug.

Generic criteria sets are given for Substance Dependence and Substance Abuse because the features of these disorders are fairly consistent across substances. However, because of attributes specific to each substance, separate criteria sets for intoxication and withdrawal symptoms are given for different substances. The code numbers for the Substance-Related Disorders vary according to the type of substance involved (e.g., 303.00 Alcohol Intoxication, 292.89 Cocaine Intoxication, 305.90 Caffeine Intoxication). You should refer to DSM-IV-TR to determine the correct code number for any particular presentation.

The category of Substance-Induced Disorders includes those characterized by symptoms that are phenomenologically similar to other categories of mental disorders but that are caused by intoxication with or withdrawal from a substance. These are presentations in which the symptoms are in excess of what would be expected given intoxication with or withdrawal from the substance and in which the symptoms are a focus of clinical attention. This means that one would diagnose 291.89 Alcohol-Induced Mood Disorder With Onset During Withdrawal rather than 291.81 Alcohol Withdrawal when the mood symptoms are a focus of treatment and go beyond what one would normally expect to find associated with Alcohol Withdrawal. If the symptoms do not go beyond what would be expected and do not form a separate focus of treatment, the appropriate intoxication or withdrawal diagnosis would be made (e.g., 291.81 Alcohol Withdrawal). To make differential diagnosis easier, these types of disorders are placed in the sections with which they share similar types of symptoms (e.g., Substance-Induced Mood Disorder is placed in the Mood Disorders section; Substance-Induced Anxiety Disorder, in the Anxiety Disorders section). A case illustrating Anticholinergic-Induced Delirium is found on p. 34, a case illustrating Cocaine-Induced Psychotic Disorder is found on p. 102, and a case illustrating Alcohol-Induced Mood Disorder is found on p. 148.

In this section, we present one case that illustrates the features of Substance Dependence and one that illustrates Substance Abuse. We focus on these diagnoses here because distinguishing between recreational use, problematic use, abuse, and dependence is one of the biggest differential diagnostic issues for this category of disorders.

Substance Dependence

❖   Case Study: A Young Mother
    Whose Drinking Is Out of Control[1]

Ms. W, a 28-year-old stockbroker, is married and the mother of a 6-year-old child. Her mother, who is a member of Alcoholics Anonymous, convinced Ms. W to come to treatment for "drinking too much" and having an "enlarged liver." Ms. W is the oldest of four girls. Her youngest sister has mental retardation and the stigmata of fetal alcohol syndrome. Both her parents, several aunts and uncles, and her grandfathers on both sides of the family are alcoholic. It is possible to trace alcoholism back for multiple generations. There is no history of mental illness in her parents; however, a great-aunt on her father's side committed suicide.

Ms. W began drinking heavily in college when she was 19 years old, along with her future husband, who was then a classmate. Her drinking progressed from weekend binges with occasional blackouts to heavy daily drinking starting in her senior year. On one morning after a heavy binge, she was shocked to find the front bumper of her car dented. She realized that she drank too much but felt that, compared to her fiancé and her mother and father, she did not have a problem. Soon after this, she married her fiancé, who had graduated from college and joined his family's plumbing business. Her husband had an enormous tolerance for alcohol and both Mr. and Ms. W had strong family histories of alcoholism, yet early in their relationship they had fun drinking together and were successful in keeping their drinking under control.

At age 22, Ms. W stopped drinking on her own for 1 year soon after she discovered that she was pregnant with her daughter. During that period, she had difficulty not drinking but "white knuckled it" out of concern for the possibility of a fetal abnormality like the one that affected her youngest sister. At about this time, Ms. W's mother left her father, who was also an alcoholic. After a brief inpatient rehabilitation, Ms. W's mother joined Alcoholics Anonymous.

Soon after the birth of her daughter, Ms. W began to feel pressured by the demands of having to care for a child and go to work and was tempted to drink with her husband again. She soon found herself stopping for a drink before coming home, consuming several cocktails with her husband in the evening, and having 5–10 drinks per day on the weekend. She became increasingly dependent on her housekeeper to care for her daughter. By age 26, her drinking had escalated to 5–10 drinks per day and to 15 per day on

---

1. Thanks go to Richard Frances, M.D., Director, Department of Psychiatry, Hackensack Medical Center for supplying the cases in this chapter.

weekends. She often called in sick on Mondays, had frequent hangovers, and developed gastritis. Her physician noted an enlarged liver and abnormalities in laboratory tests of SGOT-SGPT and MCV and strongly advised Ms. W to stop drinking. She continued to drink, however, and refused to listen to her mother's and doctor's wishes for her to get treatment. Although she has had several car accidents in the past 6 months, including one in which her daughter was in the car, she has never been arrested for driving while intoxicated. She does her best to hide her drinking from her boss but makes no such efforts at home, where her drinking is generally tolerated by her alcoholic husband. For a long time, they have been doing a good job of covering up for each other and are both talented and successful in their work. Although they both have diminishing sexual interest and have frequent battles with each other, they wish to make their marriage work for their daughter's sake.

Ms. W has found that, although she drinks less than her husband, it has greater negative effects on her health. She can no longer stop on her own and feels pained and terribly guilty about her inconsistency with and neglect of her daughter, who complains that "Mommy drinks too much." Although she has never felt close to her mother, Ms. W finally agreed to go with her to an Alcoholics Anonymous meeting and to seek help at an organized outpatient treatment program. Ms. W began smoking cigarettes at age 14 and currently smokes one pack a day but has no other history of drug use. She also has no history of an Anxiety Disorder, problems with depression, or other psychiatric problems.

Ms. W is a petite, pretty, well-dressed 28-year-old woman who appears to be deeply ashamed of herself and uncomfortable talking about her problems with the interviewer. On examination, her temperature is 99.8°F, her blood pressure is 140/90, and her pulse rate is 104. She reports insomnia, a sensation of bugs crawling on her, and a feeling of anxiety, and she appears tremulous. Ms. W has not had a drink for the previous 12 hours before the interview and is currently experiencing an extreme craving for alcohol. She talks about feeling low self-esteem and hopelessness about whether it will be possible for her to stop drinking; however, she is able to be quickly reassured when reminded of her ability to stop drinking during pregnancy and about her mother's success at remaining abstinent. Ms. W has been able to function, has not generally felt depressed, and reports that she has several close friends at work who think of her as being a lot of fun.

DSM-IV-TR Diagnosis

Axis I:	291.81	Alcohol Withdrawal, With Perceptual Disturbances
	303.90	Alcohol Dependence, With Physiological Dependence
	305.1	Nicotine Dependence, With Physiological Dependence
Axis II:	V71.09	No diagnosis
Axis III:	535.30	Alcoholic gastritis
	789.1	Hepatomegaly
Axis IV:	Recent car accident, neglect of daughter, marital stress	
Axis V:	GAF = 50	

DSM-IV-TR criteria for Substance Dependence

A maladaptive pattern of substance use, leading to clinically significant impairment or distress, as manifested by three (or more) of the following, occurring at any time in the same 12-month period:

(1) tolerance, as defined by either of the following:
   (a) a need for markedly increased amounts of the substance to achieve intoxication or desired effect
   (b) markedly diminished effect with continued use of the same amount of the substance
(2) withdrawal, as manifested by either of the following:
   (a) the characteristic withdrawal syndrome for the substance (refer to Criteria A and B of the criteria sets for Withdrawal from the specific substances)
   (b) the same (or a closely related) substance is taken to relieve or avoid withdrawal symptoms
(3) the substance is often taken in larger amounts or over a longer period than was intended
(4) there is a persistent desire or unsuccessful efforts to cut down or control substance use
(5) a great deal of time is spent in activities necessary to obtain the substance (e.g., visiting multiple doctors or driving long distances), use the substance (e.g., chain-smoking), or recover from its effects
(6) important social, occupational, or recreational activities are given up or reduced because of substance use

(continued)

DSM-IV-TR criteria for
Substance Dependence *(continued)*

---

(7)   the substance use is continued despite knowledge of having a persistent or recurrent physical or psychological problem that is likely to have been caused or exacerbated by the substance (e.g., current cocaine use despite recognition of cocaine-induced depression, or continued drinking despite recognition that an ulcer was made worse by alcohol consumption)

Specify if:
With Physiological Dependence: evidence of tolerance or withdrawal (i.e., either Item 1 or 2 is present)
Without Physiological Dependence: no evidence of tolerance or withdrawal (i.e., neither Item 1 nor 2 is present)

Course specifiers:
Early Full Remission
Early Partial Remission
Sustained Full Remission
Sustained Partial Remission
On Agonist Therapy
In a Controlled Environment

Substance Abuse

❖   Case Study: A College Student
Who Denies He Has a Drug Problem

Mr. B is a 20-year-old male college student who was recently arrested for possession of marijuana, which was detected when he was stopped for unsafe driving. He was charged with driving while intoxicated with cannabis, and his license was suspended. Mr. B is the oldest of three children and continues to live at home while attending college. His mother is a successful attorney and his father is a school administrator. He has smoked cigarettes since age 16 and currently smokes one pack a day. He drinks five drinks on occasion and has been smoking marijuana several times a week for 1 year. His usual pattern of use is to go on weekend binges, starting to smoke on Friday evenings and then again early in the day on Saturday continuing into the evening. He has had two car accidents that occurred while he was intoxicated with marijuana. During recent months, he has sometimes smoked marijuana on school nights. On the mornings after he uses marijuana, Mr. B tends to sleep in and cut class. Although he has always been a good student, his grades have begun to go down and he is not meeting his academic potential; his recreational and social interests are also limited.

Mr. B's parents detected his use of marijuana 6 months earlier, and since that time Mr. B has been in a constant struggle with his parents about his perceived "right" to smoke marijuana. When his parents first discovered his marijuana use, they insisted that he seek professional help for what they perceived to be a drug problem. Although they even threatened to call his college dean, Mr. B refused help and began to discuss quitting school. He did cut down on his use somewhat, however, and when pressed by his parents, would abstain for several weeks at a time. His parents also stopped giving him permission to drive a family car and were concerned about his influence on his younger siblings. Neither parent has any history of substance-related problems, with the exception of his mother's recovery from tobacco addiction, which began 3 years earlier. A maternal uncle was an alcoholic.

Mr. B admits that since he began smoking marijuana, his previously good and trusting relationship with his parents has soured. He has taken to hiding his use, has lied to them, and has felt increasingly negative about himself, especially as his grades have suffered and his general interests have narrowed. On one occasion, he tried cocaine and, on another, LSD, but found both experiences unpleasant. It was not until his arrest for possession that he decided that drug use was ruining his relationship with his parents and could interfere with his desire to become an attorney. He has also become gradually aware that marijuana may be affecting his motivation and schoolwork.

Mr. B was first introduced to marijuana by his girlfriend, who uses it every day and whose mother also uses marijuana. Mr. B smokes both alone and with friends; however, he would sometimes not use marijuana for weeks at a time during summer holidays and when pressed by his parents. He introduced his 17-year-old brother to marijuana, but his brother felt paranoid on that occasion and has not tried it since.

Mr. B achieved normal milestones and performed well in high school. He wanted to live away from home during college, but his parents resisted the idea because of financial pressures and a tendency to be overprotective.

Upon examination, Mr. B is a neatly dressed young man with a sarcastic manner. He appears torn between embarrassment and anger at being forced to seek help. He states that, although he has not used marijuana since he was caught, he still has doubts about its harmfulness. He says that he finds marijuana pleasurable and relaxing and that, if he could find a way not to get caught, he would like to continue using it. He believes that marijuana has helped him feel better about not achieving the high goals he had set for himself and not fulfilling the expectations his parents have for him. Mr. B shows no evidence of thought disorder. He reports that he has been unhappy at times but that this feeling has never been lasting. He has no sleeping or eating problems, suicidal ideation, history of panic attacks or agoraphobia, cognitive deficits, or learning disability.

DSM-IV-TR Diagnosis

Axis I: 305.20   Cannabis Abuse
            305.1   Nicotine Dependence
            V61.20   Parent-Child Relational Problem
Axis II: V71.09   No diagnosis
Axis III: None
Axis IV: Recent arrest, falling grades, conflicts with parents
Axis V: GAF = 70

DSM-IV-TR criteria for Substance Abuse

A. A maladaptive pattern of substance use leading to clinically significant impairment or distress, as manifested by one (or more) of the following, occurring within a 12-month period:

    (1) recurrent substance use resulting in a failure to fulfill major role obligations at work, school, or home (e.g., repeated absences or poor work performance related to substance use; substance-related absences, suspensions, or expulsions from school; neglect of children or household)

    (2) recurrent substance use in situations in which it is physically hazardous (e.g., driving an automobile or operating a machine when impaired by substance use)

    (3) recurrent substance-related legal problems (e.g., arrests for substance-related disorderly conduct)

    (4) continued substance use despite having persistent or recurrent social or interpersonal problems caused or exacerbated by the effects of the substance (e.g., arguments with spouse about consequences of intoxication, physical fights)

B. The symptoms have never met the criteria for Substance Dependence for this class of substance.

Guidelines for Differential Diagnosis of Substance Dependence and Abuse

The most important differential to consider in evaluating substance-related behaviors is whether they represent Substance Dependence, Substance Abuse, or recreational or nonpathological use. There has been a lot of controversy about whether alcohol and drug problems are an illness at all or a moral problem and about how best to define the boundaries between dependence and abuse. It can be difficult to make this distinction because behaviors associated with Substance Use occur on what many see as a continuum, ranging from recreational use at one end of the spectrum to Substance Dependence at the other end, with problematic use and Substance Abuse somewhere in between.

The DSM-III definition of Substance Dependence tended to emphasize physiological symptoms (i.e., tolerance and withdrawal) because these were much more applicable to alcohol. However, for other drugs in the section (e.g., cannabis), problems are not associated with tolerance or withdrawal but rather with psychological dependence. The definition of Substance Dependence was therefore expanded in DSM-III-R to include items reflecting compulsive use in order to make the definition applicable across all classes of substances. In DSM-III-R, Substance Abuse was included as a primarily residual category. Those developing the DSM-IV criteria for Substance Dependence and Abuse attempted to clarify the boundary between dependence and abuse and to define Substance Abuse more precisely. Although the DSM-IV Substance Dependence criteria include items that tap tolerance, withdrawal, or compulsive use, Substance Dependence is almost always also associated with adverse consequences. In contrast, the definition of Substance Abuse describes those individuals who have the adverse consequences but have never had the pattern of tolerance, withdrawal, or compulsive use that would meet criteria for Substance Dependence.

A number of factors warrant considering Substance Dependence and Abuse as mental disorders and distinguishing them from recreational and nonpathological Substance Use: the considerable morbidity and mortality associated with Substance Dependence and Abuse; the development of tolerance and withdrawal symptoms associated with Substance Dependence; and the variety of psychosocial problems associated with both Substance Dependence and Abuse that interfere with the individual's ability to fulfill important social, occupational, and legal obligations.

It should be noted that Substance Dependence and Abuse are frequently comorbid with most of the other mental disorders in DSM-IV-TR. It is therefore crucial, as part of every psychiatric evaluation, to question carefully about the presence of current or previous substance-related problems.

It is somewhat easier to evaluate for Substance Dependence than Substance Abuse because such determinations can be based on a measurement of the amount of substance used, the development of tolerance, and the presence of objectively verifiable withdrawal phenomena. There are several important issues to note in the Substance Dependence case: Ms. W has a strong family history of alcoholism, a fact that is significant because genetic and familial factors affect the development of Alcohol and Other Substance Abuse and Dependence. Ms. W's clinical course was marked by a high early tolerance and alcohol-related problems that continued to increase over time. She had blackouts early on, something that frequently occurs with very heavy drinkers. In the early stages of their drinking, both Ms. W and her husband reported enjoying it a great deal. However, the difficulties of trying to cope with her drinking and handle the increasing responsibilities of having a daughter and a job along with the increasing negative consequences of her heavy drinking (i.e., car accidents, increasing marital tension, and health problems) caused Ms. W to begin to confront the seriousness of her problem.

Another important part of the differential diagnosis in this case is to be careful that additional medical or psychiatric problems are not causing some of the symptomatology. Ms. W presents with a temperature, rapid pulse, tremulousness, and perceptual disturbances, including tactile hallucinations 12 hours after stopping drinking. Although this picture is most consistent with Alcohol Withdrawal, the clinician should also consider and rule out other possible causes (e.g., an infectious illness, an endocrine disorder, a structural brain lesion such as a tumor, withdrawal from a barbiturate or benzodiazepine, or the presence of an additional psychiatric problem such as a primary Anxiety or Depressive Disorder).

It is important also to note that, according to the DSM-IV-TR diagnostic algorithm, once an individual has met criteria for Substance Dependence for a class of substance, a diagnosis of Substance Abuse for that substance can never be given. In other words, if, after a period of remission, Ms. W were to start drinking again and have alcohol-related problems that were not severe enough to meet the full criteria for Substance Dependence, the appropriate diagnosis would be Substance Dependence in either Early Partial Remission or Sustained Partial Remission (if it had been more than a year since she met full criteria for dependence).

It may be harder to pick up the subtle and early signs of Substance Use that are causing psychosocial difficulties, such as interfering with or impairing an individual's ability to meet social, occupational, or legal obligations, because an evaluation of the level of impairment will depend in part on cultural and/or familial tolerance for patterns of Substance Use. The presence of a pattern of maladaptive behavioral changes is usually primarily responsible for the determination that someone has crossed the line from nonpathological use to abuse. Most cultures have difficulty accepting impaired control, physiological disturbances, cognitive changes, and persistence of symptoms.

Factors related to age and sex can also influence the evaluation of whether abuse is present. For example, the same amount of alcohol may have greater effects on the nervous system as one ages, causing the loss of tolerance often seen in the elderly. Men also tend to have a higher tolerance for alcohol than women, which may be a biological protective factor for women and may also contribute to higher rates of alcohol-related problems in men. Lower doses of alcohol may also have more serious consequences for women than for men.

Although Mr. B's problems are not severe enough to meet the criteria for Substance Dependence, his Substance Use has led to a number of clinically significant problems that warrant a diagnosis of Substance Abuse. He has been neglecting his schoolwork, and his grades have been falling as a result of his Cannabis Use. He has had several automobile accidents while driving under the influence of cannabis, his parents no longer allow him to use the family car, and his license was recently suspended. Finally, his Cannabis Use is causing a serious disruption in his previously positive relationship with his family. Mr. B and his parents also appear to have a number of relational problems that should probably be a focus of treatment attention because these may actually be contributing to Mr. B's substance-related problems. For this reason, we included Parent-Child Relational Problem on Axis I of the diagnosis.

The presence of certain general medical conditions, such as ulcers, liver disease, pancreatitis, or head trauma, may affect how dangerous Alcohol or Other Substance Use may be for a particular person. If you are in poor physical health, substances and Substance-Related Disorders may affect your body in different ways than when you are healthy, and this will affect where the boundary is drawn between nonpathological use and abuse for a particular individual. For example, a level of Alcohol Use that would probably not be considered abuse in a person in good health would be considered abuse in an individual with ulcers who continues to drink despite knowing that this is likely to have negative effects on his or her physical condition. If someone is in a car accident and sustains a head trauma, the sequelae of the trauma are likely to be less dangerous if the individual was not intoxicated with alcohol at the time of the accident. Alcohol can also exacerbate the symptoms of pancreatitis, and heavy drinking can be fatal for someone with hepatitis.

There are a number of interesting paradoxes concerning the effects of different substances. For example, although most Americans drink alcohol, only a small percentage drink alcoholically, with the average person being a mild to moderate user of alcohol. In contrast, users of nicotine are much more likely to be dependent; very few individuals who use nicotine would not qualify for a diagnosis of either Nicotine Abuse or Dependence. Another interesting paradox is that those who are allergic to alcohol, who feel sick as a result of even light alcohol consumption and thus have a low tolerance for it, and certain Asian people who develop an alcoholic flush are to some extent protected against developing Alcohol Dependence. In contrast, research has shown that those who can tolerate large amounts of alcohol with no ill effects and therefore have a high tolerance are more likely to have alcohol-related problems and to have a genetic predisposition to develop alcoholism. Another paradox related to alcohol is that families in which there is a high risk of alcoholism have a greater proportion of people who do not drink alcohol at all compared with the general population because they fear developing an alcohol-related problem.

When clinicians treat individuals from families that have a strong history of alcoholism, they should target prevention strategies that focus on abstinence. In our society, it is generally considered more normal to drink lightly or moderately than not to drink at all. For this reason, people who do not drink alcohol at all because of a family history of alcoholism are often considered odd by their peers, who may encourage them to begin drinking. Although the controlled use of substances, especially alcohol, by those with a history of Substance Abuse has received more attention recently and has been advocated by some, this strategy should be used very cautiously. Individuals with a history of Alcohol or Other Substance Abuse would probably be better advised not to use alcohol or drugs at all.

Treatment Planning for Substance Dependence and Abuse

In treating Ms. W for Substance Dependence, the first step is detoxification. Although it might be possible to detoxify her as an outpatient, because of the presence of delirium tremens, a brief hospitalization of 3–5 days will probably be necessary. Ms. W will probably need to receive medication, such as a benzodiazepine, during detoxification, but this should be discontinued once she is in early remission, especially with her tendency to be addictive. After detoxification, it is likely that Ms. W will do well in an organized outpatient treatment program with referral to a 12-step Alcoholics Anonymous group, with initial attention paid to getting her to see her problems clearly and accept the need for abstinence.

Mr. W's continuing drinking may complicate treatment, but the recovery of Ms. W's mother's may provide an important support. It might be helpful for Ms. W to stay with her mother part of the time during the initial phase of her outpatient treatment. Choosing a women's 12-step recovery group might also be helpful because many of these women will also have had alcoholic husbands. The clinician should carefully evaluate Ms. W's family situation and marital problems. However, unless her husband can be helped to stop drinking, it may be hard to include him in her support network. It does appear that this couple has loved each other for a long time. If they could agree to keep their house alcohol-free, it might improve their chances for a successful marriage and also have a preventive effect for their daughter, who is at high risk for developing alcoholism later.

In our society, a greater stigma is generally associated with alcoholism in women than in men. Ms. W is embarrassed and ashamed of her problem and her inability to care adequately for her own child, and she finds it hard to admit the need for help. She appears to be a person who has high expectations for herself and is likely to feel very disappointed with herself. It may be helpful for the clinician initially to help her attribute most of these problems to her drinking as a means of encouraging her to stop. As recovery progresses, Ms. W should be encouraged to take more responsibility for herself because she has been dependent on alcohol and her husband for all of her adult life. Working with a sponsor from Alcoholics Anonymous might help her to take control of her own life, which will then help to improve her self-esteem.

Some of Ms. W's guilt about her daughter may also relate to guilt she may feel about her younger sister's fetal alcohol syndrome and her inability as a child to stop her mother from drinking and damaging her sister. Although Ms. W had a poor relationship with her mother when she was growing up, she nevertheless turned out very much like her mother. She might tend to have a negative transference to a treating professional because of this early negative relationship with her mother. The clinician may need to help her work through these feelings so that she can learn to accept advice and help from others without feeling that they are trying to control her. Now that her mother is in recovery, it may be possible to use her identification with her mother in a positive way to encourage her to continue to go to Alcoholics Anonymous and remain abstinent.

Because Ms. W is intelligent and successful and has considerable coping skills, there is every reason to think that she could have an excellent prognosis. The prognosis for her marriage depends on Ms. W's husband. The couple's drinking has negatively affected their sexual relationship, and it is hard to see how this would improve if he continues drinking. Later phases of Ms. W's recovery program might emphasize helping her learn to love and care and be creative so that she can succeed in her work and important relationships with others.

Men with alcoholism are more likely to have a wife who is not an alcoholic and who is likely to be their biggest support, standing by them during their recovery and making it easier for them to maintain an alcohol-free home after recovery. Women with alcoholism are much more likely to have husbands who are also alcoholic and who may not be supportive about their wives' getting into treatment or recovering because they are codependent. Women may need to reach out to family members and friends to get help. Some women may actually be better off leaving their husbands if they are getting their lives together while the husband continues to be alcoholic. Women with alcoholism are more likely to have been abused by their husbands, are more likely to have their ability to mother their children questioned, and may fear seeking treatment because of the possibility of losing custody of their children. Many women with alcoholism especially fear inpatient treatment because of being separated from their children, a factor that clinicians should take into account when planning treatment for mothers with young children.

In treating someone like Mr. B, the real task is to get the adolescent to see that his heavy use of cannabis is affecting him adversely in a variety of ways: It is making him an unsafe driver and limiting his ability to have a car or keep his license, it is affecting his motivation and school performance, and it could lead to other psychiatric problems. The clinician should try to help Mr. B see that using cannabis should not be considered a culturally acceptable practice for adolescents. Inpatient treatment should usually be reserved for those with Substance Dependence, and less restrictive alternatives should usually be tried first. Treatment for adolescents with Substance Abuse problems can include participation in school-based groups and counseling. Adolescents can also be referred to outpatient-based practices or to programs designed for young people, which usually involve a high degree of group psychoeducation and family involvement. Exposure to other adolescents who have stopped using drugs or are in recovery in 12-step programs such as Alateen or Substance Anonymous can be helpful. It is often useful for adolescents to work with a counselor in school, or possibly a therapist, who can help them deal with denial of the problem and accept the need for abstinence to prevent lapses.

It is important that Mr. B's family be supportive but also firm about continuing to refuse to give him access to a car if he does not accept treatment. They need to be careful not to inadvertently allow the problem to continue by ignoring it. On the other hand, his parents will not be able to monitor or stop Mr. B's substance-abusing behavior unless he accepts the need to cooperate with treatment. It is important to aim for preventing relapse and for increasing the length of episodes of sobriety; however, therapists need to set reasonable treatment goals, recognizing that improvement rather than cure is often the best that can be hoped for. Improvement can mean fewer relapses; a change in attitude about use and abuse; a deepening awareness of the problem and the need for help; improvement in school or work performance; the ability to handle social, occupational, and familial obligations; and improved physical health.

Summary

Substance and medication use and abuse are ubiquitous in our society, but their effects are often missed or misdiagnosed. Substance Dependence is a pattern of tolerance, withdrawal, or compulsive use that is often also associated with adverse consequences. Substance Abuse is a maladaptive pattern of Substance Use that leads to adverse consequences but occurs with the absence of tolerance, withdrawal, or compulsive use. Symptoms associated with Substance Use can also mimic all forms of primary psychopathology (e.g., Substance-Induced Mood Disorder and Substance-Induced Psychotic Disorder). For this reason, DSM-IV-TR highlights the importance of considering the etiological role of substances in the differential diagnosis of Delirium, Dementia, Amnestic Disorders, Psychotic Disorders, Mood Disorders, Anxiety Disorders, Sexual Dysfunction, and Sleep Disorders. Clinicians must therefore assess for possible Substance Use as part of every psychiatric evaluation.

Chapter 4

Schizophrenia and Other Psychotic Disorders

S chizophrenia and a number of Other Psychotic Disorders appear in a single section in DSM-IV-TR. The disorders in this section include the following:

Schizophrenia and Other Psychotic Disorders

295.xx	Schizophrenia
.30	Paranoid Type
.10	Disorganized Type
.20	Catatonic Type
.90	Undifferentiated Type
.60	Residual Type
295.40	Schizophreniform Disorder
295.70	Schizoaffective Disorder
297.1	Delusional Disorder
298.8	Brief Psychotic Disorder
297.3	Shared Psychotic Disorder
293.xx	Psychotic Disorder Due to . . . *[Indicate the General Medical Condition]*
.81	With Delusions
.82	With Hallucinations
—.–	Substance-Induced Psychotic Disorder *(refer to Substance-Related Disorders for substance-specific codes)*
298.9	Psychotic Disorder Not Otherwise Specified

The term *psychotic symptoms* generally refers to the presence of delusions and hallucinations but may also cover very severely disorganized behavior and speech. It is important to note that psychotic symptoms also occur in the course of other disorders that are listed outside this section (i.e., delirium, dementia, Mood Disorder With Psychotic Features, and Catatonic Disorder Due to a General Medical Condition)—all of which must be considered in the differential diagnosis. The most common error in the diagnosis of psychotic symptoms is to miss or underemphasize the possible etiological role played by drugs of abuse, medication side effects, or general medical conditions. Before diagnosing one of the primary Psychotic Disorders included in this section, the clinician should always first evaluate for and rule out etiologies related to a general medical condition or Substance Use. The second most common error is to misinterpret the beliefs of someone from a different culture as psychotic when they are in fact sanctioned by the person's culture.

We will present case studies of Schizophrenia, Schizophreniform Disorder, Schizoaffective Disorder, Delusional Disorder, Brief Psychotic Disorder, and Substance-Induced Psychotic Disorder. More than one example of Schizophrenia and Delusional Disorder are presented to illustrate the various subtypes of these disorders and demonstrate the heterogeneity of the presentations that fall within these categories.

Schizophrenia

❖   Case Study: A Woman Who
    Believes She Has Telepathic Powers

Ms. A is a 26-year-old single woman who is brought in for consultation by her parents because of a recurrence of her psychotic symptoms and generally poor functioning. She lives at home with her parents and last worked 5 years earlier as a secretary, before the first of two previous hospitalizations. Two months before the present evaluation, Ms. A's trifluoperazine was reduced to 10 mg/day. Ms. A says that she can control other people's behavior through her breathing and that people can read her mind. She is convinced that she is being watched and followed, complains of feeling confused, and at times repeats any phrase she hears, even nonsense phrases. She also reports hearing multiple voices that repeatedly tell her that she will soon be killed for causing other people to commit crimes. On most days, these voices begin in the morning and continue intermittently throughout the day. She admits that she has previously heard similar threatening voices but had not reported them to her therapist. Ms. A's energy level is low, she has little motivation, and she feels resigned to being "unable to think" and "irreversibly damaged." Her condition has been deteriorating since her boyfriend decided to see less of her 2 months before this. After evaluation, Ms. A is admitted to the inpatient psychiatric unit.

Ms. A's first hospitalization followed an argument with her boyfriend. When she was admitted, Ms. A reported that she believed everyone around her knew her thoughts and that she could "telepathically" control other people's actions by looking at them and breathing in a certain way. She experienced her thoughts as "stopping in midstream" and her mind then "going blank." With antipsychotic medications, her symptoms gradually resolved over the course of 2 months.

After the first hospital discharge, Ms. A was maintained without psychosis on 25 mg of trifluoperazine daily, but she did not return to work because she felt she could not concentrate or remember things anymore. Her social life, which had previously been active, became limited to contacts with one girlfriend and her boyfriend, whom she saw once or twice a week.

Eighteen months after her first hospitalization, Ms. A was hospitalized for the second time with a recurrence of the delusion that she could control other people with her breathing, accompanied by the belief that her activities were being monitored by a television camera and that videotapes of her were being made and sold. The trifluoperazine had been discontinued 4 months before this second admission, a change that initially seemed to have had little impact on Ms. A. After the previous trifluoperazine dose was resumed, the psychotic symptoms resolved within 6 weeks. The patient then spent a year in a vocational rehabilitation program, but she never managed more than brief volunteer placements.

During her third admission, Ms. A's trifluoperazine dose is raised to 30 mg/day, and her psychotic symptoms, except for mild suspiciousness, gradually resolve. She is discharged a month after admission. Shortly after discharge, her parents bring her to the outpatient clinic again because she has begun to develop symptoms of depression. She reports feeling sad, desperate, exhausted, and unable to enjoy even simple pleasures. She says that she thinks there is nothing that anyone can like about her. She is sleeping poorly and is occasionally tearful. She blames herself for being lazy but says that, particularly in the morning, she just doesn't have enough energy to get started and prefers to lie in bed and sleep even though this behavior makes her "feel rotten." Her appetite is diminished, although her weight has not changed, and she feels chronically apprehensive. She believes herself to be incapable of working. She mostly stays at home and participates in few activities despite her parents' urging. Her only social contact besides her parents is her boyfriend.

Addendum: Although Ms. A.'s positive symptoms seemed to be well controlled while she was taking trifluoperazine, she continued to feel listless and depressed and to have great trouble concentrating. Moreover, the patient, her family, and her clinician were all concerned about the long-term risk of her developing tardive dyskinesia. Therefore, 1 year after the admission described above, the patient's physician suggested that she consider a trial of one of the newer atypical antipsychotics. The patient was gradually switched from trifluoperazine to risperidone 6 mg/day. After 6 months of risperidone treatment, the patient and her family reported that her energy was improved and that her general mood seemed much more positive. Ms. A. reported an improved ability to concentrate and had begun to work again, although only part-time, for the first time in years.

DSM-IV-TR Diagnosis

Axis I: 295.30   Schizophrenia, Paranoid Type, Episodic With
                         Interepisode Residual Symptoms
             311   Depressive Disorder Not Otherwise Specified
Axis II: V71.09   No diagnosis
Axis III: None
Axis IV: Less contact with boyfriend
Axis V: GAF = 30 (on admission to hospital); 45 (on discharge)

❖   Case Study: A Young Man Who Believes
     He Can Solve the Race Problem With Paint

Mr. D is a 24-year-old, single, unemployed college dropout who is admitted to the hospital 3 weeks after he painted everything in sight black and white, including his room, his furniture, his clothes, and, finally, even himself. He was responding to a persistent male voice that told him that his behavior would somehow solve the race problem in America and bring peace to his family.

Mr. D has been hospitalized on at least five previous occasions during the past 5 years, each time for 4–6 weeks. Each hospitalization was due to an exacerbation of his illness with some combination of command hallucinations, strange behavior, and persecutory delusions. He has always responded fairly well to treatment with antipsychotics but hates to take the medication because it makes him feel "even deader than dead." Between hospitalizations, he is likely to take medication irregularly or not at all and to miss more outpatient appointments than he keeps.

Mr. D's functioning between episodes is poor and seems to be getting worse, with increasing social withdrawal, lack of interest in the environment, anhedonia, sloppy personal hygiene, and disordered thinking. He has been arrested on three occasions as a public disturbance for indecent exposure and preaching on street corners. When on medication, however, the patient has a somewhat better appearance and speaks more coherently.

Mr. D is the fourth of five children in an extremely close-knit, guilt-provoking, and argumentative family. His mother has been hospitalized twice for hallucinations and persecutory delusions but now functions reasonably well without medication. She believes that she knows better than the doctors what is best for her son. Her other children have left the family apartment, and Ms. D has become increasingly attached to and dependent on "the only kid I have left." Mr. D responds to his mother's ministrations with annoyance and avoidance but, when they are not forthcoming, also becomes annoyed.

Mr. D spends most of his time in the apartment doing yoga and reading about Jungian archetypes and social oppression. He sleeps all day and stays up most of every night and, except when hospitalized, rarely talks to anyone outside his immediate family circle. He is afraid to go outside, especially during the day, because he believes that strangers on the street are talking to each other about him and are able to control his thoughts and actions. He is convinced that the transmission of thought commands requires solar energy and that he is safer at night. He also believes that a "right-wing, neo-Nazi" group is attempting to ruin his reputation by spreading rumors that he is one-eighth Jewish.

As usual, Mr. D responds well to antipsychotic medication during this hospitalization. He remains convinced of his delusions, but in a low-key way, and can to some extent be argued out of them. He is also able to talk to staff with less suspicion and greater coherence than when he was admitted, and his behavior is no longer overtly bizarre. He seems ready for discharge.

Mr. D's mother has had his room repainted and is eager to have him back. Mr. D's therapist has focused attention on Mr. D's resistance to taking medication and the detrimental impact that this has on his treatment and his life. Mr. D seems somewhat more insightful about this behavior than he has in the past. Because of his problem with adherence to treatment, Mr. D.'s therapist suggests that he consider depot injections of the medication he is currently taking orally, and Mr. D. agrees. Efforts to enlist his mother's cooperation have not been conspicuously successful.

DSM-IV-TR Diagnosis

Axis I: 295.90   Schizophrenia, Undifferentiated Type, Episodic
                        With Interepisode Residual Symptoms
Axis II: V71.09   No diagnosis
Axis III: None
Axis IV: None
Axis V: GAF = 25 (current); 35 (highest level past year)

DSM-IV-TR diagnostic criteria for Schizophrenia

A. *Characteristic symptoms:* Two (or more) of the following, each present for a significant portion of time during a 1-month period (or less if successfully treated):
   (1) delusions
   (2) hallucinations
   (3) disorganized speech (e.g., frequent derailment or incoherence)
   (4) grossly disorganized or catatonic behavior
   (5) negative symptoms, i.e., affective flattening, alogia, or avolition

(continued)

DSM-IV-TR diagnostic criteria for Schizophrenia *(continued)*

Note: Only one Criterion A symptom is required if delusions are bizarre or hallucinations consist of a voice keeping up a running commentary on the person's behavior or thoughts, or two or more voices conversing with each other.

B. *Social/occupational dysfunction:* For a significant portion of the time since the onset of the disturbance, one or more major areas of functioning such as work, interpersonal relations, or self-care are markedly below the level achieved prior to the onset (or when the onset is in childhood or adolescence, failure to achieve expected level of interpersonal, academic, or occupational achievement).

C. *Duration:* Continuous signs of the disturbance persist for at least 6 months. This 6-month period must include at least 1 month of symptoms (or less if successfully treated) that meet Criterion A (i.e., active-phase symptoms) and may include periods of prodromal or residual symptoms. During these prodromal or residual periods, the signs of the disturbance may be manifested by only negative symptoms or two or more symptoms listed in Criterion A present in an attenuated form (e.g., odd beliefs, unusual perceptual experiences).

D. *Schizoaffective and Mood Disorder exclusion:* Schizoaffective Disorder and Mood Disorder With Psychotic Features have been ruled out because either (1) no Major Depressive, Manic, or Mixed Episodes have occurred concurrently with the active-phase symptoms; or (2) if mood episodes have occurred during active-phase symptoms, their total duration has been brief relative to the duration of the active and residual periods.

E. *Substance/general medical condition exclusion:* The disturbance is not due to the direct physiological effects of a substance (e.g., a drug of abuse, a medication) or a general medical condition.

F. *Relationship to a Pervasive Developmental Disorder:* If there is a history of Autistic Disorder or another Pervasive Developmental Disorder, the additional diagnosis of Schizophrenia is made only if prominent delusions or hallucinations are also present for at least a month (or less if successfully treated).

Classification of longitudinal course (can be applied only after at least 1 year has elapsed since the initial onset of active-phase symptoms):

Episodic With Interepisode Residual Symptoms (episodes are defined by the reemergence of prominent psychotic symptoms); *also specify if:* **With Prominent Negative Symptoms**

Episodic With No Interepisode Residual Symptoms

(continued)

**DSM-IV-TR diagnostic criteria for
Schizophrenia *(continued)***

Continuous (prominent psychotic symptoms are present throughout the pe-
riod of observation); *also specify if:* **With Prominent Negative Symptoms**
Single Episode In Partial Remission; *also specify if:*   **With Prominent Nega-
tive Symptoms**
Single Episode In Full Remission
Other or Unspecified Pattern

Guidelines for Differential Diagnosis of Schizophrenia

The diagnosis of Schizophrenia is fairly straightforward in those individuals
who have the chronic and classic forms. Early in the course, however, the diagnosis is much more difficult. Before diagnosing Schizophrenia in younger
individuals who have had a first episode of psychotic symptoms, it is especially important to rule out Substance-Induced Psychotic Disorder, Mood
Disorder With Psychotic Features, or one of the other Psychotic Disorders
included in this section. A first onset of psychotic symptoms in an older individual may occasionally indicate late-onset Schizophrenia but is more likely
to be due to dementia or delirium, a Psychotic Disorder Due to a General Medical Condition, medication side effects, a Mood Disorder With Psychotic Features, or Delusional Disorder.

Differentiating Schizophrenia from Schizoaffective Disorder and Mood
Disorder With Psychotic Features is particularly difficult. The DSM-IV-TR
definition of Schizophrenia is narrow. Whenever psychotic symptoms occur only during a mood episode, the diagnosis is Mood Disorder With Psychotic Features and not Schizophrenia or Schizoaffective Disorder. As will
be discussed in more detail below, the diagnosis would be Schizoaffective
Disorder only if psychotic symptoms occur concurrently with a mood
episode and occur for a period of at least 2 weeks in the absence of a mood
episode and if the mood symptoms are present for a substantial portion of
the total duration of the illness. For Ms. A, the diagnosis is not Mood Disorder With Psychotic Features because her psychotic symptoms occur both
during periods of mood disturbance and during absences of mood disturbance.
Her diagnosis is Schizophrenia and not Schizoaffective Disorder because,
although she does have mood symptoms, they are not a significant part of
her presentation. The typical presentation of Schizophrenia is different in
men and women in a way that complicates the distinction between Schizophrenia and Mood Disorders. Women are likely to have a later onset of Schizo-

phrenia (late 20s versus early 20s), to have more prominent mood symptoms, and to have a better outcome.

Depressive symptoms are frequently associated with Schizophrenia and often have important implications in management. Individuals with Schizophrenia have a high rate of suicide (a 10%–20% lifetime risk). No separate diagnosis for depressive symptoms is necessary if these symptoms do not warrant separate clinical attention and do not meet criteria for a Major Depressive Episode. A separate category for postpsychotic depression of schizophrenia was proposed for inclusion in DSM-IV because depressive symptoms are a particular problem in the period after active-phase symptoms have remitted. This proposed diagnosis requires that criteria be met for a Major Depressive Episode but only during the residual phase of Schizophrenia. This was not included as an official category in DSM-IV, pending the gathering of further data, but a research criteria set for such a diagnosis is included in an appendix to DSM-IV. The official diagnostic specification for this situation in DSM-IV (and DSM-IV-TR) is Depressive Disorder Not Otherwise Specified. Although antidepressant treatment may be helpful in ameliorating the depressive symptoms associated with Schizophrenia, there is some concern that, in some individuals at least, antidepressant treatment may have a negative impact on the positive symptoms.

Neuropsychological deficits are consistently found in groups of patients with schizophrenia. Patients with schizophrenia may display a number of cognitive deficits, including problems with memory, psychomotor abilities, attention, and concentration. Cognitive problems associated with schizophrenia have attracted increasing research attention in recent years, especially given outcome studies that indicate that the severity of such problems is a relatively strong predictor of social and vocational outcome.

Ms. A's and Mr. D's symptoms have been present more or less continuously for a number of years, thus ruling out a diagnosis of Schizophreniform Disorder, in which symptoms last less than 6 months. In addition to having bizarre delusions, both also have prominent auditory hallucinations and negative symptoms, thus ruling out a diagnosis of Delusional Disorder.

In adolescents or adults, it can be difficult to distinguish between the Residual Type of Schizophrenia and a Pervasive Developmental Disorder, such as Autistic Disorder or Asperger's Disorder. To make this distinction accurately, the clinician must obtain a complete history, usually from outside informants, to establish whether the symptoms had their onset when the person was an infant or toddler—which would indicate a diagnosis of a Pervasive Developmental Disorder. Individuals with a Pervasive Developmental Disorder do not usually have prominent delusions or hallucinations. If these occur later and become a prominent part of the presentation, then both diagnoses (Pervasive Developmental Disorder and Schizophrenia) may be made.

Subtypes of Schizophrenia

The DSM-IV (and DSM-IV-TR) subtyping of Schizophrenia is meant to describe more specifically the heterogeneity of presentations that may be seen in clinical practice. This subtyping system applies to the type of presentation seen during the most recent episode and is organized in a diagnostic hierarchy so that no more than one subtype applies at any given time.

The algorithm for the subtyping of Schizophrenia is complicated. At the top of the hierarchy is the Catatonic Type, which is diagnosed whenever catatonic symptoms are prominent, regardless of other aspects of the presentation.

The Disorganized Type is next in the hierarchy. To qualify for a diagnosis of Schizophrenia, Disorganized Type, all three features—disorganized speech, disorganized behavior, and flat or inappropriate affect—must be present.

Schizophrenia, Paranoid Type, comes next in the algorithm. This type, which best describes Ms. A's symptoms, requires that there be prominent delusions and hallucinations and excludes the presence of prominent catatonic symptoms, flat affect, disorganized behavior, and disorganized speech. The paranoid subtype of Schizophrenia is similar to Delusional Disorder in its presentation and is distinguished only by the presence of hallucinations or bizarre delusions and (usually) greater impairment in social and vocational functioning.

Although pure types of Schizophrenia do occur, individuals often present with mixtures of symptoms that do not conform exactly to any of these pictures. This is the case with Mr. D, whose symptoms would be classified as Schizophrenia, Undifferentiated Type—a category that is used to describe presentations that meet the criteria for Schizophrenia but not for any of the specific subtypes. Mr. D does not display any catatonic symptoms, so the catatonic subtype would not apply. Although he does have paranoid delusions, his presentation would not fall within the paranoid subtype because it also includes prominent disorganized behavior and flat affect, which are excluded as prominent features by the definition of the paranoid subtype. Mr. D's symptoms would not warrant a diagnosis of the Disorganized Type, however, because, although he does have disorganized behavior and flat affect, disorganized speech is not prominent. All three features—disorganized speech and behavior and flat affect—must be present to warrant a diagnosis of the Disorganized Type. The Undifferentiated Type of presentation may become particularly common as the disorder progresses over time. Individuals with the Disorganized Type and the Undifferentiated Type tend to have poorer prognoses, whereas the prognosis for those with the Paranoid and Catatonic Types is better.

The Undifferentiated Type of Schizophrenia is distinguished from the

Residual Type by the continuing prominent positive symptoms of delusions, hallucinations, disorganized speech, or disorganized behavior in an
individual with the Undifferentiated Type. The diagnosis of Schizophrenia, Residual Type, is used to describe those interepisode periods in which
only negative symptoms continue to be present or during which two or more
positive symptoms are present but only in an attenuated form.

Treatment Planning for Schizophrenia

Treatment of Schizophrenia requires a combination of psychoeducation,
consistent medication management, rehabilitation, and supportive therapy to
help the individual improve performance in the activities of everyday life and
acquire increased social skills. The introduction of a number of new atypical
antipsychotics in recent years (e.g., clozapine, risperidone, olanzapine, que-
tiapine, and ziprasidone) has revolutionized the treatment of this debilitating disorder. The newer medications have a much more favorable side-effect
profile than the older traditional antipsychotics, especially since they are
much less likely to cause neurological and movement side effects. They may
also help patients who have not responded well to the older medications. Although research is still under way, it appears that the newer medications are
associated with improvements in the negative and cognitive symptoms that
can lead to such adverse social and vocational outcomes.

Intensive psychosocial interventions, such as assertive community treatment, intensive case management, or intensive outpatient treatment programs, can help patients continue to take medication and avoid the "revolving
door" cycle of repeated readmissions. Other types of psychosocial interventions, such as cognitive-behavioral therapy and skills-based training, can help
patients achieve better social and vocational outcomes.

Recent studies emphasize the crucial importance of adequate maintenance
doses of antipsychotic medications, although lower dose strategies may sometimes be necessary and feasible, particularly for those individuals who are sensitive to side effects and likely to be noncompliant with medication prescribed at
the usual maintenance doses. A major dilemma in the management of Schizophrenia is that many patients do not take their medication or may substitute
street psychopharmacology such as dopamine-enhancing drugs like cocaine. Depot antipsychotics are often necessary for patients with adherence problems.

Suicide rates among those with Schizophrenia are between 10% and 20%.
Suicides occur during acute episodes and during a demoralization or depressive phase that may begin after the psychotic symptoms have improved.
There is some evidence that antidepressants may be helpful in treating postpsychotic depression (see the discussion above), but these must be prescribed
cautiously and with adequate antipsychotic coverage.

Schizophreniform Disorder

❖ Case Study: A Promising Young
    Lawyer Makes a Satisfying Recovery

Mr. B, a 30-year-old lawyer, is brought into the emergency room in hand-cuffs. He is disheveled and shouts and struggles with the policeman who has brought him in. The patient is obviously hearing voices because he is re-sponding to them with loud and belligerent replies ("Get away from me— I won't do it"), but he denies hearing them. He has a hypervigilant stare and is easily startled by even muted sounds in the hallway outside the office. He freely admits that he expects to be killed at any moment and begs desper-ately to be allowed to run away.

Mr. B was doing well until 3 months earlier. After graduating from law school, he began a lucrative job with a prestigious law firm and was engaged to be married. People might have described Mr. B as a bit quarrelsome and complaining, but these characteristics had not handicapped his vocational or social life.

There was no intimation of impending disaster until, suddenly, the roof fell in. Mr. B's girlfriend unexpectedly decided that she did not want to continue their relationship and abruptly moved out of the apartment they shared. The patient was bewildered and outraged and felt very sorry for himself. He decided that he could win her back and began to arrange "acci-dental meetings" outside her new apartment and outside the office where she worked. When she insisted that he respect her privacy, Mr. B became preoccupied with the idea that she had jilted him for another man and be-gan following her to catch her in this act of betrayal.

Before long, Mr. B's work at his new job began to suffer. After several weeks, he was called in for a harsh scolding and told that he must improve his attendance, punctuality, and productivity. As a result, Mr. B felt enor-mous resentment toward his boss. He gradually became preoccupied with the way he had been criticized and humiliated. He could not eliminate the recurrent image of his supervisor's mocking face. Within a week, Mr. B pieced together various hints and bits of evidence and concluded that his super-visor and his former girlfriend were having an affair.

Mr. B's insight was confirmed by a male voice, probably his supervi-sor's, that jeered at him for being a "faggot" and a "jerk off." The voice com-manded that he quit his job and forget about his girlfriend. Mr. B was determined not to give his supervisor either satisfaction. He continued to work and, in the evenings, to follow his girlfriend. He became convinced that the secretaries in the office were scheming against him on their trips to the watercooler. The whole firm seemed to be in on the secret and was con-spiring to harm him. He began to suspect that his life was in danger, and he believed he needed police protection. He also considered buying a gun and striking preemptively against his tormenters.

Mr. B felt like an innocent victim throughout this episode. His sleep was interrupted by nightmares, but he could generally doze off again without difficulty. He lost no weight and had no other vegetative symptoms. His affect alternated between rage and terror. His mind was unusually alert and active, but he was not otherwise hyperactive, excessively energetic, or expansive. He did not display any disorder in the formal aspects of his thinking.

The patient was hospitalized and treated with antipsychotic medication. After several weeks of gradual improvement, his psychotic symptoms remitted altogether and he was able to return to work shortly thereafter.

DSM-IV-TR Diagnosis

Axis I: 295.40   Schizophreniform Disorder, With Good Prognostic
                        Features
Axis II: V71.09   No diagnosis
Axis III: None
Axis IV: Breakup with girlfriend
Axis V: GAF = 30 (upon admission); 60 (upon discharge);
             GAF = 90 (highest level past year)

DSM-IV-TR diagnostic criteria for
295.40 Schizophreniform Disorder

A.   Criteria A, D, and E of Schizophrenia are met.
B.   An episode of the disorder (including prodromal, active, and residual phases) lasts at least 1 month but less than 6 months. (When the diagnosis must be made without waiting for recovery, it should be qualified as "Provisional.")

Specify if:
Without Good Prognostic Features
With Good Prognostic Features: as evidenced by two (or more) of the following:
   (1)   onset of prominent psychotic symptoms within 4 weeks of the first noticeable change in usual behavior or functioning
   (2)   confusion or perplexity at the height of the psychotic episode
   (3)   good premorbid social and occupational functioning
   (4)   absence of blunted or flat affect

Guidelines for Differential Diagnosis of Schizophreniform Disorder

The concept of Schizophreniform Disorder was introduced in DSM-III to reduce the heterogeneity of outcome predicted by the category of Schizophrenia. The clinical presentation of Schizophreniform Disorder is essentially the same as that of Schizophrenia, except that 1) the duration requirement for the disorder is at least 1 month but less than 6 months and 2) there is no requirement that a deterioration in functioning take place (although it may). Mr. B's presentation clearly met these criteria because his symptoms lasted approximately 4 months and remitted very quickly after treatment. In ICD-10 (World Health Organization 1992), such short-term presentations would not be diagnosed separately from Schizophrenia. The major reason the DSM system distinguishes between Schizophreniform Disorder and Schizophrenia is prognostic significance. Individuals who have a shorter course such as Mr. B are much more likely to have a better outcome (e.g., a better response to medications, less chronicity, fewer negative symptoms, fewer symptoms of disorganization, and less likelihood of deterioration). Meeting the criteria for Schizophrenia for 6 months predicts a more chronic course and probably less responsiveness to treatment. One of the problems in diagnosing Schizophreniform Disorder is that, until the symptoms remit, it is not clear whether the episode will continue long enough to be diagnosed as Schizophrenia. Therefore, while symptoms continue and before 6 months have elapsed, the diagnosis of Schizophreniform Disorder is given only provisionally.

Mr. B's symptoms would be described as being "With Good Prognostic Features" because of their sudden onset and Mr. B's good premorbid social and occupational functioning. Good prognostic features are important to note because the more acute the symptoms, the more prominent the positive rather than negative symptoms, and the better the premorbid functioning, the more likely that the individual will recover completely from the episode and not later go on to meet criteria for Schizophrenia.

Schizophreniform Disorder would not be diagnosed if the psychotic symptoms remitted in less than 1 month. Such a presentation would be diagnosed as Brief Psychotic Disorder, which is defined as the presence of psychotic symptoms that last at least 1 day but less than 1 month. Again, the reason for making this diagnostic distinction is mostly one of prognosis. Individuals with very short psychotic episodes are more likely to have a relatively benign course.

If the psychotic symptoms occur only during a mood episode, the diagnosis would be Mood Disorder With Psychotic Features. This can be a difficult evaluation because psychotic individuals are often experiencing significant turmoil that may be confused with agitated depression or irritable mania.

Schizophrenia and Schizophreniform Disorder are distinguished from Delusional Disorder by the presence of other prominent psychotic symptoms in addition to delusions. Mr. B was experiencing hallucinations as a prominent part of his presentation, so a diagnosis of Delusional Disorder would be ruled out.

Treatment Planning for Schizophreniform Disorder

The treatment for the acute symptoms of Schizophreniform Disorder is equivalent to the treatment of the acute symptoms of Schizophrenia. The major difference in management is related to psychoeducation about the disorder and the necessity for maintenance antipsychotic medication. Although there can be optimism that at least some individuals with Schizophrenia will have a good outcome, because of psychoeducation and antipsychotics, the diagnosis of Schizophrenia does carry with it a grimness about the future that is often inappropriate for individuals who have the relatively short-term presentations of Schizophreniform Disorder. This is particularly true when the disorder is accompanied by good prognostic features, as in Mr. B's presentation.

Clear guidelines are not available for the duration of maintenance medication in Schizophreniform Disorder. This clinical judgment should take into account the severity and duration of the episode; the risk of suicidal or homicidal behaviors; the presence of previous episodes; the age at onset of previous episodes; family history; the individual's premorbid level of functioning; the impact of drug side effects; and the patient's and family's level of insight, ability to detect early signs of relapse, and preferences about choice of treatment.

Schizoaffective Disorder

❖ Case Study: A Young Woman
With a Confusing Presentation

Ms. D is a 26-year-old woman whose family brings her to the emergency room in an acutely psychotic state. Ms. D is the youngest of six siblings. She was born prematurely, weighing 4 pounds, but had no other perinatal complications. Her subsequent developmental history was normal: She did well in school, made friends, and went to work in a bank after graduating from high school. She then married (4 years before her first admission) and had two children. Ms. D has not worked outside the home since the birth of her children. There is a family history of psychotic illness in a maternal aunt and of drug abuse in two siblings.

A week before the present evaluation, Ms. D came to the psychiatric emergency clinic complaining of dizziness and trouble sleeping. She said she was also experiencing intermittent depression and felt that she was a failure as a wife and mother. An appointment at the mental health center was scheduled, but before the appointment could take place, Ms. D's family brought her into the emergency room for this evaluation, which results in Ms. D being admitted to the psychiatric unit for the second time.

Four months before this, Ms. D separated from her husband and returned home to live with her mother and two siblings. Shortly after she began living with her mother, one of her brothers was sent to jail and her boyfriend wrecked her new car. About a month after Ms. D began living with her mother, her family noticed a deterioration in her functioning that culminated in her being found in a confused state in a train station. On that day she was brought to the hospital, where she was observed to be agitated and hallucinating, with marked thought disorder. She complained of voices making both encouraging and derogatory statements about her and of command hallucinations to kill herself and her husband. Ms. D was hospitalized and treated with antipsychotic medication. She was discharged after 3 days, returned to live with her mother, and began outpatient treatment at the local mental health center.

When Ms. D is admitted for this second time, she reports that she has been having anxiety, insomnia, delusions, and auditory hallucinations for the past 3 weeks. It turns out that she has actually been experiencing hallucinations and delusions over the past 3 months, but her fear of readmission to the hospital prevented her from reporting these to her outpatient therapist. She describes paranoid delusions about her mother wanting to hurt her. She states that she believes that the television is controlling her mind and that others can read her thoughts. She is experiencing auditory control hallucinations and says that they have occurred frequently ever since her first admission.

Ms. D is also displaying prominent manic symptoms, which her mother reports began only 3 weeks before this admission. Ms. D's mother says that at that time her daughter began to go on frequent shopping sprees, suddenly seemed as if she was driven by a motor, was not sleeping, and was frequently pacing for much of the night. Three days before this admission, she became irritable and developed paranoid ideas about her teacher at the college she was attending. On returning home from school, she began to experience auditory hallucinations of God talking to her and of voices discussing her, accompanied by somatic hallucinations that someone was touching and arousing her sexually. She hardly slept for the 2 nights before she was admitted, and her family reports that she had been dancing, singing loudly, and reciting the Bible at the dinner table.

During this second admission, Ms. D is initially hostile and agitated, stating repeatedly that she believes the staff is trying to hurt her through a mirror in her room. She is hyperactive, disruptive, and excited; displays a flight of ideas; and talks nonstop. She continues to experience somatic hallucinations. She shows hypersexual behavior toward other patients and experiences grandiose delusions that she can heal them with her thoughts.

Ms. D is treated with fluphenazine in doses up to 60 mg/day. Despite 2 weeks of treatment with fluphenazine, her symptoms continue to worsen and a trial of lithium is initiated. Within 3 weeks after Ms. D achieves a therapeutic blood level of lithium, her mental status returns to normal. She is discharged on fluphenazine 15 mg at night and lithium carbonate 300 mg tid.

Her outpatient therapist helps her set simple goals for helping with small household and child-care tasks. Ms. D and her mother continue to be seen regularly in family treatment. These sessions focus on education about Ms. D's illness, recognition of early signs of relapse, reduction of tension at home, and setting of realistic goals for Ms. D during the recovery process. Over the next 6 months, Ms. D's fluphenazine dose is reduced and finally discontinued, and she regains her premorbid level of functioning and is maintained on lithium.

DSM-IV-TR Diagnosis

Axis I: 295.70   Schizoaffective Disorder, Bipolar Type
Axis II: V71.09   No diagnosis
Axis III: None
Axis IV: Boyfriend totaled her new car, two brothers in jail
Axis V: GAF = 30 (upon second admission); 70 (current)

DSM-IV-TR diagnostic criteria for 295.70 Schizoaffective Disorder

A.   An uninterrupted period of illness during which, at some time, there is either a Major Depressive Episode, a Manic Episode, or a Mixed Episode concurrent with symptoms that meet Criterion A for Schizophrenia.

(continued)

DSM-IV-TR diagnostic criteria for
295.70 Schizoaffective Disorder *(continued)*

Note: The Major Depressive Episode must include Criterion A1: depressed mood.

B. During the same period of illness, there have been delusions or hallucinations for at least 2 weeks in the absence of prominent mood symptoms.

C. Symptoms that meet criteria for a mood episode are present for a substantial portion of the total duration of the active and residual periods of the illness.

D. The disturbance is not due to the direct physiological effects of a substance (e.g., a drug of abuse, a medication) or a general medical condition.

Specify type:

Bipolar Type: if the disturbance includes a Manic or a Mixed Episode (or a Manic or a Mixed Episode and Major Depressive Episodes)

Depressive Type: if the disturbance only includes Major Depressive Episodes

Guidelines for Differential Diagnosis of Schizoaffective Disorder

Certain presentations lie on a continuum between Schizophrenia and Mood Disorder With Psychotic Features. The category of Schizoaffective Disorder fills this gap in the system, but unfortunately it does not do its job very well because the presentations are so varied and its definition is vague. Clinicians find it very hard to agree on this boundary diagnosis, and Schizoaffective Disorder is probably the least reliable diagnosis in DSM-IV. This should probably not be too surprising. It is always most difficult to get agreement on the diagnosis of confusing boundary conditions. The area of greatest disagreement in diagnosing Schizoaffective Disorder is whether the mood symptoms are of sufficient duration and severity to warrant a diagnosis of Schizoaffective Disorder rather than Schizophrenia. It is also often difficult to determine whether the psychotic symptoms occur only within the context of a mood episode, in which case the diagnosis would be Mood Disorder With Psychotic Features rather than Schizoaffective Disorder. (For a more detailed discussion of the differential of Bipolar I Disorder, see p. 132).

Ms. D's presentation is indeed confusing. During her first admission, her presentation was characterized by florid psychotic symptoms that appeared to develop in response to a series of stressors. These psychotic symptoms seemed to respond rapidly and completely to antipsychotic treatment, and the apparent diagnosis was Brief Psychotic Disorder because her symptoms were reported to have lasted for less than 1 month. However, it turned out that Ms. D was doing her best to appear as healthy as possible and, in fact, her psychotic symptoms did not fully resolve. In the period before Ms. D developed manic symptoms, the appropriate diagnosis would have been Schizophreniform Disorder (if her psychotic symptoms had been known). Once the substantial mood symptoms developed, however, the diagnosis would become Schizoaffective Disorder because the three essential conditions for that disorder were satisfied: 1) an overlap of mood and psychotic symptoms, 2) a period of psychotic symptoms without mood symptoms, and 3) mood symptoms that were a prominent and enduring part of the clinical picture. A diagnosis of Schizoaffective Disorder applies only to a given episode of illness, not to the lifetime course experienced by the individual. This leads to the probably unfortunate possibility that, during the course of a lifetime, a given patient may have episodes that are variously labeled as Schizophrenia, Schizoaffective Disorder, and Mood Disorder With Psychotic Features. These changes in diagnosis for episodes occurring during the course of a lifetime undoubtedly reflect a limitation in the diagnostic system rather than the presence of a number of distinct disorders.

Treatment Planning for Schizoaffective Disorder

The treatment of Schizoaffective Disorder has not been, and probably never will be, well studied. Because the diagnosis is so unreliable, it does not provide a convenient subject for research or allow for clear treatment guidelines. It is therefore usually necessary to treat the target symptoms and determine empirically what seems to be most helpful in the acute and maintenance phases of treatment for a particular patient. The acute management tends to be fairly straightforward, with antipsychotic medication used to treat the acute psychotic symptoms, lithium or another mood stabilizer for manic or mixed symptoms, and an antidepressant for depressive symptoms. What is much less clear is how to manage the continuation and maintenance phases of treatment. Should Ms. D remain on lithium and/or antipsychotics for 6 months, 1 year, 2 years, or 5 years? Different clinicians and different patients would have varying preferences in this regard. The psychoeducational tips regarding the identification of early symptoms, reduction of stress, and medication compliance that are useful in Mood Disorders and Schizophrenia may be helpful here as well.

Delusional Disorder

We provide several different case examples to illustrate some of the different subtypes of Delusional Disorder.

❖   Case Study: A Restaurant Owner Under Siege

Mr. C is a 44-year-old unmarried restaurant owner who comes for treatment because he has been charged with assault and battery. He spent a week in jail before making bail and has become depressed while awaiting trial. The charges are the result of a fight Mr. C had with his butcher, whom he accused of trying to destroy his business by supplying him with poisoned meat. He became convinced of this after a customer complained of becoming ill after eating in the restaurant, but even before this he had been concerned that his butcher was conspiring with other suppliers to price gouge and drive him out of business in order to buy him out.

Mr. C is completely preoccupied with his business, works 16 hours a day, is constantly fearful that he is being taken advantage of, and has very frequent verbal and sometimes physical altercations with his waiters and cooks. He has accused the waiters of stealing food, dishes, and hardware. He is convinced his staff is sabotaging the food and that they are in the pay of the butcher. He is also convinced that there is something wrong with the heating system and that there is a dangerous contaminant in the air that no one else can smell. When he goes to the market, he thinks that everyone is looking at him and thinking of him as that "jerk" who is always cheated. This most recent delusional episode has lasted for 3 months, but Mr. C has a history of these sorts of problems that goes back many years. These symptoms began in his late 20s when he developed persecutory ideas and delusions of reference. These episodes lasted only for several months and sometimes remitted spontaneously but usually required treatment with antipsychotics. These periods alternated with periods when he was not delusional but continued to exhibit marked paranoid traits, always feeling that people were taking advantage of him. Mr. C is also a perfectionist who is very demanding.

DSM-IV-TR Diagnosis

Axis I: 297.1   Delusional Disorder, Persecutory Type
Axis II: Rule out 301.0 Paranoid Personality Disorder (premorbid)
             Rule out 301.4 Obsessive-Compulsive Personality Disorder
Axis III: None
Axis IV: Financial difficulties
Axis V: GAF = 50 (current); 65 (highest level in past year)

❖   Case Study: A Woman With an Infestation

Ms. W, a 49-year-old woman, is referred by a dermatologist who could find no objective evidence of skin disease, although the patient insists that she is plagued with insects. She says that the "infestation" began nearly 12 years earlier when she developed a skin itch that spread all over her body. She is convinced that the itch is due to "bugs." She believes that the bugs have burrowed under her skin, and, although she has never seen them, she says she can feel the subcutaneous lumps and feel pain from bites. She has consulted numerous physicians over the past 12 years, especially dermatologists, and she is distressed and angry that no one has been able to help her.

Just before the onset of her complaint, she had been undergoing a very stressful divorce. When the skin symptoms appeared, she became more and more preoccupied with them and washed herself and her clothes frequently. When treatment from various family physicians and dermatologists, which included tricyclics, antipsychotics, and benzodiazepines, was unavailing, she resorted to assorted applications (e.g., bleach) that burned her skin. She used to gouge out the "lumps" from under her skin but now prevents herself from doing so. During the previous 10 years, she has taken two serious overdoses because she felt so wretched. She gave up work, withdrew socially, and habitually sleeps very poorly.

Ms. W had a severely unstable and unhappy childhood, and she has been nervous throughout her life. At age 10, she took an overdose of pills and, at about the same time, suffered a skull fracture in a fall. One sister committed suicide, and one of her own three children took a serious overdose on one occasion.

During the interview, Ms. W is agitated, very unhappy, and almost totally preoccupied with the "bugs." She has marked ideas of reference, especially that people are avoiding her because she is "dirty." However, when diverted from the topic of her "infestation," she appears to think rationally and to be a charming and engaging woman who can converse intelligently on a number of topics. Ms. W is angry about being referred to a psychiatrist, however, and insists that her problems are physical.

A mental status examination reveals an illness characterized by a single delusion that is accompanied by very severe anxiety. The delusion has virtually taken over Ms. W's life, yet many aspects of her personality are well preserved. She gives no convincing evidence of hallucinations and has no marked thought disorder. There is no evidence of a major Mood Disorder, Schizophrenia, or a general medical condition that might be responsible for her symptoms.

DSM-IV-TR Diagnosis

Axis I:	297.1	Delusional Disorder, Somatic Type
	311	Depressive Disorder Not Otherwise Specified
Axis II:	V71.09	No diagnosis
Axis III:	900.9	Head injury at age 10: no obvious neurological sequelae
Axis IV:		Social isolation, inability to work, constant fear that others regard her as unclean
Axis V:		GAF = 30 (current); 40 (highest level in past year)

❖　Case Study: A Victim of Love

Ms. T is a 25-year-old second-year law student who comes in at the insistence of one of her professors. She is convinced that this law professor, a 45-year-old married man, is secretly in love with her. Ms. T says she first began to suspect his feeling for her because of the way he looked at her and the friendly manner in which he answered her questions after class. She came to believe that his corrections to her legal briefs were coded love messages. She responded to this by sending him cards and bringing him small gifts such as ties and books. At first he accepted these but very soon began returning the gifts saying that it was not appropriate to their professional relationship for him to be receiving them. Instead of discouraging her interest, this caused her to be even more convinced that he was deeply in love with her and was fighting very hard not to declare his intentions. She began calling him to ask questions about her law school work when there was no need to do so. She then began calling him at home and engaged his wife in conversations that convinced Ms. T that her professor and his wife no longer loved each other.

Finally, one day she could contain her feelings no longer and declared herself in his office at the law school. Shocked, embarrassed, and surprised, he disavowed any romantic attraction or intention toward her. Ms. T then grew angry and accused him of leading her on, nevertheless declaring that despite the shabby way he had treated her, she would love him forever. She told him that she was sure that he secretly loved her and was only staying with his wife and family out of a misplaced sense of loyalty, and she challenged him to follow his heart. When she began leaving long and suggestive messages on his answering machine, the professor became seriously alarmed and warned Ms. T that she could be arrested for such behavior. He told her that he would call the police and have her taken out of his class if she did not seek professional help.

During the initial evaluation, Ms. T maintains that she is not the crazy one but is only coming to treatment to satisfy her "lover's" condition so that she can stay in his class and be near the man she loves and who, she is convinced, really loves her despite his denials. She says that she believes that he calls her and hangs up, follows her around the campus, and has tapped her phone.

Ms. T had two previous such episodes of being loved by someone who "refused to admit it": The first involved one of her high school teachers and the second, her father's business partner while she was in college. When this second episode ended in a very humiliating way, Ms. T attempted suicide with an overdose of 40 aspirin. These two previous occasions were the only times in her life Ms. T has ever felt that she was in love or that someone else was in love with her. With the exceptions of these three incidents, Ms. T has otherwise functioned very well.

DSM-IV-TR Diagnosis

Axis I: 297.1   Delusional Disorder, Erotomanic Type
Axis II: V71.09   No diagnosis
Axis III: None
Axis IV: None
Axis V: GAF = 50 (initial evaluation); 70 (highest level in past year)

DSM-IV-TR diagnostic criteria for 297.1 Delusional Disorder

A. Nonbizarre delusions (i.e., involving situations that occur in real life, such as being followed, poisoned, infected, loved at a distance, or deceived by spouse or lover, or having a disease) of at least 1 month's duration.

B. Criterion A for Schizophrenia has never been met. **Note:** Tactile and olfactory hallucinations may be present in Delusional Disorder if they are related to the delusional theme.

C. Apart from the impact of the delusion(s) or its ramifications, functioning is not markedly impaired and behavior is not obviously odd or bizarre.

D. If mood episodes have occurred concurrently with delusions, their total duration has been brief relative to the duration of the delusional periods.

E. The disturbance is not due to the direct physiological effects of a substance (e.g., a drug of abuse, a medication) or a general medical condition.

Specify type (the following types are assigned based on the predominant delusional theme):

Erotomanic Type: delusions that another person, usually of higher status, is in love with the individual

Grandiose Type: delusions of inflated worth, power, knowledge, identity, or special relationship to a deity or famous person

(continued)

**DSM-IV-TR diagnostic criteria for
297.1 Delusional Disorder *(continued)***

Jealous Type: delusions that the individual's sexual partner is unfaithful

Persecutory Type: delusions that the person (or someone to whom the person is close) is being malevolently treated in some way

Somatic Type: delusions that the person has some physical defect or general medical condition

Mixed Type: delusions characteristic of more than one of the above types but no one theme predominates

Unspecified Type

Guidelines for Differential Diagnosis of Delusional Disorder

For several reasons, determining that a person is delusional is much harder than clinicians might first imagine. First, the person's beliefs, however strange, may indeed reflect the reality of the situation. However implausible it may seem, the individual may in fact be in real physical danger, may have a real illness, or may be loved by someone who has not yet declared that love. Second, although false, the beliefs may not be held with absolute delusional conviction and may be amenable to change (e.g., as with the false beliefs or overvalued ideas that characterize Obsessive-Compulsive Disorder, Social Phobia, or Hypochondriasis). Third, the beliefs may be part of a cultural system with which the clinician is not familiar but for which such beliefs are sanctioned and appropriate. We discuss how to evaluate for each of these possibilities in more detail below.

To evaluate whether a person's beliefs are based in reality, the clinician must first learn as much as possible about the real situation. To obtain accurate information, other sources, such as family members, friends, physicians, and co-workers, should be consulted whenever possible. It is also helpful to examine the patient's history to discover whether previous delusional episodes have occurred.

The distinction between beliefs that are delusional and those that are merely strongly held is based on whether the individual can admit that there is a possibility that the belief may not be correct. When an individual persistently denies that any other explanation could possibly account for the occurrences described, it strongly suggests that the person is delusional. The clinician must judge that the patient's adherence to the belief does not reflect momentary argumentativeness or oppositionalism. This issue may be complicated because the strength with which the beliefs are held may vary over time, even during the course of a given clinical interview.

When the clinician is evaluating those whose backgrounds are unfamiliar, it is especially important to consider whether beliefs that seem delusional may actually reflect cultural or religious beliefs. In such cases, it may be helpful for the clinician to consult someone who is more familiar with the individual's culture or belief system. Overdiagnoses of Delusional Disorder occur most often because of misunderstandings caused by the cultural naiveté of the clinician.

After establishing that delusions are indeed present, the clinician must determine whether they are due to the use of substances (e.g., Substance-Induced Psychotic Disorder) or a general medical condition (e.g., Psychotic Disorder Due to a General Medical Condition). In younger people, it is especially important to consider drugs of abuse; whereas, in older people, alcohol, a general medical condition, or the side effects of a medication are common causes of delusions. When the delusions occur during a delirium or dementia, a separate diagnosis of Delusional Disorder is not necessary.

After establishing that delusions are present and related to a primary mental disorder rather than to a substance or general medical condition, the next step is to determine which primary disorder best accounts for the presentation (e.g., Schizophrenia, Schizophreniform Disorder, Schizoaffective Disorder, Mood Disorder With Psychotic Features, Delusional Disorder, or Brief Psychotic Disorder).

Delusional Disorder is distinguished from Schizophrenia by the absence of characteristic symptoms such as prominent hallucinations, bizarre delusions, disorganized speech, grossly disorganized or catatonic behavior, and negative symptoms. The delusions that characterize Delusional Disorder are, by definition, nonbizarre—that is, they involve situations that occur in real life and are usually encapsulated, plausible, and systematized. Transient hallucinations may occur in Delusional Disorder, but these are not common and, when they are present, are limited to ideas that are related to the delusional theme (e.g., Ms. W might experience the occasional feeling that the bugs are crawling on her). In contrast to the patient with Schizophrenia, the individual can maintain excellent functioning in areas that don't touch on the delusional belief system, although marked impairment may result from reactions to the delusions. Ms. W shows considerable impairment that is directly related to her delusional beliefs, having given up work and become withdrawn socially because she believes that people are avoiding her for being "dirty." On subjects other than her delusions, however, Ms. W does not show any disturbance in her thinking. Although social withdrawal is frequently present in Schizophrenia, it tends to occur as a result of the characteristic negative symptoms. The social withdrawal that may occur in Delusional Disorder is more likely to be a consequence of the delusional belief. For example, as mentioned above, Ms. W's social withdrawal is a result of her belief that others think she is "dirty." Those with the delusion that people are plotting to kill them may avoid eating in a restaurant for fear of being poisoned. To make an accurate diagnosis, therefore, the clinician needs to determine not only what types of behaviors are present but what is causing those behaviors.

Many experts believe that Schizophrenia and Delusional Disorder are on a continuum, have a shared pathogenesis, and should perhaps be considered as part of one disorder. Some evidence, however, shows that Delusional Disorder is characterized by different family loading (i.e., it breeds true), course, prognosis, and treatment response.

The most complicated differential may be with Mood Disorders. Many individuals with Delusional Disorder have associated mood symptoms, as Mr. C did when he came for treatment after his arrest. Even if delusions are present, the appropriate diagnosis would be Mood Disorder With Psychotic Features if the delusions occur only during mood episodes. However, prominent mood symptoms may also be present as a secondary aspect of Delusional Disorder (e.g., Mr. C's demoralization about his business going bad) and either could be considered an associated feature requiring no separate diagnosis or diagnosed as Depressive Disorder Not Otherwise Specified.

Delusional Disorder may co-occur with Paranoid Personality Disorder but is distinguished from it by the presence of persistent delusions. If an individual with Paranoid, Schizoid, or Schizotypal Personality Disorder later develops either Delusional Disorder or Schizophrenia, this is noted on Axis II by listing the Personality Disorder followed by "(premorbid)."

Subtypes of Delusional Disorder

A number of different subtypes may be assigned to the diagnosis of Delusional Disorder based on what is the most prominent delusional theme. These subtypes also differ in which disorders are most important to consider in the differential: For the Somatic Type, the most common differential is with a Somatoform Disorder, such as Body Dysmorphic Disorder or Hypochondriasis; for the persecutory and jealous subtypes, the most important differential is with the Paranoid Type of Schizophrenia; for the erotomanic subtype, the main differential is with genuine unrequited love and with Schizophrenia and Mood Disorder With Psychotic Features; and for the grandiose subtype, the main differential is with Mood Disorders With Psychotic Features and Personality Disorders.

Ms. W's symptoms clearly warrant a diagnosis of Delusional Disorder, Somatic Type. She is convinced that she is suffering from a physical disorder, an infestation of insects, and she holds this belief with delusional intensity, insisting that she does not need to see a psychiatrist but should be treated for a real physical problem.

Ms. T does not display any prominent mood symptoms and is convinced, despite much evidence to the contrary, that her love for her professor is returned; therefore, her symptoms warrant a diagnosis of Delusional Disorder, Erotomanic Type. Individuals with Delusional Disorder, Erotomanic Type, such as Ms. T, often also develop persecutory feelings. They may come to believe that the alleged lover is following or stalking them or tapping their phone. When erotomanic symptoms predominate, however, even if persecutory symptoms are also present, the erotomanic subtype takes precedence.

Mr. C does not have any of the other characteristic symptoms of Schizophrenia and therefore receives a diagnosis of Delusional Disorder, Persecutory Type. It may sometimes be difficult, however, to decide whether disorganized speech, disorganized behavior, or negative symptoms are present to a degree that would warrant switching the diagnosis from Delusional Disorder to Schizophrenia. We adhere to a high threshold in making these determinations. For example, a subtle "loosening of associations" does not count for a diagnosis of Schizophrenia because less than completely logical speech is fairly ubiquitous, especially when people are under stress. "Disorganized behavior" must really be disorganized, not merely social awkwardness or difficulty making eye contact. Finally, the loss of motivation that comes with a sense that one must avoid danger or escape persecution does not count as a negative symptom.

Treatment Planning for Delusional Disorder

Because Delusional Disorder is relatively rare and does not lend itself to controlled trials, it has not been studied in any systematic fashion. Although case reports suggest that Delusional Disorder does respond to antipsychotics, the choice among these medications remains unclear, and patients often do not comply with treatment. When prominent mood symptoms accompany the delusions, it may be necessary to use an antidepressant medication.

There is also controversy in the literature concerning the appropriate psychotherapeutic approach to a patient with delusions. Many authors counsel against confronting the unreality of the delusions on the grounds that this may impair the therapeutic relationship, increase anxiety, and promote further decompensation. On the other hand, not confronting the delusion is often taken by the patient as tacit confirmation that his or her fears are indeed real, and this may be even more terrifying. Gentle probing sometimes results in dramatically improved reality testing. For example, the clinician asked Ms. T what could prove to her that she might have gone overboard in her imagination and that her "lover" was not really in love with her. Ms. T replied that she would reevaluate her notion "if he looks me in the eye and tells me flat out that he doesn't love me." A meeting was arranged for later that day in which the professor said, with considerable sensitivity but flat out and looking her straight in the eye, that he did not love her, that such thoughts had never occurred to him, and that her romantic attentions made him uncomfortable. The patient was able to accept this and temporarily to give up her symptoms. Several months later, however, Ms. T began to feel that her male therapist had fallen in love with her.

Brief Psychotic Disorder

❖ Case Study: A Recent Graduate Is Overwhelmed

Mr. Y is a 26-year-old recent business school graduate who just landed his first job with a prestigious firm and is making a salary three times higher than his father had ever earned. Mr. Y was surprised at his success because he had attended a small, relatively uncompetitive college and business school. This new job required that he move from the small town where he grew up to a much larger city. For the past 3 weeks, Mr. Y has been taking a summer management training course sponsored by the firm for their 30 new recruits before they start work in the fall. Almost as soon as he began the course, Mr. Y began to feel completely out of step. It seemed to him that everyone else was able to grasp everything immediately, whereas he felt lost. He began to develop anxiety symptoms and had trouble sleeping. About a week after beginning the course, Mr. Y became convinced that the other students in the class were talking about him pejoratively and conspiring to have him fail. When he lost some important class notes, he was sure that some of the other students had stolen them to ensure his failure. He has been hearing strange clicks on his phone and is convinced that the firm has tapped his phone to find a reason to let him go. Three weeks after beginning the course, he comes for evaluation because he has been unable to sleep or function adequately in the course and is terrified of failing. Within 1 week of beginning treatment with an antipsychotic, Mr. Y's psychotic symptoms are completely gone. He is able to finish the course, although he describes feeling "slowed down" by the medication. Although Mr. Y did experience sleeplessness and agitation during this episode, no other symptoms of mania were present. However, it is of note that his maternal aunt has had a classical course of Bipolar Disorder with many hospitalizations.

DSM-IV-TR Diagnosis

Axis I: 298.8   Brief Psychotic Disorder
Axis II: V71.09   No diagnosis
Axis III: None
Axis IV: New and very stressful employment situation, move from
            small home town to larger city
Axis V: GAF = 45 (at presentation for treatment); 90 (highest level in
            past year)

DSM-IV-TR diagnostic criteria for
298.8 Brief Psychotic Disorder

A. Presence of one (or more) of the following symptoms:
    (1) delusions
    (2) hallucinations
    (3) disorganized speech (e.g., frequent derailment or incoherence)
    (4) grossly disorganized or catatonic behavior

Note: Do not include a symptom if it is a culturally sanctioned response pattern.

B. Duration of an episode of the disturbance is at least 1 day but less than
    1 month, with eventual full return to premorbid level of functioning.
C. The disturbance is not better accounted for by a Mood Disorder With Psy-
    chotic Features, Schizoaffective Disorder, or Schizophrenia and is not due
    to the direct physiological effects of a substance (e.g., a drug of abuse, a
    medication) or a general medical condition.

Specify if:
With Marked Stressor(s) (brief reactive psychosis):   if symptoms occur shortly
    after and apparently in response to events that, singly or together, would be
    markedly stressful to almost anyone in similar circumstances in the per-
    son's culture
Without Marked Stressor(s):   if psychotic symptoms do *not* occur shortly af-
    ter, or are not apparently in response to events that, singly or together,
    would be markedly stressful to almost anyone in similar circumstances in
    the person's culture
With Postpartum Onset: if onset within 4 weeks postpartum

Guidelines for Differential Diagnosis of Brief Psychotic Disorder

The DSM-IV (and DSM-IV-TR) category of Brief Psychotic Disorder replaces what was called "Brief Reactive Psychosis" in DSM-III-R. The concept was broadened to include all psychotic presentations that last less than 1 month, whether the result of a stressor or not, that are not better accounted for by another mental disorder (e.g., a Mood Disorder With Psychotic Features) or by the effects of a general medical condition or substance. When, as is often the case, a brief psychotic episode is precipitated by a marked stressor, such as beginning a new school or job or joining the military, this can be indicated by using the subtype "With Marked Stressor." At times, the stressor can be an experience that would generally be considered a positive occurrence (e.g., landing a really good job, achieving an impressive promotion, having a new baby). Brief Psychotic Disorder is generally characterized by good premorbid functioning and a good prognosis.

The duration of symptoms required to diagnose Brief Psychotic Disorder is at least 1 day but less than 1 month. This is a change from the DSM-III-R definition in which symptoms that were present for only a few hours were included. If the clinician wants to diagnose the very brief symptoms that sometimes occur in association with a Schizotypal, Paranoid, or Borderline Personality Disorder, the category Psychotic Disorder Not Otherwise Specified may be used.

A diagnosis of Brief Psychotic Disorder may not be given provisionally (i.e., before the psychotic symptoms have remitted) but is assigned after the individual has recovered in less than 1 month. For example, when Mr. Y first presented for treatment, it would have been impossible to determine whether his subsequent course would conform to this disorder, Schizophreniform Disorder, Delusional Disorder, or a Mood Disorder, and therefore the appropriate diagnosis would have been Psychotic Disorder Not Otherwise Specified.

Treatment Planning for Brief Psychotic Disorder

Brief psychotic episodes are generally treated with a combination of antipsychotic medication and psychotherapy aimed at helping the individual cope with, or escape from, the stressor (if one is present). The most difficult question often concerns how long medication treatment should be maintained once the psychotic symptoms are in remission. The answer depends on the duration of the symptoms and their severity, whether suicidal or homicidal impulses were associated with them, whether the patient and family are likely to be able to respond to early signs of relapse, and whether there are concerns about the presence of a Mood Disorder.

The most difficult question in treating Mr. Y is whether the appropriate diagnosis is indeed Brief Psychotic Disorder or whether this is a first and somewhat atypical presentation of what will go on to become Bipolar Disorder. This differential diagnosis would have profound treatment implications because a diagnosis of Bipolar Disorder would suggest that there will almost certainly be subsequent recurrent episodes that will require long-term maintenance with mood-stabilizing medication. Mr. Y and his family were informed of the possibility that he might be vulnerable to repeat episodes of Bipolar Disorder and encouraged to take the stress-reducing and life-stabilizing steps outlined in the discussion of the treatment of Bipolar I Disorder on p. 134. Mr. Y was also placed on maintenance lithium for 1 year.

Substance-Induced Psychotic Disorder

❖ Case Study: A College Student Has a Very Bad Trip

Mr. K is a 19-year-old college sophomore who was functioning reasonably well until finals week, when he began using large amounts of crack cocaine because he felt unprepared to take the tests. He began having the delusional belief that he was being watched by the police and that his parents were having him followed by a detective. Mr. K became convinced that his roommate was an informer for the college president and developed the idea that the college president was giving nightly reports to his parents on his study habits, performance in class, and drug use. Finally, one night about a week after these delusional symptoms began, Mr. K became extremely excited and agitated and threatened to hurt his roommate if he continued to inform on him. Mr. K's roommate became seriously alarmed at Mr. K's behavior and called campus security. This action reinforced Mr. K's conviction that his roommate was a hostile spy who had been observing him and informing on him.

The patient is brought into the emergency room by the dean of students who was called by campus security. During the emergency room evaluation, the patient reports sleeplessness and auditory hallucinations that keep suggesting that he blow up the registrar's office. He is very agitated and paces continuously. After admission to the hospital, the patient is given low doses of antipsychotics and sleeping medication and recovers in 3 days. Mr. K has only a vague dreamy memory of the episode. When his parents come, they report no history of such symptoms, although they do report that the patient has used marijuana and cocaine in the past. A drug screen for cocaine performed on admission to the hospital is positive.

DSM-IV-TR Diagnosis

Axis I: 292.11   Cocaine-Induced Psychotic Disorder,
                     With Delusions
Axis II: V71.09   No diagnosis
Axis III: None
Axis IV: Worry concerning examinations
Axis V: GAF = 30 (upon admission); 85 (highest level in past year)

DSM-IV-TR diagnostic criteria for Substance-Induced Psychotic Disorder

A. Prominent hallucinations or delusions.   **Note:** Do not include hallucinations if the person has insight that they are substance induced.
B. There is evidence from the history, physical examination, or laboratory findings of either (1) or (2):
    (1) the symptoms in Criterion A developed during, or within a month of, Substance Intoxication or Withdrawal
    (2) medication use is etiologically related to the disturbance
C. The disturbance is not better accounted for by a Psychotic Disorder that is not substance induced. Evidence that the symptoms are better accounted for by a Psychotic Disorder that is not substance induced might include the following: the symptoms precede the onset of the substance use (or medication use); the symptoms persist for a substantial period of time (e.g., about a month) after the cessation of acute withdrawal or severe intoxication, or are substantially in excess of what would be expected given the type or amount of the substance used or the duration of use; or there is other evidence that suggests the existence of an independent non-substance-induced Psychotic Disorder (e.g., a history of recurrent non-substance-related episodes).
D. The disturbance does not occur exclusively during the course of a delirium.

Note: This diagnosis should be made instead of a diagnosis of Substance Intoxication or Substance Withdrawal only when the symptoms are in excess of those usually associated with the intoxication or withdrawal syndrome and when the symptoms are sufficiently severe to warrant independent clinical attention.

Code [Specific Substance]–Induced Psychotic Disorder:
(291.5 Alcohol, With Delusions; 291.3 Alcohol, With Hallucinations; 292.11 Amphetamine [or Amphetamine-Like Substance], With Delusions; 292.12 Amphetamine [or Amphetamine-Like Substance], With Hallucinations; 292.11 Cannabis, With Delusions; 292.12 Cannabis, With Hallu-

(continued)

DSM-IV-TR diagnostic criteria for
Substance-Induced Psychotic Disorder *(continued)*

---

cinations; 292.11 Cocaine, With Delusions; 292.12 Cocaine, With Hallucinations; 292.11 Hallucinogen, With Delusions; 292.12 Hallucinogen, With Hallucinations; 292.11 Inhalant, With Delusions; 292.12 Inhalant, With Hallucinations; 292.11 Opioid, With Delusions; 292.12 Opioid, With Hallucinations; 292.11 Phencyclidine [or Phencyclidine-Like Substance], With Delusions; 292.12 Phencyclidine [or Phencyclidine-Like Substance], With Hallucinations; 292.11 Sedative, Hypnotic, or Anxiolytic, With Delusions; 292.12 Sedative, Hypnotic, or Anxiolytic, With Hallucinations; 292.11 Other [or Unknown] Substance, With Delusions; 292.12 Other [or Unknown] Substance, With Hallucinations)

Specify if:

With Onset During Intoxication: if criteria are met for Intoxication with the substance and the symptoms develop during the intoxication syndrome

With Onset During Withdrawal: if criteria are met for Withdrawal from the substance and the symptoms develop during, or shortly after, a withdrawal syndrome

Guidelines for Differential Diagnosis of Substance-Induced Psychotic Disorder

The differential diagnosis of Substance-Induced Psychotic Disorder requires three items: first, confirmation that a substance has been used; second, a judgment that the psychotic symptoms go beyond those that might be expected from uncomplicated intoxication with or withdrawal from the substance; and third, evidence that the substance is the direct physiological cause of the psychotic symptoms. The DSM-IV-TR criteria for Substance-Induced Psychotic Disorder give some guidance in making the determination of whether the Substance Use should be considered causal. The psychotic symptoms are more likely to be primary and not due to Substance Use if 1) the symptoms were present before the Substance Use began, 2) the symptoms persisted for a substantial period of time (such as 4 weeks) after the end of acute withdrawal or intoxication, 3) the development of psychotic symptoms is not characteristic given the type or amount of substance used, and 4) there is a family history of a primary Psychotic Disorder. If the symptoms are no more severe than would be expected when someone is intoxicated with cocaine (transient fears that the police are coming that last only an hour or two), no separate diagnosis of psychotic symptoms would be made and a diagnosis of Cocaine Intoxication would adequately describe the symptoms. It is also important to determine whether withdrawal symptoms or an underlying general medical condition is present and should be treated.

The determination that Mr. K's delusions and hallucinations resulted from drug use seems relatively straightforward because his psychotic symptoms appeared only after he began using large amounts of crack cocaine and remitted very quickly after he discontinued using cocaine. In clinical practice, however, such determinations can be much more difficult, especially when the psychotic symptoms persist. For example, it is often difficult to determine whether psychotic symptoms are due to drug use or Schizophrenia because many individuals with Schizophrenia have an early onset of symptoms and a continuous course and often may be using substances in a remarkably persistent fashion. If possible, the clinician needs to put the individual in a drug-free situation for 1 month to 6 weeks to determine whether this helps to eliminate the psychotic symptoms. Certain findings from a physical examination, such as pupillary dilatation and tachycardia, can also help distinguish cocaine-related psychosis from other psychoses.

It is also often unclear to what degree a substance may have triggered a psychotic episode in someone who was already vulnerable to having one. This differential may be particularly difficult in cases involving LSD because recurrent flashbacks are sometimes a feature of such presentations.

If the psychotic symptoms occur only during a delirium, you diagnose only the delirium and treat the symptoms as a medical emergency.

Treatment Planning for Substance-Induced Psychotic Disorder

The first priority in treating someone who presents with substance-induced psychotic symptoms is to deal with the possible risks associated with the psychotic beliefs and to detoxify the individual. If possible, the individual should be removed from an environment in which substances are available. The clinician should also be mindful that the symptoms of Substance Withdrawal can sometimes be confounded with psychotic symptoms and be sure that withdrawal symptoms that should be treated are not missed. Short-term antipsychotic medication is often necessary. Finally, precautions should be taken to prevent patients from hurting themselves or others in response to the delusions or hallucinations.

Summary

Before diagnosing a primary Psychotic Disorder, the clinician must rule out a Mood Disorder With Psychotic Features. DSM-III introduced (and DSM-IV has retained) the narrowest definitions of Schizophrenia and Schizoaffective Disorder ever created. In DSM-IV, the diagnosis of Mood Disorders takes precedence over the diagnosis of Schizoaffective Disorder whenever the psychotic symptoms occur exclusively during mood episodes. Many individuals who in the ICD-10 system would be diagnosed as having Schizoaffective Disorder would be considered to have a Mood Disorder With Psychotic Features according to the DSM-IV classification.

Given the widespread availability of drugs, the clinician should also consider the possibility of substance-induced symptoms when evaluating any psychotic presentation. This is especially true when such symptoms occur in individuals who have no previous history of psychotic symptoms. In younger individuals, the most likely substance to cause a Psychotic Disorder is a drug of abuse; whereas, in older individuals, it is more likely to be caused by alcohol, a medication side effect, or a general medical condition. The presence of drug use, however, does not necessarily mean that the substance is causing the psychotic symptoms because individuals with an established history of a primary psychosis also frequently use drugs. Moreover, some individuals develop an uncharacteristically persistent psychotic episode after using substances that usually cause more transient psychotic symptoms. In such situations, it is difficult to determine the degree to which drug use is implicated in the etiology of the psychotic symptoms or is merely incidental or partly contributory in an individual who was already vulnerable to having a psychotic episode.

These questions about etiology can often be answered only by careful evaluation over time to determine the role in the clinical presentation of mood symptoms or Substance Use. After determining that a primary Psychotic Disorder is present, there are a number of important points to keep in mind in determining which primary psychotic diagnosis is most appropriate.

Schizophreniform Disorder is not distinguished from Schizophrenia in ICD-10. This distinction is made in DSM-IV to guide prognosis and treatment planning, but the clinician should not be too surprised if a patient who, early in the course, has a diagnosis of Schizophreniform Disorder, later meets criteria for a diagnosis of Schizophrenia.

Delusional Disorder is something of a residual category describing a persistent pattern of nonbizarre delusions that are not better accounted for by Schizophrenia, Schizophreniform Disorder, a Substance-Induced Psychotic Disorder, or a Psychotic Disorder Due to a General Medical Condition.

Brief Psychotic Disorder describes episodes lasting less than 1 month and must be distinguished from Mood Disorder With Psychotic Features.

In treating Schizophrenia, clinicians must strive to achieve a combination of medication and psychotherapy approaches to achieve the most effective control of positive symptoms while helping patients improve their social and vocational functioning. The newer antipsychotics, which not only have a better side-effect profile than the older medications but also appear to be associated with improvements in negative and cognitive symptoms, have ushered in a new era in the treatment of Schizophrenia. Current research on the treatment of Schizophrenia is increasingly focusing on functional outcomes as well as symptom control. In addition to medication, most patients will need a variety of psychosocial interventions in order to achieve the best possible outcome.

Substance abuse continues to be a serious complicating problem for patients with Schizophrenia that can seriously interfere with effective treatment. In recent years, research efforts have focused on developing integrated treatment programs for patients with dual diagnoses.

Although Schizophrenia continues to be one of the most devastating psychiatric disorders, great strides have been made in developing more effective medications and psychosocial interventions that hold great promise for improved outcomes for patients with Schizophrenia.

Chapter 5

Mood Disorders

T he Mood Disorders section at first glance may seem long, cumbersome, and confusing; however, it is really very easy to use once you are familiar with it. For purposes of convenience, the section begins by providing text and criteria sets for the "building blocks" used in defining the Mood Disorders. Four types of episodes are included: major depressive, manic, mixed, and hypomanic. Although "criteria sets" are given for these episodes, they are not themselves codable disorders. The types of episodes present and the configuration in which they occur determine which specific Mood Disorder diagnosis is most appropriate.

The second part of the section provides text and criteria for the codable Mood Disorders, which are divided into the "unipolar" disorders (Major Depressive Disorder and Dysthymic Disorder), the Bipolar Disorders (Bipolar I and II Disorders and Cyclothymic Disorder), and those that have an established etiology (Mood Disorder Due to a General Medical Condition and Substance-Induced Mood Disorder). Mood Disorder Due to a General Medical Condition and Substance-Induced Mood Disorder are placed here to alert clinicians to consider these frequently encountered and important etiologies in the differential diagnosis of all mood presentations. Note that mood symptoms may also occur as associated features of many other disorders listed in other sections of the manual (e.g., Adjustment Disorder and Schizophrenia).

The third part of the section provides text and criteria for the Mood Disorder specifiers. The criteria sets for the Mood Disorders are broad enough to allow a fairly heterogeneous group of patients to receive each diagnosis. For example, the diagnosis of Major Depressive Disorder can be used to describe patients with relatively mild depression and little impairment and is also applicable to patients with the most severe and persisting mental disorders. Both cross-sectional and longitudinal specifiers have been included in DSM-IV to allow the clinician to describe more specifically individual presentations in a way that will assist with treatment planning and determining prognosis.

Depressive Disorders

Depressive Disorders

296.2x   Major Depressive Disorder, Single Episode
296.3x   Major Depressive Disorder, Recurrent
300.4   Dysthymic Disorder
311   Depressive Disorder Not Otherwise Specified

In this section, we present three cases that illustrate Major Depressive Disorder (one With Psychotic Features, one With Melancholic Features, and one With Atypical Features) and one case illustrating Dysthymic Disorder.

Major Depressive Disorder

❖   Case Study: A Woman Whose Dead Parents
     Keep Telling Her to Kill Herself

During her initial evaluation, Ms. C, a 38-year-old mother of three, has a look of dread on her face. Her hands pick restlessly at the enlarging sores on her arms. For several weeks before this consultation, she has become increasingly withdrawn, and during this interview responds only with grunts and nods. Ms. C's husband, who accompanied her for this visit, is extremely alarmed by his wife's symptoms. He reports that she says she is hearing voices that keep her from communicating with "outsiders." Her mother, who has been dead for 5 years, is insisting that she kill herself so that they can be reunited. Her father is also appearing in visual as well as auditory hallucinations, calling her a "freaking, dumb whore" and threatening to kill her if she doesn't kill herself first. In addition, a medley of unrecognizable and tormenting voices are mocking the patient, voices which she told her husband she could silence only by banging her head sharply against the wall, although she usually doesn't have the energy to do this. Ms. C also believes that she has cancer and that her children are also gravely ill. She told her husband that she feels a mission to kill everyone in her family so they can all be together after death.

This episode of depression began insidiously with a feeling of increasing despair and emptiness. At night, Ms. C could not fall asleep because of the painful, recurring thought that she was a damaged and damaging creature. She blamed herself for her mother's death and felt that she was a witch who deserved burning. After awakening early each morning, she would sit shivering on the bathroom floor so that she would not disturb her husband. She wished that she had the will and courage to kill herself and played listlessly with razor blades. Ms. C felt hopeless about herself, and she was also convinced that nuclear war would soon end all life on the planet. She was retarded in her thoughts and actions and looked like a lifeless shell of a person.

Ms. C had been hospitalized five times during the previous 9 years. One hospitalization 6 years ago was characterized by symptoms very much like her current ones. Her other hospitalizations were necessitated by severe depression and suicidal thoughts but were not accompanied by psychotic symptoms. Her previous treatments included electroconvulsive therapy (ECT) (three separate regimens), antidepressants, and a combination of a tricyclic antidepressant and antipsychotic medication. Ms. C generally improved during her hospitalizations and was able to return home within 6–8 weeks.

Ms. C does not function very well between her major episodes, and her functioning before her first episode was also poor. There are only brief periods—days or occasionally weeks—when she finds life worth living and feels that she can approach responsibilities with reasonable energy and confidence. For the most part, she is a withdrawn and despairing person who spends many hours alone, feeling empty and sad. Because she only occasionally feels up to preparing meals or shopping, her husband employs a housekeeper to run the house and care for the children. Ms. C has only one friend, whom she sees rarely. The patient loves her children but also avoids them. Close contact with them often infuriates her, and she worries that someday she may lose control and kill them.

Sometimes the patient has transient and self-limited hallucinatory experiences (her parents' voices) that last no longer than a day or two. Sometimes she is able to test their reality and sometimes not. The voices do not seem related to an exacerbation of her depression. The voices appear when Ms. C feels unusual stress—most commonly after a fight with her husband—and disappear when he has agreed to stay home more or reduce demands on her. Ms. C finds her husband most concerned and helpful when she is most disturbed. She accuses herself of making up voices to gain his attention.

DSM-IV-TR Diagnosis

Axis I: 296.34   Major Depressive Disorder, Recurrent, With Mood-
                      Congruent Psychotic Features, Without Full Inter-
                      episode Recovery, superimposed on Dysthymic
                      Disorder
            300.4   Dysthymic Disorder
Axis II: V71.09   No diagnosis
Axis III: None
Axis IV: None
Axis V: GAF = 30 (current); 50 (highest level in past year)

DSM-IV-TR criteria for Major Depressive Episode

A. Five (or more) of the following symptoms have been present during the
    same 2-week period and represent a change from previous functioning; at
    least one of the symptoms is either (1) depressed mood or (2) loss of in-
    terest or pleasure.

    Note: Do not include symptoms that are clearly due to a general medi-
    cal condition, or mood-incongruent delusions or hallucinations.

    (1) depressed mood most of the day, nearly every day, as indicated by ei-
         ther subjective report (e.g., feels sad or empty) or observation made
         by others (e.g., appears tearful).   **Note:** In children and adolescents,
         can be irritable mood.
    (2) markedly diminished interest or pleasure in all, or almost all, activi-
         ties most of the day, nearly every day (as indicated by either subjec-
         tive account or observation made by others)
    (3) significant weight loss when not dieting or weight gain (e.g., a change
         of more than 5% of body weight in a month), or decrease or increase
         in appetite nearly every day.   **Note:** In children, consider failure to
         make expected weight gains.
    (4) insomnia or hypersomnia nearly every day
    (5) psychomotor agitation or retardation nearly every day (observable by
         others, not merely subjective feelings of restlessness or being slowed
         down)
    (6) fatigue or loss of energy nearly every day
    (7) feelings of worthlessness or excessive or inappropriate guilt (which
         may be delusional) nearly every day (not merely self-reproach or
         guilt about being sick)
    (8) diminished ability to think or concentrate, or indecisiveness, nearly
         every day (either by subjective account or as observed by others)

(continued)

DSM-IV-TR criteria for
Major Depressive Episode *(continued)*

---

(9) recurrent thoughts of death (not just fear of dying), recurrent suicidal ideation without a specific plan, or a suicide attempt or a specific plan for committing suicide

B. The symptoms do not meet criteria for a Mixed Episode.

C. The symptoms cause clinically significant distress or impairment in social, occupational, or other important areas of functioning.

D. The symptoms are not due to the direct physiological effects of a substance (e.g., a drug of abuse, a medication) or a general medical condition (e.g., hypothyroidism).

E. The symptoms are not better accounted for by Bereavement, i.e., after the loss of a loved one, the symptoms persist for longer than 2 months or are characterized by marked functional impairment, morbid preoccupation with worthlessness, suicidal ideation, psychotic symptoms, or psychomotor retardation.

DSM-IV-TR diagnostic criteria for
296.3x Major Depressive Disorder, Recurrent

A. Presence of two or more Major Depressive Episodes.

Note: To be considered separate episodes, there must be an interval of at least 2 consecutive months in which criteria are not met for a Major Depressive Episode.

B. The Major Depressive Episodes are not better accounted for by Schizoaffective Disorder and are not superimposed on Schizophrenia, Schizophreniform Disorder, Delusional Disorder, or Psychotic Disorder Not Otherwise Specified.

C. There has never been a Manic Episode, a Mixed Episode, or a Hypomanic Episode. **Note:** This exclusion does not apply if all of the manic-like, mixed-like, or hypomanic-like episodes are substance or treatment induced or are due to the direct physiological effects of a general medical condition.

If the full criteria are currently met for a Major Depressive Episode, *specify* its current clinical status and/or features:

Mild, Moderate, Severe Without Psychotic Features/
    Severe With Psychotic Features
Chronic
With Catatonic Features
With Melancholic Features

(continued)

> ## DSM-IV-TR diagnostic criteria for 296.3x
> ## Major Depressive Disorder, Recurrent *(continued)*
>
> ---
>
> With Atypical Features
> With Postpartum Onset
>
> If the full criteria are not currently met for a Major Depressive Episode, *specify* the current clinical status of the Major Depressive Disorder or features of the most recent episode:
> **In Partial Remission, In Full Remission**
> **Chronic**
> **With Catatonic Features**
> **With Melancholic Features**
> **With Atypical Features**
> **With Postpartum Onset**
>
> *Specify:*
> **Longitudinal Course Specifiers (With and Without Interepisode Recovery)**
> **With Seasonal Pattern**

Guidelines for Differential Diagnosis of Major Depressive Disorder With Psychotic Features

One of the most fundamental and useful distinctions in diagnosing Mood Disorders is the division between the Depressive, or unipolar, Disorders (Major Depressive Disorder, Dysthymic Disorder, Depressive Disorder Not Otherwise Specified) and the Bipolar Disorders (Bipolar I Disorder, Bipolar II Disorder, Cyclothymic Disorder, Bipolar Disorder Not Otherwise Specified). This distinction predicts very different patterns of family loading, course, and response to treatment. Whenever a clinician is evaluating someone for a possible Major Depressive Disorder, it is also necessary to evaluate for a history of Manic, Mixed, or Hypomanic Episodes to determine whether the condition falls within the bipolar spectrum. It is also important to inquire whether the family has a history of Bipolar Disorder because this may increase the risk of the patient subsequently developing Bipolar Disorder. Approximately 10%–15% of those with Recurrent Major Depressive Disorder will later develop a Manic or Mixed Episode, thus changing the diagnosis to Bipolar I Disorder.

   Perhaps the most dramatic change introduced in DSM-III was the priority given to Mood Disorders over Schizoaffective Disorder or Schizophrenia. If psychotic symptoms are present only during the course of a mood episode, a Mood Disorder With Psychotic Features is diagnosed instead of Schizophrenia or Schizoaffective Disorder, regardless of the nature of the psychotic symptoms. This is in contrast to the prevailing practice in the United States before DSM-III and to the guidelines in ICD-10, which allow the diagnosis of Schizoaffective Disorder if the particular psychotic symptoms occurring during a mood episode are especially bizarre.

The available literature supports the view that there are no pathognomonic symptoms of Schizophrenia and that the differential diagnosis of psychotic symptoms should depend instead on the course (i.e., the presence or absence of a mood episode occurring concurrently with the psychotic symptoms). The major problem in assessment is that it is not always easy to determine the exact temporal relationship between the development of the psychotic and the mood symptoms. Moreover, it is not uncommon for individuals with Schizophrenia to become depressed. The diagnosis depends on how persistent the psychotic symptomatology outside the mood episode is. The criteria for Schizoaffective Disorder require that symptoms that meet criteria for a Major Depressive, Manic, or Mixed Episode exist concurrently with symptoms that meet the A criterion for Schizophrenia and that delusions or hallucinations are present for at least 2 weeks during the same period of illness in the absence of prominent mood symptoms. Ms. C's psychotic symptoms occur only with her mood symptoms; therefore, a diagnosis of Schizoaffective Disorder would not be appropriate.

Another problem in making this diagnosis is determining where to draw the line in deciding that an individual is delusional. Many individuals have feelings of worthlessness or guilt, ideas of reference, or somatic concerns that are on the boundary between "overvalued ideas" and delusions. For more details about the issues involved in making these distinctions, see the discussion of Delusional Disorder on p. 95.

It is of some interest that Ms. C had visual as well as auditory hallucinations. Although visual hallucinations are completely compatible with a diagnosis of Mood Disorder With Psychotic Features, they should alert the clinician to the possibility of an etiology that includes Substance Use or a general medical condition.

Mood Disorders Specifiers

DSM-IV-TR includes longitudinal course specifiers that allow the clinician to note whether subthreshold mood symptoms are present between episodes that meet full criteria for Major Depressive Disorder or Bipolar Disorder. These specifiers also allow the clinician to note whether preexisting Dysthymic Disorder was present. This information on course is helpful in determining the most appropriate treatment and making a more accurate prognosis. The four possible course patterns for Recurrent Major Depressive Disorder are as follows:

1. Full remission between episodes and no preexisting Dysthymic Disorder. This pattern has the best prognosis.

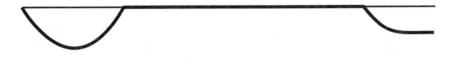

2. Only partial remission between episodes and no preexisting Dysthymic Disorder. This pattern would indicate the need for more aggressive treatment of the acute episode.

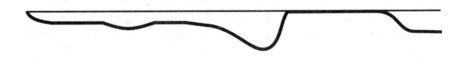

3. Full remission between episodes, but with a history of Dysthymic Disorder. This pattern is rare, occurring in only 3% of those with Major Depressive Disorder, although it may become more common as more aggressive antidepressant treatment is provided to those who are chronically depressed.

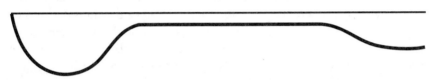

4. Only partial remission between episodes of Major Depressive Disorder, superimposed on preexisting Dysthymic Disorder. This pattern is often termed *double depression* and occurs in approximately 20%–25% of those with Major Depressive Disorder. The chronic form of Major Depressive Disorder, in which symptoms are present for at least 2 years, occurs in only about 10%–20% of those with the disorder.

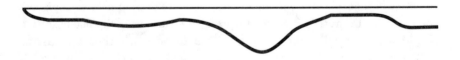

Ms. C's course followed the fourth pattern (double depression).

Treatment Planning for Major Depressive Disorder With Psychotic Features

Major Depressive Disorder accompanied by psychotic features can be a dangerous situation with an appreciable suicide risk. Hospitalization or very careful observation outside the hospital is often necessary. Clinicians should consider the seriousness of the suicidal thoughts; whether definite plans have been made; the means available to the patient; and the history of previous suicidal ideation, suicide attempts, or suicide by other family members.

In determining appropriate treatment modalities, it is important to note that antidepressants alone and antipsychotics alone are helpful only for a quarter to a third of patients with delusional depression. A combined treatment with antidepressants and antipsychotics is much more effective, with response rates of about two-thirds. ECT is the most effective treatment for psychotic depression, with response rates of more than 90%.

❖   Case Study: A Businesswoman
Who Feels She Has Failed Everyone

Ms. D, a 55-year-old business executive, has previously had several relatively brief (up to 1 month) episodes of depression. These episodes each followed a psychosocial stressor but remitted after cognitively oriented psychotherapy without any need for medication or hospitalization. The current depression also began in the context of a possible business reversal, but, unlike the previous depressions, it did not improve as business did. Instead, the depression gradually deepened and became more severe and pervasive. Within 6 weeks, the patient became unable to work. She spent her day lying in bed facing a blank wall.

Upon evaluation, the patient reports that, although she is usually able to fall asleep easily, she often awakens in the early morning hours and paces and becomes very agitated. She says that, although she does not feel very good during the day, the worst time for her is shortly before sunrise, when she sometimes feels like killing herself. Ms. D appears dehydrated and reports that she has lost between 15 and 20 pounds. (Physical and laboratory testing revealed no significant abnormalities.) Her face shows no emotion, and she states convincingly that she finds nothing pleasurable and has even lost her sense of humor, which has always been a mainstay for her. She says that even when her grandchildren arrived on a visit she was able to summon up only a temporary smile. She quickly returned to feeling blank and empty and didn't have the energy to play with the children as she always had in the past. The patient describes feeling overwhelming guilt but does not have bizarre delusional beliefs. She says that she feels like a failure at work and as a wife and grandmother and is constantly apologizing to everyone for not getting better. She feels that she is letting people down and that the business will collapse without her.

Ms. D describes her overall mood as feeling dead inside. Although she has experienced depression before, she says it was never anything like this, not even when she lost her mother to whom she was very close. She says that it is very difficult to describe her feelings and that she has an emotional ache that is "horrid beyond words."

DSM-IV-TR Diagnosis

Axis I: 296.33   Major Depressive Disorder, Recurrent, Severe
                          Without Psychotic Features, With Melancholic
                          Features, With Full Interepisode Recovery
Axis II: V71.09   No diagnosis
Axis III: None
Axis IV: Recent business problems
Axis V: GAF = 45 (current); 90 (highest level in past year)

DSM-IV-TR criteria for Melancholic Features Specifier

Specify if:

With Melancholic Features (can be applied to the current or most recent Major Depressive Episode in Major Depressive Disorder and to a Major Depressive Episode in Bipolar I or Bipolar II Disorder only if it is the most recent type of mood episode)

A. Either of the following, occurring during the most severe period of the current episode:
    (1) loss of pleasure in all, or almost all, activities
    (2) lack of reactivity to usually pleasurable stimuli (does not feel much better, even temporarily, when something good happens)

B. Three (or more) of the following:
    (1) distinct quality of depressed mood (i.e., the depressed mood is experienced as distinctly different from the kind of feeling experienced after the death of a loved one)
    (2) depression regularly worse in the morning
    (3) early morning awakening (at least 2 hours before usual time of awakening)
    (4) marked psychomotor retardation or agitation
    (5) significant anorexia or weight loss
    (6) excessive or inappropriate guilt

Guidelines for Differential Diagnosis of Major Depressive Disorder With Melancholic Features

In using the Mood Disorders specifiers, the clinician must first establish that the basic criteria for a Major Depressive Episode have been met. The clinician must then determine whether the episode is the first one or is recurrent and which specifiers apply to the symptoms that are present in the current episode. For example, although Ms. D has had Recurrent Major Depressive Episodes, only the current episode would appear to meet the criteria for the specifier "With Melancholic Features." During this most recent episode of depression, she has felt no pleasure or interest in anything, and even a visit from her grandchildren, something she normally greatly enjoyed, did not cause her mood to brighten. She described a distinct quality to her depressed mood (saying she felt sort of dead inside) and reported that she had never felt anything like this even when her mother died. Her depression was clearly worse in the morning, and she frequently experienced early morning awakening and psychomotor agitation. She had lost her appetite and lost weight and felt constant guilt about being a failure in all roles in her life. Ms. D's symptoms therefore appear to meet all the criteria for the melancholic features specifier.

This specifier may also be used to describe symptoms in a Major Depressive Episode that occurs in the course of Bipolar I or II Disorders. If Ms. D had ever had a Manic or Hypomanic Episode, her diagnosis would be considered Bipolar I Disorder, Most Recent Episode Depressed With Melancholic Features.

During any given episode of depression, the patient's symptomatology may change. The clinician should assign the diagnosis based on the most severe symptoms present during the episode. This can be a matter of clinical judgment because the criteria for the melancholic features specifier do not require that the symptoms be present for any specific length of time. If a person meets criteria for melancholia for only a day or two, however, the presentation probably wouldn't warrant this specifier. But if melancholic features developed and persisted for several weeks during the current depressive episode, even if it had started out relatively mildly, the assignment of the specifier "With Melancholic Features" would probably be appropriate.

At least nine methods for defining melancholia have been proposed over the last 20 years, none of which is clearly superior to the others. The DSM-IV (and DSM-IV-TR) description is a best approximation that attempts to capture symptom descriptions that have been included in many of the other formulations. The nature of the relationship between melancholic features and the severity of the depression remains controversial. Is melancholia just

a severe form of depression or is it categorically distinct and capable of occurring in milder forms? This has been difficult to study because most individuals
with melancholia do indeed have severe depressions. Many laboratory studies
have attempted to establish a relationship between melancholia and particular biological markers, particularly the dexamethasone suppression test and
sleep laboratory measures of rapid eye movement (REM) sleep latency. Although none of these measures have yet proved to be sufficiently sensitive or
specific to be included as diagnostic criteria, they may sometimes be helpful
in management, particularly in predicting those who are at risk for relapse and
require continued maintenance treatment.

Treatment Planning for Major Depressive Disorder With Melancholic Features

One of the main reasons for including a melancholic features specifier in
DSM-IV was that it helps in treatment planning. Individuals with melancholic features are less likely to respond to a trial of placebo medication and
consequently are more likely to require active antidepressant treatment. Individuals with melancholia usually have a severe illness in which the risk of
suicide must always be considered. Hospitalization is sometimes necessary if
there is accompanying suicidal ideation, a need for ECT, or serious medical
comorbidity.

❖   Case Study:
An Unhappy Teenager

Ms. G is a 17-year-old high school senior who is referred for evaluation after she attempted suicide with an overdose of pills. Earlier on the night of
the suicide attempt, she had a fight with her mother over a request to order
pizza. The patient remembers her mother saying that she was a "spoiled brat"
and asking whether she would be happier living elsewhere.

The patient, feeling rejected and despondent, went to her room and
wrote a note saying that she was having a mental breakdown and that she
loved her parents but could not communicate with them. She added a request that her favorite glass animals be given to a particular friend. The parents, who had gone out to a movie, returned home later that evening to find
their daughter comatose and immediately rushed her to the hospital emergency room.

During the last couple of months, Ms. G has been crying frequently
and has lost interest in her friends, school, and social activities. She has
been eating more and more and has recently begun to gain weight, which
her mother is very unhappy about. Ms. G says that her mother is always
harping about "taking care of herself," and, in fact, the argument on the

night of her suicide attempt was about Ms. G's desire to order a pizza that her mother did not think she needed. Ms. G's mother reports that all her daughter seems to want to do is sleep and that she never wants to go out with her friends or help around the house. When questioned about changes in her sleep habits, Ms. G admits that she has been feeling very tired lately and that she often feels as if there is nothing to make it worth getting out of bed. She does mention that she is excited about an upcoming visit from her boyfriend, who attends a college a considerable distance away and has not been home for several months.

Upon evaluation, it is apparent that this teenager, the third of three children of upper-middle-class and very intelligent parents, is struggling with a view of herself as less bright, clever, and attractive than her two siblings. She feels ignored and essentially rejected by her hard-working father and in hostile conflict with her well-organized and seemingly omnipresent mother. The daughter is having difficulty developing a sense of separation from her mother and an image of her individual identity. She experiences her mother's directives as interference with her efforts to express autonomy and independence.

DSM-IV-TR Diagnosis

Axis I:	296.22	Major Depressive Disorder, Single Episode, Moderate, With Atypical Features
Axis II:	V71.09	No diagnosis
Axis III:	None	
Axis IV:	Conflict with mother	
Axis V:	GAF = 35 (current); 80 (highest level in past year)	

DSM-IV-TR criteria for Atypical Features Specifier

Specify if:

With Atypical Features (can be applied when these features predominate during the most recent 2 weeks of a Major Depressive Episode in Major Depressive Disorder or in Bipolar I or Bipolar II Disorder when a current Major Depressive Episode is the most recent type of mood episode, or when these features predominate during the most recent 2 years of Dysthymic Disorder; if the Major Depressive Episode is not current, it applies if the feature predominates during any 2-week period)

A. Mood reactivity (i.e., mood brightens in response to actual or potential positive events)

(continued)

> **DSM-IV-TR criteria for Atypical Features Specifier *(continued)***
> _____
>
> B. Two (or more) of the following features:
>   (1) significant weight gain or increase in appetite
>   (2) hypersomnia
>   (3) leaden paralysis (i.e., heavy, leaden feelings in arms or legs)
>   (4) long-standing pattern of interpersonal rejection sensitivity (not lim-
>   ited to episodes of mood disturbance) that results in significant so-
>   cial or occupational impairment
> C. Criteria are not met for With Melancholic Features or With Catatonic
>   Features during the same episode.

Guidelines for Differential Diagnosis of Major Depressive Disorder With Atypical Features

Although the term *atypical* is used in DSM-IV-TR to describe this subtype of depression, this is misleading because this presentation is much more frequently seen in outpatient practice than is the melancholic type. The term atypical is a relic of the fact that most early studies of depression were conducted on inpatients who were more likely to present with melancholic features.

The symptom presentation of Major Depressive Disorder With Atypical Features is almost the opposite of the presentation of Major Depressive Disorder With Melancholic Features. Atypical depressions are characterized by the reverse vegetative symptoms of overeating and hypersomnia in contrast to melancholic depressions, which are characterized by anorexia and insomnia. Other symptoms that may be present in atypical depressions are a sensation of leaden paralysis and a long-standing pattern of interpersonal rejection sensitivity. Also in contrast to melancholia, atypical depressions are characterized by mood reactivity (i.e., pleasurable stimuli such as good news or opportunities for fun cause the individual to brighten). For example, although Ms. G is depressed, her mood definitely brightens when her parents apologize or when her boyfriend comes to visit.

Treatment Planning for Major Depressive Disorder With Atypical Features

The atypical features modifier was introduced in DSM-IV because of its possible utility in guiding treatment. Individuals "With Atypical Features" may have a poorer response to traditional tricyclic antidepressants but often do well with serotonin reuptake inhibitors and monoamine oxidase inhibitors. These individuals also often have comorbid Personality Disorder diagnoses, which may become a focus of treatment or a major factor in the management of the depression. Psychotherapy may be helpful, particularly in teaching the individual new skills for dealing with interpersonal loss.

Dysthymic Disorder

❖   Case Study: Nowhere Man

Mr. A, a 28-year-old unmarried accountant, seeks consultation because "I feel I am going nowhere with my life." Problems with his career and girlfriend have been escalating and are causing him increasing distress. Mr. A recently received a critical job review. Although he is reliable and his work accurate, his productivity is low, his management skills are poor, and he has conflicts with his boss over minor issues.

The patient's fiancée recently postponed their wedding date. She said that, although she respects and loves him, she is ambivalent because on many occasions he tends to be remote and critical and he is often uninterested in sex.

Mr. A describes himself as a pessimist who has difficulty experiencing pleasure or happiness. He says that, as far back as he can remember, he has always been aware of an undercurrent of hopelessness, feeling that his life is hard and not worth living. Mr. A grew up in a suburban community and attended public schools. His mother is a quiet person, periodically "moody," remote, and depressed. Shortly after the birth of Mr. A's sister, 3 years his junior, his mother became very depressed and was hospitalized. She responded well to ECT and had no further psychiatric care. Mr. A's father, now deceased, was successful in business but was also overbearing, critical, and intimidating and drank to excess. Mr. A says that he respected him but never felt they were close.

The patient did well academically in high school and college. He participated in some social activities but was shy and was considered gloomy and not fun to be with by most of his classmates.

In college, Mr. A benefited from counseling after breaking up with his first girlfriend. During this time an internist gave him amitriptyline for migraine headaches, which provided good relief from both the headaches and the feelings of hopelessness. In retrospect, he feels that this was a very good period of his life. He began a new job and relationship, functioned well, and almost seemed to enjoy life. However, when he discontinued the medication after 3 months, he seemed to slip slowly and insidiously back into his previous state of pessimism and hopelessness.

Although he is usually depressed, he has never had depressive episodes that met criteria for a Major Depressive Disorder: He has never been suicidal or had prominent suicidal ideation and has not experienced significant problems with weight loss, insomnia, or psychomotor activity. For months at a time, however, Mr. A's energy levels are diminished and his ability to concentrate impaired. He views himself negatively, feeling he has little to offer. He is always surprised when others like and respect him. When he is depressed, his sex drive is reduced and he has difficulty maintaining an erection, which frightens him.

Mr. A has periods when he withdraws from friends and social activities, but with effort he always goes to work. Some weekends, he stays in bed in a state of profound inertia. In the past, he would sometimes drink excessively but now has only an occasional glass of wine. He does not recall ever having periods of excessive energy or elation. Mr. A says that he recognizes his strong need to please others, to obtain approval, and to avoid conflicts. He feels extremely anxious when forced to deal directly with a hostile situation. He takes pride in his acknowledged perfectionistic traits.

Mr. A appears early for his appointment, is conservatively dressed, and initially appears outgoing and affable. As the interview progresses, however, he becomes tearful as he discusses his problems and acknowledges his depressed mood. There is no evidence of a thought disorder or of hallucinations or delusions. His insight is impaired by his tendency to deny and repress emotionally laden material. His judgment is intact, as are his orientation and recent memory. His intelligence appears to be high-average.

DSM-IV-TR Diagnosis

Axis I: 300.4   Dysthymic Disorder, Early Onset
Axis II: Obsessive-compulsive personality traits
Axis III: None
Axis IV: Problems with work, troubles with his fiancée
Axis V: GAF = 60 (current)

DSM-IV-TR diagnostic criteria for 300.4 Dysthymic Disorder

A.   Depressed mood for most of the day, for more days than not, as indicated either by subjective account or observation by others, for at least 2 years.   **Note:** In children and adolescents, mood can be irritable and duration must be at least 1 year.

(continued)

DSM-IV-TR diagnostic criteria for
300.4 Dysthymic Disorder *(continued)*

B. Presence, while depressed, of two (or more) of the following:
    (1) poor appetite or overeating
    (2) insomnia or hypersomnia
    (3) low energy or fatigue
    (4) low self-esteem
    (5) poor concentration or difficulty making decisions
    (6) feelings of hopelessness
C. During the 2-year period (1 year for children or adolescents) of the disturbance, the person has never been without the symptoms in Criteria A and B for more than 2 months at a time.
D. No Major Depressive Episode has been present during the first 2 years of the disturbance (1 year for children and adolescents); i.e., the disturbance is not better accounted for by chronic Major Depressive Disorder, or Major Depressive Disorder, In Partial Remission.

    Note: There may have been a previous Major Depressive Episode provided there was a full remission (no significant signs or symptoms for 2 months) before development of the Dysthymic Disorder. In addition, after the initial 2 years (1 year in children or adolescents) of Dysthymic Disorder, there may be superimposed episodes of Major Depressive Disorder, in which case both diagnoses may be given when the criteria are met for a Major Depressive Episode.

E. There has never been a Manic Episode, a Mixed Episode, or a Hypomanic Episode, and criteria have never been met for Cyclothymic Disorder.
F. The disturbance does not occur exclusively during the course of a chronic Psychotic Disorder, such as Schizophrenia or Delusional Disorder.
G. The symptoms are not due to the direct physiological effects of a substance (e.g., a drug of abuse, a medication) or a general medical condition (e.g., hypothyroidism).
H. The symptoms cause clinically significant distress or impairment in social, occupational, or other important areas of functioning.

Specify if:
Early Onset: if onset is before age 21 years
Late Onset: if onset is age 21 years or older

Specify (for most recent 2 years of Dysthymic Disorder):
With Atypical Features

Guidelines for Differential
Diagnosis of Dysthymic Disorder

Dysthymic Disorder is characterized by less severe but chronic depressive symptoms that may continue for years. To diagnose Dysthymic Disorder, the dysthymic symptoms must have been present for at least 2 years and no Major Depressive Episode can have occurred during the first 2 years of the dysthymic symptoms. In contrast, Major Depressive Disorder may be either episodic or chronic. It is sometimes difficult to distinguish between Dysthymic Disorder and the forms of Major Depressive Disorder that present with long-term symptoms (i.e., Chronic Major Depressive Disorder and Major Depressive Disorder in Partial Remission).

To further complicate the issue, individuals very frequently begin by having Dysthymic Disorder and then later develop a Major Depressive Episode and meet criteria for Major Depressive Disorder. If a Major Depressive Episode develops after 2 years of Dysthymic Disorder, both diagnoses are noted (i.e., double depression or Major Depressive Disorder with preexisting Dysthymic Disorder). The DSM-IV convention that describes double depression as two separate disorders is somewhat misleading because it might be better conceptualized as no more than variations in symptom severity occurring during the course of a single chronic Depressive Disorder.

There is also a lack of agreement about which features best define Dysthymic Disorder. The criteria given in DSM-III-R and continued in DSM-IV (and DSM-IV-TR) place more emphasis on somatic symptoms (i.e., appetite, sleep, and energy level). Recent studies, including the DSM-IV Mood Disorders Field Trial, have suggested that Dysthymic Disorder may be better described by criteria that place greater emphasis on the cognitive and interpersonal symptoms of depression. For this reason, an alternative criterion B was included in the DSM-IV appendix for diagnoses and criteria sets requiring further study in order to encourage more investigation of this question (see below).

Alternative DSM-IV-TR Research
Criterion B for Dysthymic Disorder

B. Presence, while depressed, of three (or more) of the following:
    (1) low self-esteem or self-confidence, or feelings of inadequacy
    (2) feelings of pessimism, despair, or hopelessness
    (3) generalized loss of interest or pleasure

(continued)

Alternative DSM-IV-TR Research Criterion B for Dysthymic Disorder (continued)

(4)   social withdrawal
(5)   chronic fatigue or tiredness
(6)   feelings of guilt, brooding about the past
(7)   subjective feelings of irritability or excessive anger
(8)   decreased activity, effectiveness, or productivity
(9)   difficulty in thinking, reflected by poor concentration, poor memory, or indecisiveness

Mr. A's symptoms appear to meet the DSM-IV-TR criteria for Dysthymic Disorder and also to fit the description in the alternative B criterion. His depressive mood is long-standing, going back to his early childhood (he can't remember when he didn't have a feeling of hopelessness). His energy level is low, he often has difficulty concentrating, and he feels worthless and unlikable. Mr. A also displays some additional symptoms from the list in the alternative B criterion such as social withdrawal, irritability, and decreased productivity. Mr. A did not appear to meet full criteria for a Major Depressive Episode at the time of the evaluation.

The clinician must also rule out any chronic medical condition or Substance-Related Disorder that might account for the symptoms, especially drug or Alcohol Abuse or thyroid problems. Such etiologies would be more likely when the depressive symptoms have an onset later in life.

The fact that many dysthymic symptoms can be traced back to childhood and follow a persistent life-long course raises the question of whether early-onset depressive symptoms should be considered "depressive personality disorder." This proposed diagnosis could be related to Axis I Major Depressive Disorder the way Schizotypal Personality Disorder is related to Schizophrenia. Depressive personality disorder is included as an example of Personality Disorder Not Otherwise Specified, and research criteria for this personality disorder are included in an appendix to DSM-IV (and DSM-IV-TR) to encourage further study of this question.

Treatment Planning for Dysthymic Disorder

Evidence suggests that approximately half of patients with Dysthymic Disorder have a good response to medication. This far exceeds the 10% placebo response rate for Dysthymic Disorder, which is much lower than for most Mood Disorders. The low placebo response rate probably is a reflection that individuals who are chronically depressed are pretty much immune to feeling hopeful. Although it has not been systematically studied, clinical experience suggests that a number of different forms of psychotherapy may also be helpful and that combinations of psychotherapy and medication are often necessary. Frequently, patients relapse when taken off treatment; therefore, fairly prolonged maintenance medication and psychotherapy are often required.

Bipolar Disorders

Bipolar Disorders

296.xx	Bipolar I Disorder
.0x	Single Manic Episode
.40	Most Recent Episode Hypomanic
.4x	Most Recent Episode Manic
.6x	Most Recent Episode Mixed
.5x	Most Recent Episode Depressed
.7	Most Recent Episode Unspecified
296.89	Bipolar II Disorder
301.13	Cyclothymic Disorder
296.80	Bipolar Disorder Not Otherwise Specified

In this section, we present cases that illustrate Bipolar I Disorder, Bipolar II Disorder, and Cyclothymic Disorder.

Bipolar I Disorder

❖   Case Study: A Young Woman on
an Emotional Roller Coaster

Ms. A, a 30-year-old unmarried schoolteacher, is dragged to the hospital by her parents, each pulling one of her arms. When the clinician enters the consultation room, the patient is restlessly pacing and loudly singing "The Battle Hymn of the Republic." When introduced to the doctor, Ms. A notices his green tie and assumes that his name is Dr. Green. She consoles him for having brown, rather than green, eyes but assures him that he can change their color if he only wishes hard enough. Her attention immediately switches to something else, and Ms. A covers eight different topics in the first 2 minutes.

Although Ms. A is at first friendly and flirtatious, offering to show the doctor a bruise on her upper thigh, when the clinician suggests hospitalization, she becomes furious and threatens to hit him. She screams that her parents have bribed him to railroad her into the hospital so they can collect her disability insurance. She shouts that she has friends in the Mafia whom she will instruct to wipe out both the doctor and her parents.

This episode began suddenly 10 days earlier, shortly after Ms. A broke up with her most recent boyfriend. Since that time, she has been sleeping only a few hours a night, has lost 8 pounds, has ordered several thousand dollars worth of special textbooks for her students, and has made dozens of long-distance calls. At the time of the initial evaluation, Ms. A is actually booked on a flight to the West Coast that is scheduled to take off in a few hours.

The patient has been hearing voices, both male and female, which suggest that she kill herself and persist in calling her a "dumb whore." She believes the voices are inspired by her parents but says she does not know how they transmit them. She has also come to believe that her thoughts can influence the course of future events and that her dreams are appearing in a disguised form in the daily newspaper.

Two observers disagreed on how best to characterize Ms. A's disordered thinking. One described her racing thoughts as flight of ideas; the other found them more disconnected and called them pattern derailment. Both agreed that Ms. A was occasionally incoherent.

Ms. A has had three previous episodes during the past 2 years, each of which began in a similar manner and then progressed to a depression that lasted 4–8 weeks. Between episodes, the patient was not delusional, hallucinating, or thought disordered. She drinks a bit too much alcohol and uses pot several times a week, but these activities do not seem to be related to the onset of this episode.

The patient is an only child who has always been her parent's pampered darling. Since early childhood, she has been difficult to please, subject to frequent temper tantrums, pervasively bitter, and extremely covetous of possessions (but bored when they are acquired). She has never married in spite of her great desire to do so and her considerable beauty and charm.

In her relationships with men, there is initially an intense mutual attraction that soon deteriorates into an equally great mutual hatred. She generally blames each new man for disappointing her and turning out to be "a selfish S.O.B. just like all the rest." She also blames her parents for being "middle class" and not exposing her to "country club" opportunities. Her relationships with men end in stormy displays of emotion, and several times she has made exhibitionist suicide attempts with pills. On occasion, she becomes promiscuous and was once severely beaten by a man she picked up in a bar.

Ms. A often feels hollow and unreal, unconnected to the strange reflection that appears in the mirror, as if she is watching herself go through the motions of life like a two-dimensional cardboard figure. These feelings are intermittent and can be interrupted by stimulus seeking (e.g., sex, drugs, or loud music). Although she tends to be pessimistic, unhappy, tearful, and suicidal, these feelings lift immediately when she meets a new man. She does not have vegetative symptoms of depression, except during her acute episodes. With all her difficulties, Ms. A has nonetheless been a relatively steady worker, supports herself, and is able to live alone.

DSM-IV-TR Diagnosis

Axis I:	296.44	Bipolar I Disorder, Most Recent Episode Manic, With Mood-Congruent Psychotic Features
Axis II:	V71.09	No diagnosis
Axis III:	None	
Axis IV:	Breakup with boyfriend	
Axis V:	GAF = 35 (current); 70 (highest level in past year)	

DSM-IV-TR criteria for Manic Episode

A. A distinct period of abnormally and persistently elevated, expansive, or irritable mood, lasting at least 1 week (or any duration if hospitalization is necessary).

B. During the period of mood disturbance, three (or more) of the following symptoms have persisted (four if the mood is only irritable) and have been present to a significant degree:
  (1) inflated self-esteem or grandiosity
  (2) decreased need for sleep (e.g., feels rested after only 3 hours of sleep)
  (3) more talkative than usual or pressure to keep talking
  (4) flight of ideas or subjective experience that thoughts are racing
  (5) distractibility (i.e., attention too easily drawn to unimportant or irrelevant external stimuli)
  (6) increase in goal-directed activity (either socially, at work or school, or sexually) or psychomotor agitation
  (7) excessive involvement in pleasurable activities that have a high potential for painful consequences (e.g., engaging in unrestrained buying sprees, sexual indiscretions, or foolish business investments)

C. The symptoms do not meet criteria for a Mixed Episode.

(continued)

DSM-IV-TR criteria for Manic Episode *(continued)*

D. The mood disturbance is sufficiently severe to cause marked impairment in occupational functioning or in usual social activities or relationships with others, or to necessitate hospitalization to prevent harm to self or others, or there are psychotic features.
E. The symptoms are not due to the direct physiological effects of a substance (e.g., a drug of abuse, a medication, or other treatment) or a general medical condition (e.g., hyperthyroidism).

Note: Manic-like episodes that are clearly caused by somatic antidepressant treatment (e.g., medication, electroconvulsive therapy, light therapy) should not count toward a diagnosis of Bipolar I Disorder.

DSM-IV-TR diagnostic criteria for Bipolar I Disorder

A. Currently (or most recently) in a Hypomanic (296.40), Manic (296.4x), Mixed (296.6x), or Major Depressive Episode (296.5x). If the criteria are met for one of these episodes except for duration, the episode is considered unspecified (296.7).

Note: An *x* in the diagnostic code indicates that a fifth digit indicating severity is required.

B. There has previously been at least one Manic or Major Depressive Episode.
C. The mood episodes in A and B are not better accounted for by Schizoaffective Disorder and are not superimposed on Schizophrenia, Schizophreniform Disorder, Delusional Disorder, or Psychotic Disorder Not Otherwise Specified.

If the full criteria are currently met for a Manic, Mixed, or Major Depressive Episode, *specify* its current clinical status and/or features:
**Mild, Moderate, Severe Without Psychotic Features/
    Severe With Psychotic Features**
Chronic
With Catatonic Features
With Melancholic Features
With Atypical Features
With Postpartum Onset

If the full criteria are not currently met for a Manic, Mixed, or Major Depressive Episode, *specify* the current clinical status of the Bipolar I Disorder and/or features of the most recent Manic, Mixed, or Major Depressive Episode:

(continued)

DSM-IV-TR diagnostic criteria for Bipolar I Disorder *(continued)*

In Partial Remission/In Full Remission
Chronic
With Catatonic Features
With Melancholic Features
With Atypical Features
With Postpartum Onset

Specify:
Longitudinal Course Specifiers (With and Without Interepisode Recovery)
With Seasonal Pattern (applies only to the pattern of Major Depressive Episodes)
With Rapid Cycling

Note: This a summary of five criteria sets.

Guidelines for Differential Diagnosis of Bipolar I Disorder

The distinction between unipolar Depressive Disorder and Bipolar Disorder is especially important because it has a considerable effect on choice of treatment (e.g., whether to use a mood stabilizer such as lithium or divalproex on a maintenance basis and to restrict antidepressants to reduce the risk of inducing a Manic Episode and rapid cycling) and on prognosis (e.g., recurrences are almost certain to occur in Bipolar I Disorder). Consider also that some individuals who are chronically depressed may misinterpret a period of normal euthymia as abnormal elevation of mood. The clinician should therefore use caution in diagnosing a Manic Episode in such individuals, unless the symptoms are sufficient in severity, duration, and impairment.

Although a diagnosis of Bipolar I Disorder requires the presence of only one Manic or Mixed Episode, in practice, this tends to be the most recurrent of disorders, with 90%–95% of those who have had one Manic or Mixed Episode going on to have repeated mood episodes. In contrast, the course of Major Depressive Disorder is far more variable, with a 50% chance of having another episode after one Major Depressive Episode, a 70% chance after two episodes, and a 90% chance after three episodes. Once an individual is diagnosed with Bipolar I Disorder because of the presence of one documented Manic or Mixed Episode, the diagnosis always remains Bipolar Disorder.

Two important issues related to Substance Use may affect the diagnosis of Bipolar I Disorder. First, manic-type symptoms that are indistinguishable from primary manic symptoms may occur in association with Substance Use.

If an individual has a positive urine drug screen and the symptoms developed in close temporal relationship with the drug use, or the symptoms quickly remit when the person is drug-free, this could suggest that the symptoms are substance-induced and not part of a primary Manic Episode. However, also remember that during a Manic Episode many individuals have a tendency toward hedonic activity that leads them to use stimulant drugs: The mania may be causing the drug use rather than vice versa. A past history or family history of Bipolar Disorder would suggest that a primary Manic Episode is the more likely diagnosis.

Another issue regarding the relationship between substances and Mood Disorders is whether treatment-induced Manic Episodes occurring in someone who otherwise has only depressive episodes should count toward a diagnosis of Bipolar Disorder. Certain antidepressant medications, light therapy, and ECT can sometimes induce mania. The question that faced the developers of DSM-IV was whether they should retain the DSM-III-R convention that such episodes count toward a diagnosis of Bipolar I Disorder and therefore the occurrence of a single treatment-induced Manic Episode would result in a change from a diagnosis of Major Depressive Disorder to a lifetime diagnosis of Bipolar I Disorder. Because it is not well established whether individuals who have treatment-induced Manic Episodes proceed to a more bipolar or a more unipolar course, the DSM-IV Task Force decided to exclude such treatment-induced Manic Episodes from the definition of Bipolar I Disorder. They instead advised clinicians to use two diagnoses, Major Depressive Disorder and Substance-Induced Mood Disorder With Manic Features, to describe this situation.

Manic symptoms can also develop as a result of a general medical condition—a possibility the clinician should consider, especially when the manic symptoms have their onset later in life. Bipolar Disorder usually has an early onset, sometime before the mid-20s. Any late onset of manic symptoms warrants a complete workup for a general medical condition or substance or medication use.

Ms. A's diagnosis is fairly straightforward. A drug or alcohol etiology does not seem likely because Ms. A has had previous mood episodes and because there does not appear to be any evidence of sufficient drug or Alcohol Use to account for the severity of her symptoms.

Psychotic Disorders (e.g., Schizoaffective Disorder, Schizophrenia, and Delusional Disorder) can share a number of symptoms with Bipolar Disorder (e.g., grandiose or persecutory delusions, agitation, and irritability). However, when the psychotic symptoms occur only during the course of the mood episodes, a diagnosis of Bipolar Disorder takes priority. When the psychotic symptoms persist even after the mood symptoms have remitted, a diagnosis of Schizoaffective Disorder should be considered.

The clinician should be cautious in diagnosing a Personality Disorder when a comorbid Mood Disorder is present. Many of the behaviors that seem to suggest the presence of a Personality Disorder (e.g., irritability, obnoxiousness, instability, or anger) may actually be a function of the mood symptoms. State features may be misinterpreted as trait features that are characteristic of a person's previous functioning. The diagnosis of a Personality Disorder requires observation over time after the mood symptoms have been successfully treated.

DSM-IV introduced the specifier "With Rapid Cycling" to describe a particularly difficult-to-treat type of Bipolar Disorder in which at least four mood episodes occur in a 12-month period. Although Ms. A's presentation would not qualify as rapid cycling because she has had only four mood episodes in the past 2 years, the clinician should be watchful for and should alert the family to the possibility that her episodes could occur more frequently and should take steps to prevent this. Risk factors that tend to predispose to this rapid cycling pattern include being female, a high level of previous exposure to antidepressants, hypothyroidism, and a positive family history. This pattern has important prognostic and treatment implications. Bipolar Disorder With Rapid Cycling is associated with increased morbidity and suicide risk, management problems, and a poor lithium response that often requires clinicians to try additional or alternative mood-stabilizing medications or high-dose thyroid replacement.

Treatment Planning for Bipolar I Disorder

In treating Bipolar I Disorder, prevention of future mood episodes is a crucial part of management. Bipolar I Disorder is almost always recurrent; therefore, the patient and family should be given adequate psychoeducation on the ways in which medication and changes in life-style may be helpful in avoiding recurrences. The clinician should emphasize the importance of continuing long-term maintenance of mood-stabilizing medication, reducing stress, maintaining a stable pattern of sleep, and avoiding Substance Use and overstimulation. The family and patient should also be cautioned to be alert to early warning signs of a relapse, especially a reduction in sleep. There is an elevated risk of suicide with Bipolar I Disorder, especially early in the course. For this reason, clinicians in recent years have tended to treat Bipolar Disorder more aggressively and persistently by using long-term maintenance treatment with mood stabilizers (e.g., lithium, divalproex) after one episode to avert suicide risk and recurrences. The clinician should, of course, carefully monitor the patient's thyroid function, because it may be compromised in patients who take lithium, which may predispose to rapid cycling. As mentioned earlier, because a rapid cycling pattern is often associated with a poor response to lithium, this pattern should alert the clinician to consider treatment alternatives such as mood-stabilizing drugs other than lithium and high-dose thyroid replacement.

Bipolar II Disorder

❖ Case Study: A Man Who Is Convinced He Is Dying

Mr. Z is a 45-year-old married business administrator who is admitted to a psychiatric unit at a teaching hospital for evaluation. He has had two psychiatric hospitalizations elsewhere for depression and suicidal ideation during the preceding 2 years. At the time of this admission, as in his earlier admissions, he denies having any psychiatric illness but claims that he is dying from a mysterious disease of aging that no one has been able to diagnose. His admission complaints include, "I'm dying," "I'm mentally retarded," "I'm going blind," "My bowels are shut down," "My skin is coming off in clumps," and "I'm losing my hair." During the 2 weeks before this admission, Mr. Z has spent most of his time lying in bed ("because of his illness") and has refused to go to work or participate in his family's life in any way. His wife reports that his mood has been persistently gloomy and pessimistic and that he has frequently become irritable with her when she suggested possible courses of action that might be helpful to him.

According to his wife, throughout their marriage Mr. Z has always fluctuated between periods of dejection and depression in which he seems to have a hard time doing anything and sudden bursts of excessive energy that usually last from a few days to several weeks. During his energetic periods, he stays late at work, often keeping several secretaries busy with his productivity. He also plunges into volunteer activities—most recently, writing speeches for local politicians—and designs and begins elaborate exercise programs. During some of these episodes, Mr. Z has suddenly announced that he has planned an exotic and elaborate family vacation for which they are to leave almost immediately. Although his wife and daughter almost always agree to accompany him on these jaunts, he vacations at such a vigorous pace—mountain climbing in Europe or scuba diving in the Caribbean—that his family struggles unsuccessfully to keep up with him. It was after returning from one of these whirlwind vacations that Mr. Z impulsively bought an expensive piece of land because it was similar to an Austrian farm he had admired. Mr. Z's wife estimates that he has five or six Hypomanic Episodes a year, each lasting between 3 days and 2 weeks. She also reports that this pattern of behavior was already established when she first met Mr. Z in college. He did fairly well in school but would fluctuate between irritable "glum" periods, when he would sleep in and miss classes, and marathon 2- or 3-day study binges.

Mr. Z's wife says that his brief bursts of energy tend to vanish as suddenly as they come and that Mr. Z then lets his projects lapse, often becoming gloomy and pessimistic about them. Beginning when he was 32 years old, Mr. Z has been treated on four occasions for a full Major Depressive Episode, each of which lasted approximately 4–5 months. He was hospitalized for two of these episodes in the past 2 years, on one occasion following a serious car accident that was judged to be a suicide attempt, although he denied this.

His wife reports that his severe depressions have always occurred in the fall and winter, whereas his really energetic periods have been especially common in spring and summer. She says that she has come to dread the winter, which she associates with the possibility of her husband having yet another depressive episode.

When questioned about his energetic periods, Mr. Z says that, although he realizes that he sometimes goes too far and loses control, he much prefers these times because he feels so intensely alive, has so much fun, and accomplishes so much. He says that he can remember having such brief bursts of productivity since he was in his early teens or even earlier and that he has always been a flighty person whose moods fluctuate quickly.

DSM-IV-TR Diagnosis

Axis I:	296.89	Bipolar II Disorder, Depressed, Severe, With Seasonal Pattern, With Rapid Cycling, With Interepisode Recovery
Axis II:	Narcissistic personality traits	
Axis III:	None	
Axis IV:	Marital- and job-related stress	
Axis V:	GAF = 40 (upon admission); 70 (highest level in past year)	

DSM-IV-TR criteria for Hypomanic Episode

A.   A distinct period of persistently elevated, expansive, or irritable mood, lasting throughout at least 4 days, that is clearly different from the usual nondepressed mood.

B.   During the period of mood disturbance, three (or more) of the following symptoms have persisted (four if the mood is only irritable) and have been present to a significant degree:

   (1)   inflated self-esteem or grandiosity

   (2)   decreased need for sleep (e.g., feels rested after only 3 hours of sleep)

   (3)   more talkative than usual or pressure to keep talking

   (4)   flight of ideas or subjective experience that thoughts are racing

(continued)

DSM-IV-TR criteria for Hypomanic Episode *(continued)*

    (5) distractibility (i.e., attention too easily drawn to unimportant or irrelevant external stimuli)

    (6) increase in goal-directed activity (either socially, at work or school, or sexually) or psychomotor agitation

    (7) excessive involvement in pleasurable activities that have a high potential for painful consequences (e.g., the person engages in unrestrained buying sprees, sexual indiscretions, or foolish business investments)

C. The episode is associated with an unequivocal change in functioning that is uncharacteristic of the person when not symptomatic.

D. The disturbance in mood and the change in functioning are observable by others.

E. The episode is not severe enough to cause marked impairment in social or occupational functioning, or to necessitate hospitalization, and there are no psychotic features.

F. The symptoms are not due to the direct physiological effects of a substance (e.g., a drug of abuse, a medication, or other treatment) or a general medical condition (e.g., hyperthyroidism).

Note: Hypomanic-like episodes that are clearly caused by somatic antidepressant treatment (e.g., medication, electroconvulsive therapy, light therapy) should not count toward a diagnosis of Bipolar II Disorder.

DSM-IV-TR diagnostic criteria for 296.89 Bipolar II Disorder

A. Presence (or history) of one or more Major Depressive Episodes.

B. Presence (or history) of at least one Hypomanic Episode.

C. There has never been a Manic Episode or a Mixed Episode.

D. The mood symptoms in Criteria A and B are not better accounted for by Schizoaffective Disorder and are not superimposed on Schizophrenia, Schizophreniform Disorder, Delusional Disorder, or Psychotic Disorder Not Otherwise Specified.

E. The symptoms cause clinically significant distress or impairment in social, occupational, or other important areas of functioning.

Specify current or most recent episode:

Hypomanic: if currently (or most recently) in a Hypomanic Episode

Depressed: if currently (or most recently) in a Major Depressive Episode

(continued)

DSM-IV-TR diagnostic criteria for
296.89 Bipolar II Disorder *(continued)*

If the full criteria are currently met for a Major Depressive Episode,
   specify its current clinical status and/or features:
Mild, Moderate, Severe Without Psychotic Features/
   Severe With Psychotic Features
Chronic
With Catatonic Features
With Melancholic Features
With Atypical Features
With Postpartum Onset

If the full criteria are not currently met for a Hypomanic or Major Depressive
   Episode, *specify* the clinical status of the Bipolar II Disorder and/or fea-
   tures of the most recent Major Depressive Episode (only if it is the most
   recent type of mood episode):
In Partial Remission/In Full Remission
Chronic
With Catatonic Features
With Melancholic Features
With Atypical Features
With Postpartum Onset

Specify:
Longitudinal Course Specifiers (With and Without Interepisode Recovery)
With Seasonal Pattern (applies only to the pattern of Major Depressive Episodes)
With Rapid Cycling

Guidelines for Differential Diagnosis of Bipolar II Disorder

This disorder is at the boundary between the unipolar and the Bipolar Disorders. The combination of Major Depressive Episodes and Hypomanic Episodes is included in DSM-IV (and DSM-IV-TR) as Bipolar II Disorder
because studies indicate that this pattern has a course, family loading, and
a treatment response that are more similar to the Bipolar than the unipolar
Mood Disorders. It is important to recognize this pattern of mood episodes
in order to take steps to prevent the development of Bipolar I Disorder and a
rapid-cycling pattern, particularly because prolonged exposure to high doses
of antidepressant medication, especially in the absence of accompanying
mood stabilizers, may provoke manic symptoms in susceptible individuals.
Note that the Major Depressive Episodes in Bipolar II Disorder may occur in
a seasonal pattern, as did Mr. Z's episodes.

Because the diagnosis of a single Hypomanic Episode in an individual with Major Depressive Disorder will bring about a lifetime change of diagnosis to Bipolar II Disorder, with all the treatment and prognostic consequences associated with Bipolar Disorders, it is very important that the clinician carefully distinguish a normal euthymic state in someone with chronic depression from an actual Hypomanic Episode. The C and D criteria for a Hypomanic Episode are included to help raise the threshold for making this determination, requiring that "an unequivocal change in functioning that is uncharacteristic of the person when not symptomatic" be present and that the "disturbance in mood and the change in functioning" be "observable by others." It can be difficult to evaluate for hypomania in someone who is accustomed to being chronically depressed and who may misinterpret a normal nondepressed mood as hypomania. Any single 4-day episode of seemingly hypomanic symptoms could represent no more than a period of a normal very good mood in someone who is usually depressed. Despite the definition requiring only one Hypomanic Episode, in most cases it is probably wisest to first establish a recurrent pattern of Hypomanic Episodes before changing the diagnosis from Major Depressive Disorder to Bipolar II Disorder. At the same time, because of the marked differences in treatment and prognosis for Bipolar Disorders, whenever clinicians evaluate someone for a Major Depressive Disorder, they should be sure to ask whether the patient has any history of Hypomanic Episodes or whether there is a history of manic or hypomanic symptoms in family members.

The same considerations discussed earlier (see p. 132) concerning substances and Bipolar I Disorder also apply here. The issue of treatment- induced hypomanic symptoms is even more germane to the diagnosis of Bipolar II Disorder. When hypomanic symptoms are triggered in an individual with Major Depressive Disorder by antidepressant treatment (e.g., medications, light therapy, or ECT), the diagnosis remains Major Depressive Disorder and an additional diagnosis of Medication-Induced Mood Disorder With Manic Features would be given. To make a correct determination as to the cause of the hypomanic symptoms, the clinician should evaluate the status of the patient when off the substance or medication and should also consider whether there is a family history of Bipolar Disorder.

Some people make the error of assuming that Bipolar II Disorder is less severe than Bipolar I Disorder because Hypomanic Episodes may occur without any distress or impairment. However, this disorder can have the most devastating effects because many people with Bipolar II Disorder have extremely severe and incapacitating depressive episodes. For example, although Mr. Z enjoyed and preferred his hypomanic periods, which were times of great productivity and creativity for him, his depressive periods were severe enough to have led to suicide attempts and repeated hospitalizations.

Treatment Planning for Bipolar II Disorder

The major reason that Bipolar II Disorder was included as a formal disorder for the first time in DSM-IV is its potential significance in treatment planning. Because over a 5-year period approximately 5%–15% of those with Bipolar II Disorder will go on to develop a Manic Episode and because patients with Bipolar II Disorder may develop rapid cycling, a diagnosis of Bipolar II Disorder strongly suggests that the clinician should use caution when prescribing antidepressants and that a maintenance regimen of mood-stabilizing medications may be needed. Patients and their families should receive psychoeducation about the nature of the disorder and training in life-stabilizing techniques and recognizing early signs of relapse.

Cyclothymic Disorder

❖   Case Study: Up and Down

Mr. F, a 27-year-old single man, comes for evaluation at the insistence of his girlfriend because he has been irritable, jumpy, excessively energetic, unable to sleep, and dissatisfied with the humdrum nature of his work and life. He has had many such episodes that usually last for a few days but sometimes for as long as a few weeks and that usually alternate with slightly longer periods (weeks to months) of feeling dejected, hopeless, and worn out and wanting to die. He describes himself as an "emotional roller coaster" and says that his moods may shift as many as 20 or 30 times in a year. Mr. F reports that he has been this way for as long as he can remember. He has never been treated for this behavior in spite of two impulsive suicide attempts with alcohol and sleeping pills. However, his symptoms have never met full criteria for either a Major Depressive Episode or a Manic Episode, nor has he ever had psychotic or prominent vegetative symptoms. Mr. F denies using drugs and claims that he drinks alcohol only minimally in order to relax.

Mr. F has had a chaotic life. He was brought up by a succession of aunts and uncles, none of whom were very pleased with the task. He was an irresponsible and trouble-making child, frequently running away, being absent from school, and committing small thefts. At 16, Mr. F hitched a ride to a distant city and never returned or called home. Since that time, he has drifted around the country working irregularly as a car washer or night watchman, on a road construction crew, and at other unskilled jobs. He gets restless and then moves on to other jobs. He forms friendships quickly but then gives them up just as quickly.

DSM-IV-TR Diagnosis

Axis I: 301.13   Cyclothymic Disorder
Axis II: V71.09   No diagnosis
Axis III: None
Axis IV: Problems at work, lack of social supports
Axis V: GAF = 55

DSM-IV-TR diagnostic criteria for 301.13 Cyclothymic Disorder

A. For at least 2 years, the presence of numerous periods with hypomanic symptoms and numerous periods with depressive symptoms that do not meet criteria for a Major Depressive Episode. **Note:** In children and adolescents, the duration must be at least 1 year.

B. During the above 2-year period (1 year in children and adolescents), the person has not been without the symptoms in Criterion A for more than 2 months at a time.

C. No Major Depressive Episode, Manic Episode, or Mixed Episode has been present during the first 2 years of the disturbance.

Note: After the initial 2 years (1 year in children and adolescents) of Cyclothymic Disorder, there may be superimposed Manic or Mixed Episodes (in which case both Bipolar I Disorder and Cyclothymic Disorder may be diagnosed) or Major Depressive Episodes (in which case both Bipolar II Disorder and Cyclothymic Disorder may be diagnosed).

D. The symptoms in Criterion A are not better accounted for by Schizoaffective Disorder and are not superimposed on Schizophrenia, Schizophreniform Disorder, Delusional Disorder, or Psychotic Disorder Not Otherwise Specified.

E. The symptoms are not due to the direct physiological effects of a substance (e.g., a drug of abuse, a medication) or a general medical condition (e.g., hyperthyroidism).

F. The symptoms cause clinically significant distress or impairment in social, occupational, or other important areas of functioning.

Guidelines for Differential Diagnosis of Cyclothymic Disorder

Cyclothymic Disorder is not often encountered in clinical practice and will probably be diagnosed even less often with the introduction in DSM-IV of the new diagnosis of Bipolar II Disorder. To diagnose Cyclothymic Disorder, the periods of hypomanic or depressive symptoms must be present for at least 2 years and, during the first 2 years of cyclothymic symptoms, there must not be any Major Depressive, Manic, or Mixed Episodes. If a Manic or Mixed Episode occurs during those first 2 years, the diagnosis would be Bipolar I Disorder. If a Major Depressive Episode occurs in addition to the hypomanic symptoms, the diagnosis would be Bipolar II Disorder. After the first 2 years have elapsed, if the patient experiences a Manic or Mixed Episode, both Bipolar I Disorder and Cyclothymic Disorder may be diagnosed; if the patient has a Major Depressive Episode after the first 2 years, then Bipolar II Disorder and Cyclothymic Disorder may both be diagnosed.

One of the more interesting questions in clinical practice concerns the relationship between this disorder and Borderline Personality Disorder because both tend to have labile mood shifts, early onset, long duration, and a pervasive impact on a person's functioning. Some researchers have suggested that many individuals who are considered to have Borderline Personality Disorder would be better diagnosed as having Cyclothymic Disorder. This is a question that needs more study.

In making this diagnosis, it is important to rule out etiologies related to Substance Abuse and Dependence because these are often also characterized by marked mood lability. Mr. F's problems are long standing and do not appear to be related to a Substance Use problem.

Treatment Planning for Cyclothymic Disorder

Because this disorder is rarely encountered and is somewhat difficult to study, little systematic information has been gathered to guide treatment decisions. Mood-stabilizing drugs and/or antidepressants are often prescribed. Psychoeducational approaches may also be helpful, focusing on encouraging the patient to lead a more stable life, eliminate excessive external stimulation, maintain a regular sleep pattern, and avoid Substance Use. One of the ways to deal with the tendency toward internal mood swings is to keep the external world as stable and predictable as life and the individual's personality allow and to avoid Substance Use.

Mood Disorder Due to a
General Medical Condition

❖   Case Study: I'm Tired[1]

Mrs. J, a 65-year-old widow of 2 years, visits her medical doctor because of increasing fatigue, lethargy, and depression that have developed over the past 6 months. These symptoms began gradually, but over the past month have worsened to the point that she is having trouble getting out of bed in the morning, quit her volunteer job at the local hospital, and stopped a number of her usual social activities at church. She does not seem to have any motivation, and it has become a chore to perform even the most basic activities of daily living, such as cooking and housekeeping. Mrs. J reports that she has been sleeping too much (sometimes 10–12 hours per day) and has gained weight (15 pounds over the past month) because of inactivity. She also complains of diffuse aches and pains, difficulty staying warm, and a range of other physical discomforts. Other family members have recently remarked about how tired and fatigued she looks. Mrs. J's daughter is very concerned because her mother has dropped out of so many activities that she formerly enjoyed and does not even show much interest in spending time with her two young grandchildren, to whom she has always been devoted. Mrs. J is very upset about feeling so tired all the time. She reports that she is frequently tearful and is beginning to feel that she is a burden on the daughter with whom she lives. Most of the household chores that she used to help with now fall on her daughter, who also cares for her two small children and husband. Mrs. J says she has started wondering whether she wouldn't be better off dead so that "I wouldn't be a burden on everyone." Mrs. J reports that her concentration has worsened over the past couple of months, that she frequently misplaces things, and that she even has difficulty following the plot of television programs.

Mrs. J has no history of depression, excessive Alcohol Use, or problems with memory before 6 months ago. She has never been hospitalized for psychiatric problems, nor is there any family history of such problems. She has seen a mental health professional only once for a short period of psychotherapy following the death of her husband. She says that she thinks of her husband often and continues to miss him because they were happily married for 48 years and had a satisfying and fulfilling relationship. Mrs. J says that she had just begun to feel some relief from that loss when this feeling of fatigue and "the blues" started. She has also experienced a number of new physical health problems since her husband's death and has been diagnosed with both diabetes and hypertension within the past year. Mrs. J is currently taking glyburide 5 mg/day for diabetes and hydrochlorothiazide 50 mg/day for hypertension. Over the past 6 months, she has also experienced worsening constipation for which she takes a stool softener (docusate sodium 100 mg) twice a day and occasionally gives herself an enema to obtain relief.

Upon physical examination, Mrs. J is afebrile with a pulse of 55, blood pressure of 120/80, and respirations of 14 per minute. Her face appears a

---

1. Thanks to Harold Koenig, M.D., of the Psychiatry Department of Duke University Medical Center for supplying this case.

bit swollen, and there is edema in both lower extremities. Neurological exam is nonfocal, and reflexes are symmetrical but slowed. Otherwise, the physical exam is normal.

During the initial interview, Mrs. J appears tired, listless, and older than her stated age. She describes her mood as depressed and discouraged. She says this is because she is so tired and can't do the things she used to be able to do. Her affect is somewhat constricted and depressed, but her eye contact is good and she relates well to the therapist. Her speech is slowed but spontaneous and friendly in tone. Her thought processes are goal directed and logical. Her thought content is characterized by ruminations about her fatigue and difficulty with usual activities, but no hallucinations or delusions are present. Mrs. J's concentration is mildly impaired on formal testing, but the impairment is not as severe as she initially indicated. Her judgment, ability to abstract, and insight are all intact. Initial laboratory testing reveals normal electrolytes, blood glucose, complete blood count, and vitamin B_{12} level. Her electrocardiogram and a head magnetic resonance imaging (MRI) scan are also normal.

The clinician initially concludes that Mrs. J is depressed over the loss of her husband and her physical health problems and places her on fluoxetine 20 mg/day. However, when she returns in 1 month, she says that she does not feel any better and that, although she is sleeping less, she is also feeling shaky and anxious. The fluoxetine is reduced to 10 mg/day, and a thyroid panel is drawn. Later that week, the thyroid studies reveal a T-4 of 3.5 and a TSH of 15.

Mrs. J is then placed on a dose of levothyroxine 0.05 mg/day, which is increased to 0.1 mg/day after 2 weeks. After 1 month of treatment, Mrs. J begins noticing her energy returning and a gradual improvement in her mood and outlook. She resumes her volunteer work at the hospital and her previous activities at church. After 3 months of treatment, Mrs. J is back to her usual self. The fluoxetine is then discontinued and, when followed up 2 years later, Mrs. J has not experienced any recurrence of symptoms.

DSM-IV-TR Diagnosis

Axis I:	293.83	Mood Disorder Due to Hypothyroidism, With Major Depressive-Like Episode
Axis II:	V71.09	No diagnosis
Axis III:	244.9	Hypothyroidism
	250.00	Diabetes mellitus, noninsulin dependent
	401.9	Hypertension
Axis IV:	Inability to perform day-to-day social and housework activities	
Axis V:	GAF = 40 (at time of initial evaluation); 80 (at follow-up)	

DSM-IV-TR diagnostic criteria for 293.83 Mood Disorder Due to . . . *[Indicate the General Medical Condition]*

A. A prominent and persistent disturbance in mood predominates in the clinical picture and is characterized by either (or both) of the following:
    (1) depressed mood or markedly diminished interest or pleasure in all, or almost all, activities
    (2) elevated, expansive, or irritable mood
B. There is evidence from the history, physical examination, or laboratory findings that the disturbance is the direct physiological consequence of a general medical condition.
C. The disturbance is not better accounted for by another mental disorder (e.g., Adjustment Disorder With Depressed Mood in response to the stress of having a general medical condition).
D. The disturbance does not occur exclusively during the course of a delirium.
E. The symptoms cause clinically significant distress or impairment in social, occupational, or other important areas of functioning.

Specify type:
With Depressive Features: if the predominant mood is depressed but the full criteria are not met for a Major Depressive Episode
With Major Depressive-Like Episode: if the full criteria are met (except Criterion D) for a Major Depressive Episode
With Manic Features: if the predominant mood is elevated, euphoric, or irritable
With Mixed Features: if the symptoms of both mania and depression are present but neither predominates

Coding note: Include the name of the general medical condition on Axis I, e.g., 293.83 Mood Disorder Due to Hypothyroidism, With Depressive Features; also code the general medical condition on Axis III.

Coding note: If depressive symptoms occur as part of a preexisting Vascular Dementia, indicate the depressive symptoms by coding the appropriate subtype, i.e., 290.43 Vascular Dementia, With Depressed Mood.

Guidelines for Differential Diagnosis of a Mood Disorder Due to a General Medical Condition

One of the most difficult tasks that clinicians face is differentiating psychiatric symptoms from medical symptoms in patients with physical illness. Mrs. J presents with a combination of symptoms that might be due to a general medical condition or to a Depressive Disorder or both. Mrs. J has a classic case of hypothyroidism, which is found in up to 6% of older women. Symptoms of this disorder typically include weakness, fatigue, cold intolerance, weight gain, constipation, hair loss, menstrual irregularities, hoarseness, and muscle aches and pains, many of which could also be due to depression. Physical findings include bradycardia, dry skin, facial puffiness, slow speech, peripheral edema, and delayed deep tendon reflexes. These symptoms and signs are a direct physiological consequence of hypothyroidism, and they are completely relieved (as in this case) by thyroid replacement. Although clinicians may find differentiating the symptoms of a general medical condition from a Depressive Disorder to be a demanding task, certain guidelines may help with this process:

1. Take a careful medical history, including a drug and medication history, being alert to any conditions or substances that are known to physiologically induce a depressive-like state. Careful physical and neurological examinations should follow, along with a complete laboratory evaluation that includes thyroid studies, serum vitamin B_{12} level, serum chemistries, a complete blood count, and, if indicated, tests for syphilis and acquired immunodeficiency syndrome (AIDS). A head MRI may be helpful in cases of head injury, when the neurological exam is positive, or of an elderly patient with a new onset of psychopathology with no history of psychiatric symptoms.

2. Be alert to the time course of depressive symptoms in relationship to the onset of the physical illness. Symptoms that represent a direct physiological consequence of the medical illness usually (but not always) appear either just before physical manifestations of the disease (as with pancreatic cancer) or concurrently with the physical health problem (hypothyroidism). Depressive symptoms that are a reaction to a medical illness often manifest themselves after exacerbation of the medical condition and resolve with improvements in functional status. If a primary Depressive Disorder is present, depressive symptoms will usually persist even after the medical illness improves. It should be noted that depressive symptoms may sometimes precede the onset of a "primary" medical illness, and the symptoms may persist after it has been treated.

3. When depressive symptoms appear in the setting of physical illness, give greater weight to the presence of the affective or cognitive symptoms of depression, which are less likely to be confused with the somatic symptoms of a general medical illness. Examples of affective or cognitive

symptoms include depressed mood, loss of interest, diminished ability to experience pleasure, insomnia, feelings of worthlessness or being a burden, tearfulness or crying, irritability, social withdrawal, feeling punished, or wanting to die. Somatic symptoms that should receive less attention because they are often caused by a general medical condition include anorexia or weight loss, weight gain, fatigue, difficulty concentrating, hypersomnia, and psychomotor slowing. These symptoms are present in 30%–50% of patients with medical illness alone.

4. Ask patients whether they are experiencing stress in their personal life, having problems with family members, undergoing role changes, or struggling with unmet personal goals. If this is the case, then the likelihood of a psychological component to the depression is increased. However, this is fairly nonspecific because stress and psychological factors are ubiquitous and do not rule out or even reduce the likelihood of a medical illness.

5. Is there a personal or family history of problems with depression, "nerves," or alcoholism? If so, these patients are at increased risk for depression during the stress of physical illness.

Remember that a Mood Disorder Due to a General Medical Condition should be diagnosed only when the mood symptoms are the direct physiological consequence of the general medical condition and are severe enough to cause clinically significant distress or impairment that warrants clinical attention. If Mrs. J were experiencing only fatigue, lethargy, and the other physical symptoms associated with hypothyroidism, without prominent mood symptoms that required separate attention, only the hypothyroidism would be diagnosed.

In addition, although approximately 10%–15% of patients with a general medical condition experience significant depressive symptoms, most depressive symptoms are not due to the direct physiological effects of an underlying general medical condition. Instead, these depressive states often represent difficulties the individual is having adjusting to changes in functional capacity caused by a general medical condition.

Treatment Planning for a Mood Disorder Due to a General Medical Condition

The first step in the treatment of a Mood Disorder Due to a General Medical Condition is to attempt to correct the underlying medical illness responsible for the problem. However, at times, such treatment is not completely successful in relieving the general medical condition or the consequent

Mood Disorder. In these instances, an appropriate psychotropic drug—anti-depressant or mood stabilizer—may be helpful. Most people in the field to-day believe that depression is probably underdiagnosed and undertreated in the medically ill.

Alcohol-Induced Mood Disorder

❖   Case Study: A Quart a Day

Ms. R is a 40-year-old married businesswoman with four children who is ad-mitted for treatment of her alcoholism at the insistence of her family. She has been drinking a quart of gin a day and having frequent severe fights with her husband. She has been awakening very early in the morning and "lies there thinking about how everyone would be better off if I were dead." She has always prided herself on being well groomed and nicely dressed ("well put together"), but lately she has felt too tired and demoralized to care what she wears or how she looks. Her family reports that she bursts into tears when confronted with the most minor problems or at a hint of criti-cism.

Ms. C's heavy drinking began 10 years ago, soon after she discovered her husband was having an affair. She says that ever since she discovered his disloyalty, her predominant feeling for her husband has been one of great contempt. Nevertheless, she feels unable to leave the marriage because she and her husband are business partners and she continues to feel dependent on him to make certain decisions and handle aspects of the business that have always been his responsibility. Although Ms. C's capabilities make her indispensable to the family business, she has become increasingly unde-pendable, often missing work, making major errors in judgment, and creat-ing scenes. Her daughter complains that her mother's behavior has become an embarrassment to the entire family.

During the past 2 years, she began drinking in the morning and has had periods of memory loss for recent events. On one occasion she was arrested for driving while intoxicated. She denies using other substances.

Upon initial evaluation, the patient is cognitively intact. She has an un-steady gait, is wearing no makeup, and is dressed in a baggy business suit. On physical exam, she is tremulous, with rapid pulse, elevated blood pres-sure, and enlarged liver. Her SGOT, SGPT, and LDH are elevated.

Ms. R expresses a wish to die but says she does not have the courage to commit suicide. Although she is embarrassed at needing help, she has tried many times unsuccessfully to stop drinking, both on her own and with her internist's help. She knows that at home she would surely drink but at the same time is furious at her husband and children for forcing her to seek help. She begins crying at several points during the interview and repeatedly describes herself as being a burden on everyone.

A year ago, Ms. R spent a month in a freestanding alcohol treatment program, where she appeared to make rapid progress through alcohol counseling and Alcoholics Anonymous (AA). Her family reports that as soon as Ms. R recovered from the acute effects of Alcohol Withdrawal, her mood improved and she began to present a much brighter outlook and to make optimistic plans for the future. She planned to stop drinking, to continue in AA, to reduce her involvement with the business, and to consider marital counseling or, if that was not successful, separating from her husband. Unfortunately, within 2 months Ms. R had fallen back into the same old pattern. She resumed a full work load, stopped attending AA meetings, began battling with her husband, and started drinking heavily again. Her depressive symptoms returned and intensified, and, during the past 10 months, she has experienced increasing hopelessness, inability to concentrate, weight gain, and early morning awakening.

Ms. R is the third of four children. She has a strong family history of alcoholism, including an alcoholic father who was violent with her mother. Throughout her childhood, she felt embarrassed and humiliated by her father, whom she both loved and despised. At age 16 she eloped with her present husband and soon became pregnant. Although he was abusive and tyrannical, she felt trapped in the marriage and proceeded to have three more children.

DSM-IV-TR Diagnosis

Axis I:	291.89	Alcohol-Induced Mood Disorder, With Depressive Features, With Onset During Intoxication
	303.90	Alcohol Dependence
	291.81	Symptoms of Alcohol Withdrawal
Axis II:	V71.09	No diagnosis
Axis III:	571.2	Cirrhosis, alcoholic
Axis IV:	Marital problems, alcohol's effect on marriage and job performance	
Axis V:	GAF = 50 (current)	

DSM-IV-TR diagnostic criteria for
Substance-Induced Mood Disorder

A. A prominent and persistent disturbance in mood predominates in the clinical picture and is characterized by either (or both) of the following:
    (1) depressed mood or markedly diminished interest or pleasure in all, or almost all, activities
    (2) elevated, expansive, or irritable mood
B. There is evidence from the history, physical examination, or laboratory findings of either (1) or (2):
    (1) the symptoms in Criterion A developed during, or within a month of, Substance Intoxication or Withdrawal
    (2) medication use is etiologically related to the disturbance
C. The disturbance is not better accounted for by a Mood Disorder that is not substance induced. Evidence that the symptoms are better accounted for by a Mood Disorder that is not substance induced might include the following: the symptoms precede the onset of the substance use (or medication use); the symptoms persist for a substantial period of time (e.g., about a month) after the cessation of acute withdrawal or severe intoxication or are substantially in excess of what would be expected given the type or amount of the substance used or the duration of use; or there is other evidence that suggests the existence of an independent non-substance-induced Mood Disorder (e.g., a history of recurrent Major Depressive Episodes).
D. The disturbance does not occur exclusively during the course of a delirium.
E. The symptoms cause clinically significant distress or impairment in social, occupational, or other important areas of functioning.

Note: This diagnosis should be made instead of a diagnosis of Substance Intoxication or Substance Withdrawal only when the mood symptoms are in excess of those usually associated with the intoxication or withdrawal syndrome and when the symptoms are sufficiently severe to warrant independent clinical attention.

Code [Specific Substance]–Induced Mood Disorder:
(291.89 Alcohol; 292.84 Amphetamine [or Amphetamine-Like Substance]; 292.84 Cocaine; 292.84 Hallucinogen; 292.84 Inhalant; 292.84 Opioid; 292.84 Phencyclidine [or Phencyclidine-Like Substance]; 292.84 Sedative, Hypnotic, or Anxiolytic; 292.84 Other [or Unknown] Substance)

(continued)

DSM-IV-TR diagnostic criteria for
Substance-Induced Mood Disorder *(continued)*

Specify type:
With Depressive Features: if the predominant mood is depressed
With Manic Features: if the predominant mood is elevated, euphoric, or irritable
With Mixed Features: if symptoms of both mania and depression are present and neither predominates

Specify if:
With Onset During Intoxication: if the criteria are met for Intoxication with the substance and the symptoms develop during the intoxication syndrome
With Onset During Withdrawal: if criteria are met for Withdrawal from the substance and the symptoms develop during, or shortly after, a withdrawal syndrome

---

Guidelines for Differential Diagnosis of Substance-Induced Mood Disorder

One of the major features of DSM-IV (and DSM-IV-TR) is the increased emphasis on all of the substance-induced forms of psychopathology. Instead of being placed in a section by themselves, these disorders are included with the disorders with which they share symptoms (e.g., Substance-Induced Mood Disorder is included with the Mood Disorders and Substance-Induced Anxiety Disorder with the Anxiety Disorders). This was done to improve differential diagnosis by alerting clinicians to consider the frequent role of substances in causing psychopathology.

Two conditions must be met to diagnose a Substance-Induced Mood Disorder. The clinician must first judge that the mood symptoms are due to the direct effects of the substance. For example, in evaluating a patient with mood symptoms that the clinician suspects may be related to a substance, the first step, as with Ms. R, is to evaluate for substance use through history, physical examination, and laboratory workup. Ms. R's family reported that she had recently been drinking a quart of gin a day and that she had a history of being treated in an alcohol detoxification program. Her laboratory results are consistent with a long-term history of Alcohol Dependence, and there is a family history of alcoholism—the patient's father. The patient does not have a history of a preexisting Mood Disorder: Her depression began after her Substance Use. When she was successfully detoxified for a period of time, the patient and her family reported that her mood improved. If Ms. R's depressive symptoms had preceded her Alcohol Use or continued unchanged for more than a month after detoxification, a primary Mood Disorder rather than a Substance-Induced Disorder would have been suspected. Although depressive symptoms similar to those described here can also be caused by a general medical condition, such as Ms. R's liver disease, it appears more likely that Ms. R's change in mood is more closely linked with her alcohol dependence. It should also be noted that the late onset of manic symptoms usually suggests that the symptoms are due to a substance or a general medical condition rather than to a primary Mood Disorder.

Once it is established that a substance is etiological to mood symptoms, the second step is to determine whether the mood symptoms go beyond what is usually seen with Alcohol Intoxication and Withdrawal (both of which are frequently associated with mood symptoms). Ms. R's symptoms appear to be severe: She is experiencing increasing hopelessness, an inability to concentrate, weight gain, early morning insomnia, and thoughts of death and suicide. An integral part of the family business, she has begun to make mistakes and become undependable because of her alcohol-related problems. Socially, she has become an embarrassment to her family and herself. Ms. R's symptoms would therefore be diagnosed as Alcohol-Induced Mood Disorder, and an additional diagnosis of Alcohol Intoxication would not be given.

The subtyping depends on the symptom presentation and allows for greater specificity. Although Ms. R is also experiencing some anxiety symptoms, her depressive symptoms are clearly most prominent; therefore, the subtype "With Depressive Features" is used.

Treatment Planning for Substance-Induced Mood Disorder

The first step in treating a patient with a Substance-Induced Mood Disorder is to determine whether hospitalization is necessary to treat the condition (e.g., the clinician must determine whether any of the following are present: prominent suicidal ideation, serious withdrawal complications, complications from a general medical condition, or an inability to detoxify in another setting). The initial treatment efforts should generally be targeted to the Substance Abuse or Dependence, although the presence of prominent mood symptoms may warrant close observation, medication treatment, and psychotherapy. Most individuals with Alcohol-Induced Mood Disorder show a dramatic reduction of depressive symptoms when they are successfully detoxified. Psychopharmacological treatment may be helpful if the Mood or Anxiety Disorder persists for more than a month, which it does in a large minority of alcoholic patients.

Summary

Two fundamental distinctions should be made in deciding how to categorize a Mood Disorder presentation: 1) whether the symptoms are primary or are the result of the direct physiological effects of a general medical condition or a substance and 2) whether the symptoms are unipolar (Major Depressive Disorder, Dysthymic Disorder) or bipolar (Bipolar I and II Disorders, Cyclothymic Disorder) in nature.

The unipolar/bipolar distinction has extremely important ramifications for treatment choice and prognosis. Bipolar Disorders are much more likely to be recurrent and are much more homogeneous in their clinical presentations, genetic loading, and treatment recommendations. In contrast, Depressive Disorders include a much more heterogeneous group of presentations, with treatment recommendations varying according to the specific type of depressive presentation.

A system of specifiers is provided to help increase the specificity of Mood Disorder diagnosis and assist in treatment planning and predicting prognosis. For example, Major Depressive Disorder With Melancholic Features is not responsive to a placebo and usually requires somatic treatment; Major Depressive Disorder With Atypical Features tends not to respond very well to the traditional tricyclic antidepressants; and antidepressants should be used with caution in treating individuals with rapid-cycling Bipolar Disorder. Bright light therapy may be particularly helpful for individuals with Seasonal Mood Disorders, and ECT may be particularly helpful for those with Mood Disorders With Catatonic Features.

Finally, since DSM-III, the DSM diagnostic system has employed an inclusive definition of Mood Disorders and a narrow definition of Schizophrenia, Schizoaffective Disorder, and the other Psychotic Disorders. If psychotic symptoms occur only during mood episodes, a Mood Disorder diagnosis takes priority, no matter how severe, prominent, or bizarre the psychotic symptoms.

Chapter 6

Anxiety Disorders

Anxiety Disorders are among the most frequently encountered psychiatric disorders. They are also among the most frequently missed or misdiagnosed disorders. This is especially unfortunate because fairly well-defined and effective treatments exist for all the Anxiety Disorders (with the possible exception of Generalized Anxiety Disorder). The disorders in this section include the following:

Anxiety Disorders

300.01	Panic Disorder Without Agoraphobia
300.21	Panic Disorder With Agoraphobia
300.22	Agoraphobia Without History of Panic Disorder
300.29	Specific Phobia
300.23	Social Phobia
300.3	Obsessive-Compulsive Disorder
309.81	Posttraumatic Stress Disorder
308.3	Acute Stress Disorder
300.02	Generalized Anxiety Disorder
293.84	Anxiety Disorder Due to . . . *[Indicate the General Medical Condition]*
—.–	Substance-Induced Anxiety Disorder *(refer to Substance-Related Disorders for substance-specific codes)*
300.00	Anxiety Disorder Not Otherwise Specified

We will discuss cases illustrating Panic Disorder both With and Without Agoraphobia, Specific and Social Phobias, Obsessive-Compulsive Disorder, Posttraumatic Stress Disorder, and Generalized Anxiety Disorder.

Panic Disorder Without Agoraphobia

❖   Case Study: A Businesswoman Fights Panic Attacks

Ms. B is a 27-year-old businesswoman with a 3-year history of panic attacks. Her first panic attack occurred suddenly when Ms. B was home watching television. This was about 3 months after her paternal grandfather died and 1 month after she announced her marriage plans. The attack began with the sensation of an electric shock going up her spine and a feeling of terror. Her heart raced, her hands tingled, and she could barely catch her breath. She felt hot, shaky, and disoriented and was convinced she was having a stroke and would soon die.

Although barely able to talk, Ms. B placed an emergency call to her family physician. By the time the doctor returned her call 10 minutes later, the sensation of terror had passed and the other symptoms had abated, but she still felt weak and fearful. A subsequent thorough medical workup indicated that she was a healthy young woman with low blood pressure (100/60) and normal resting heart rate (78 beats per minute). She had a soft heart murmur. An echocardiogram diagnosis of a slight mitral valve prolapse was made. Laboratory test results were normal, although they showed a mild reduction of plasma bicarbonate level.

During the next week the patient had five more panic episodes that occurred unexpectedly in different situations. The episodes were characterized by a rapid onset of electrical feelings in her spine, heart palpitations, dizziness, tingling in her fingers, fear of going crazy, and a sense of unreality.

Ms. B accepted a prescription for a benzodiazepine, but she refused to see the psychiatrist recommended by her family doctor. She was convinced that psychiatrists had never helped her agoraphobic mother and could not help her and that seeing a psychiatrist would prove that she was losing control. Determined not to let her symptoms interfere with her life, she forced herself to continue working.

After a few weeks, the attacks began to diminish in frequency and intensity, but Ms. B continued to experience intermittent episodes of panic several times a month for the next 2 years. These usually occurred when she was on a crowded subway or bus, was exercising on a stationary bike, was anticipating an interpersonal confrontation, or was relaxing in bed at night. On several occasions she awakened at night in the middle of a panic attack.

After a recent promotion at work, the frequency of Ms. B's panic attacks increased to several times a week. She began spending 14 hours a day at her job but felt that her anxiety was making her indecisive and reducing her efficiency. She worried constantly that her incompetence would be discovered and she would be fired. She also hated her boss and believed that he hated her, even though he had recommended her promotion. Although she is often uncomfortable in crowded stores, movies, and restaurants, Ms. B has forced herself to continue going to these places; however, she does avoid subways and driving by herself through a tunnel.

Ms. B is a meticulous worker who takes her job very seriously. She is friendly but distant to co-workers and feels contempt for others who are less careful or waste their time gossiping or doing personal errands. Although she is engaged to be married and has several close women friends, she is generally isolated and tends to avoid people because she is afraid of being criticized, rejected, or burdened by other people's problems.

Ms. B comes in for consultation because her symptoms have worsened and because her fiancé read that new treatment methods were available for panic symptoms. Nevertheless, she appears to be an unwilling participant in the evaluation process. Guarded and mistrustful, she frequently replies to questions with "Why do you need to know that?" She seems sensitive to criticism and says she is fearful that discussing her problems with a therapist will only increase her anxiety.

DSM-IV-TR Diagnosis

Axis I: 300.01   Panic Disorder Without Agoraphobia
Axis II: Avoidant and compulsive personality traits
Axis III: 424.0   Possible mitral valve prolapse
Axis IV: Job promotion, impending marriage
Axis V: GAF = 60 (current); 85 (highest level in past year)

DSM-IV-TR criteria for Panic Attack

Note: A Panic Attack is not a codable disorder. Code the specific diagnosis in which the Panic Attack occurs (e.g., 300.21 Panic Disorder With Agoraphobia).

A discrete period of intense fear or discomfort, in which four (or more) of the following symptoms developed abruptly and reached a peak within 10 minutes:

(continued)

DSM-IV-TR criteria for Panic Attack *(continued)*

(1) palpitations, pounding heart, or accelerated heart rate
(2) sweating
(3) trembling or shaking
(4) sensations of shortness of breath or smothering
(5) feeling of choking
(6) chest pain or discomfort
(7) nausea or abdominal distress
(8) feeling dizzy, unsteady, lightheaded, or faint
(9) derealization (feelings of unreality) or depersonalization (being detached from oneself)
(10) fear of losing control or going crazy
(11) fear of dying
(12) paresthesias (numbness or tingling sensations)
(13) chills or hot flushes

DSM-IV-TR diagnostic criteria for
300.01 Panic Disorder Without Agoraphobia

A. Both (1) and (2):
   (1)   recurrent unexpected Panic Attacks
   (2)   at least one of the attacks has been followed by 1 month (or more) of one (or more) of the following:
      (a) persistent concern about having additional attacks
      (b) worry about the implications of the attack or its consequences (e.g., losing control, having a heart attack, "going crazy")
      (c) a significant change in behavior related to the attacks
B. Absence of Agoraphobia.
C. The Panic Attacks are not due to the direct physiological effects of a substance (e.g., a drug of abuse, a medication) or a general medical condition (e.g., hyperthyroidism).
D. The Panic Attacks are not better accounted for by another mental disorder, such as Social Phobia (e.g., occurring on exposure to feared social situations), Specific Phobia (e.g., on exposure to a specific phobic situation), Obsessive-Compulsive Disorder (e.g., on exposure to dirt in someone with an obsession about contamination), Posttraumatic Stress Disorder (e.g., in response to stimuli associated with a severe stressor), or Separation Anxiety Disorder (e.g., in response to being away from home or close relatives).

Guidelines for Differential Diagnosis
of Panic Disorder Without Agoraphobia

The most important feature to be considered here is the nature of Ms. B's panic attacks. "Recurrent unexpected panic attacks" must be present to diagnose Panic Disorder. An unexpected panic attack occurs spontaneously and "out of the blue." Two other kinds of panic attacks occur. A situationally bound panic attack is one that always occurs when a person is exposed to a specific triggering situation (e.g., when someone with a phobia about cats sees a cat). This type of attack is more characteristic of Specific or Social Phobia, Obsessive-Compulsive Disorder, or Posttraumatic Stress Disorder. A situationally predisposed attack is one that is more likely to, but doesn't always, occur when a person is exposed to the situational trigger. This type of panic attack is most commonly part of the evolution of Panic Disorder as the individual develops a conditioned response and begins avoiding situations in which he or she is likely to have an attack. Agoraphobia may result as the number of these situations increases.

Ms. B's original attacks were classic panic attacks that developed abruptly, quickly reached a peak, and were accompanied by nearly all the typical somatic symptoms listed in the criteria for a panic attack (i.e., she felt a sensation of terror; her heart raced; her hands tingled; she felt hot, shaky, dizzy, and disoriented; and she thought she was having a stroke and would soon die). The original attacks occurred unexpectedly and were not related to a specific social or situational cue. In addition, on several occasions Ms. B awoke from sleep in the middle of a panic attack. Nocturnal panic attacks are especially characteristic of Panic Disorder. It is not clear whether (or how) mitral valve prolapse is an etiological factor contributing to the development of Panic Disorder, and its presence does not appear to affect choice of treatment or treatment response. The relationship between Panic Disorder and mitral valve prolapse is controversial, but the DSM-IV (and DSM-IV-TR) convention is to diagnose Panic Disorder when criteria are met even in the presence of mitral valve prolapse.

To diagnose Ms. B's symptoms as Panic Disorder, we must also rule out a general medical condition or Substance Use as possible causes for the symptoms. A thorough medical evaluation performed at the time of the original attacks appears to have ruled out a general medical condition, and there is no indication that Substance Use is an issue here. An important point about Panic Disorder is the tendency for individuals who are having somatic symptoms during the attack to present in general medical settings where the correct diagnosis is often missed. In the medical emergency room, the patient's complaints are likely either to be dismissed as not warranting clinical attention or, more often, to result in excessively detailed and invasive medical workups that could have been avoided had the Panic Disorder been diagnosed accurately.

After establishing that Ms. B's attacks should probably be diagnosed as Panic Disorder, it must be determined whether the diagnosis should be Panic Disorder With or Without Agoraphobia. The main feature of agoraphobia is avoidance of, or extreme distress in, a variety of situations because of fear of having a panic attack. Although the DSM-IV-TR criteria for Panic Disorder With Agoraphobia and Panic Disorder Without Agoraphobia make it seem as if two distinct "brands" of Panic Disorder occur, real life is more complicated. Many patients, like Ms. B, have symptoms that seem to lie at the boundary. She has some avoidance that she did not have before the panic attacks began, but she still manages to do most of the things she needs to do. In many cases, it is a question of how to interpret criterion B for agoraphobia, especially the phrase, "are endured with marked distress." The clinician must evaluate the level of distress and impairment to decide which diagnosis is more appropriate in a given case. Although Ms. B has some agoraphobic tendencies (e.g., her discomfort in crowded stores, movies, and restaurants and her avoidance of tunnels and subways), the impairment and distress associated with these tendencies are probably not severe enough to warrant a diagnosis of Panic Disorder With Agoraphobia at the time of this evaluation.

Treatment Planning for
Panic Disorder Without Agoraphobia

Probably the most important treatment hint is not to miss this diagnosis. Because the symptoms of panic attacks very often appear in slightly atypical ways (e.g., rage attacks, dissociative episodes, and disinhibition), this disorder may be misdiagnosed, particularly in primary care, emergency room, and consultation-liaison settings. Individuals with Panic Disorder are often concerned that their somatic symptoms are evidence of serious physical illness (especially a "heart attack") or that their depersonalization is evidence of a serious mental disorder (a "nervous breakdown").

Once the disorder is identified, psychoeducation is very helpful in reducing such fears and also sets the stage for enlisting the patient's cooperation in other specific treatments that are often necessary. Fortunately, a wide variety of treatments are available. Many of the symptoms of a Panic Disorder are probably caused or exacerbated by hyperventilation. Breathing retraining may reduce hyperventilation and help patients to understand that many of their symptoms are no more than the transient result of the ratio of oxygen to carbon dioxide in their blood supply and do not indicate some catastrophic general medical condition. Cognitive approaches focus on reducing the individual's misinterpretation of bodily sensations. Behavioral approaches encourage exposure to situations that are likely to provoke panic attacks, hyperventilation, and other somatic symptoms. Their purpose is to desensitize the patient and make it easier for him or her to take part in activities and enter situations that have provoked panic attacks in the past. Teaching the patient distraction techniques may also be helpful (i.e., learning to focus attention on other thoughts may help the individual to avert or reduce the severity of a panic attack). A number of different medications (e.g., tricyclic antidepressants, serotonin reuptake inhibitors, monoamine oxidase inhibitors, and high-potency benzodiazepines) are effective in the treatment of Panic Disorder. In many cases, combinations of cognitive-behavior therapy and medication are particularly helpful. Longer term psychodynamic treatment to explore the unconscious triggers of panic symptoms (usually separation fears) may also be useful once the target symptoms are under control.

Panic Disorder With Agoraphobia

❖ Case Study: A Young Man
Who Is Scared to Leave the House

Mr. A is a 28-year-old unemployed accountant who has become increasingly incapacitated by panic attacks, agoraphobia, and somatic preoccupations to the point that he can no longer tolerate being alone and cannot go out without a companion. The patient has had similar symptoms on and off for many years, but his symptoms worsened 3 months ago when his girlfriend suddenly left him because of his "passivity." He fears that he is losing his mind and experiencing a schizophrenic deterioration. The patient is now spending most of his time at his parents' home, where he behaves and is treated like an invalid.

The patient is the only child of parents who were already in their late 30s and expected to be childless when he was conceived. As an infant, Mr. A had considerable separation anxiety and could not be left with baby-sitters. He developed into a shy boy who was subject to many minor illnesses and was much more comfortable with adults than in the rough-and-tumble of peer relationships. Mr. A developed mild school refusal in the first and fourth grades and was never willing to try summer camp. He attended college and business schools locally so that he could continue to live at home; he then went into the family business. He was interested in dating but was usually too shy to initiate his own relationships with women and depended on his mother to serve as matchmaker.

Mr. A's symptoms have waxed and waned throughout his 20s. On occasion he has tried to establish his separateness in various ways: taking trips overseas, dating a girl of his own choosing, and even quitting his father's firm and finding a job on his own. Each effort has ended in failure and humiliation because Mr. A becomes anxious, ruminates that he is doing the wrong thing, and finally gives up and returns to the "family routine."

The patient feels especially bound to his physically ailing mother, worries that she will die soon, and is troubled by the thought that she gets lonely without him, just as he feels lonely without her. Mr. A's mother is equally bound to him. She cannot tolerate his "suffering" and is willing to sacrifice her relationship with her husband and her social life to be with him. When apart, Mr. A and his mother call each other several times a day. At the same time, Mr. A is angry at both parents and blames them for his difficulties, for not loving him enough and also for loving him too much, for not taking care of him, and for making him dependent. He is particularly contemptuous of his father, who also has some mild phobias.

Mr. A feels defective and inferior. He expects to be criticized by others and is sensitive to rejection. He is also highly critical of others and feels constantly let down. He has had close friends in the past but is now too embarrassed to call them.

Mr. A has been in psychotherapy on several occasions, each of which lasted for about a year. Typically, he becomes increasingly demanding and then becomes disappointed and disillusioned with his therapist and decides that things are going nowhere. He has a strong tendency toward addiction to minor tranquilizers and shows little ability to use them within the recommended dosage. He has used antipsychotics with poor results, and antidepressants in low dosages have not been helpful. He is bright and perceptive about his motivations and behavior but seems unable to change them.

DSM-IV-TR Diagnosis

Axis I:	300.21	Panic Disorder With Agoraphobia
	309.21	Separation Anxiety Disorder (prior history)
Axis II:	301.82	Avoidant Personality Disorder
	301.6	Dependent Personality Disorder
Axis III:	None	
Axis IV:	Losing girlfriend, unemployment	
Axis V:	GAF = 50 (current); 60 (highest level in past year)	

DSM-IV-TR criteria for Agoraphobia

Note: Agoraphobia is not a codable disorder. Code the specific disorder in which the Agoraphobia occurs (e.g., 300.21 Panic Disorder With Agoraphobia or 300.22 Agoraphobia Without History of Panic Disorder).

A. Anxiety about being in places or situations from which escape might be difficult (or embarrassing) or in which help may not be available in the event of having an unexpected or situationally predisposed Panic Attack or panic-like symptoms. Agoraphobic fears typically involve characteristic clusters of situations that include being outside the home alone; being in a crowd or standing in a line; being on a bridge; and traveling in a bus, train, or automobile.

Note: Consider the diagnosis of Specific Phobia if the avoidance is limited to one or only a few specific situations, or Social Phobia if the avoidance is limited to social situations.

B. The situations are avoided (e.g., travel is restricted) or else are endured with marked distress or with anxiety about having a Panic Attack or panic-like symptoms, or require the presence of a companion.

C. The anxiety or phobic avoidance is not better accounted for by another mental disorder, such as Social Phobia (e.g., avoidance limited to social situations because of fear of embarrassment), Specific Phobia (e.g., avoidance limited to a single situation like elevators), Obsessive-Compulsive Disorder (e.g., avoidance of dirt in someone with an obsession about contamination), Posttraumatic Stress Disorder (e.g., avoidance of stimuli associated with a severe stressor), or Separation Anxiety Disorder (e.g., avoidance of leaving home or relatives).

DSM-IV-TR diagnostic criteria for 300.21 Panic Disorder With Agoraphobia

A. Both (1) and (2):
   (1) recurrent unexpected Panic Attacks
   (2) at least one of the attacks has been followed by 1 month (or more) of one (or more) of the following:
       (a) persistent concern about having additional attacks
       (b) worry about the implications of the attack or its consequences (e.g., losing control, having a heart attack, "going crazy")
       (c) a significant change in behavior related to the attacks

(continued)

**DSM-IV-TR diagnostic criteria for
300.21 Panic Disorder With Agoraphobia** *(continued)*

B. The presence of Agoraphobia.
C. The Panic Attacks are not due to the direct physiological effects of a sub-
    stance (e.g., a drug of abuse, a medication) or a general medical condition
    (e.g., hyperthyroidism).
D. The Panic Attacks are not better accounted for by another mental disor-
    der, such as Social Phobia (e.g., occurring on exposure to feared social sit-
    uations), Specific Phobia (e.g., on exposure to a specific phobic situation),
    Obsessive-Compulsive Disorder (e.g., on exposure to dirt in someone
    with an obsession about contamination), Posttraumatic Stress Disorder
    (e.g., in response to stimuli associated with a severe stressor), or Separa-
    tion Anxiety Disorder (e.g., in response to being away from home or close
    relatives).

Guidelines for Differential Diagnosis of Panic Disorder With Agoraphobia

The discussion of panic attacks on p. 160 is relevant here. Unlike Ms. B, Mr. A's symptoms clearly included both panic attacks and agoraphobia. At the time of this evaluation, he was unable to be alone, could not go out without a companion, and was spending most of his time at his parents' house being treated like an invalid. Mr. A was not working or functioning at all well. His impairment was clearly severe enough to warrant a diagnosis of Panic Disorder With Agoraphobia.

Mr. A's history demonstrates a pattern that is often seen in individuals who develop Panic Disorder With Agoraphobia. Such patients often have evidence of childhood Separation Anxiety Disorder and avoidant and dependent personality features. These individuals are particularly likely to develop avoidant behavior after the onset of panic attacks. In other individuals, however, the avoidance and dependency develop only as a consequence of the Panic Disorder. In such cases, the avoidant and dependent features would not be considered evidence of a Personality Disorder because they don't have an early onset and a course that are independent of the Axis I condition. As always, however, life is more complicated than DSM-IV algorithms. Especially when individuals develop Panic Disorder in their late teens or early adulthood and have a chronic course, it may be impossible to distinguish which behaviors are the consequence of a Personality Disorder and which are the consequence of panic attacks.

It can also be difficult to establish the diagnostic boundary between Panic Disorder With Agoraphobia and a Specific or Social Phobia. Mr. A is unwilling to be alone and will not go out without a companion because he is afraid of having a panic attack in a situation in which he will be without help. Fear of panic attacks has caused him to change his behaviors. Although someone with Social Phobia may also avoid going out in public, this is not so much because of fear of having a panic attack but rather because of fear of being embarrassed or humiliated. A person with Social Phobia may nevertheless have a panic attack when forced to be in a social situation that triggers fear. Likewise, a person with a Specific Phobia involving automobiles may avoid going out in a car or riding in a taxi, but this is because of fear of being in that specific situation. Again, such a person may have a panic attack when forced to ride in a car, but the attack is triggered by the specific situation rather than the fear of having a panic attack. In contrast, Mr. A has panic attacks that are not as closely related to specific cues. His fear of having a panic attack causes him to avoid many situations in which he feels unsafe or likely to be embarrassed.

Another consideration in the differential diagnosis of panic attacks is that the cued panic attacks that characterize Social and Specific Phobias are more likely to occur immediately upon exposure to the phobic stimulus (e.g., when a person with fear of heights is forced to climb to the top of a tower or when a person with a phobia of snakes encounters a snake), whereas the panic attacks that categorize Panic Disorder With and Without Agoraphobia may not occur immediately upon exposure to a stressful situation but after a period of time (e.g., a panic attack occurring after a person with Panic Disorder has been riding on the subway for 20 minutes without any special anxiety).

Treatment Planning for Panic Disorder With Agoraphobia

The treatment modalities previously discussed for Panic Disorder Without Agoraphobia also apply here. The main target of treatment for most individuals with this disorder remains psychoeducation, the alleviation of panic attacks with medication, and teaching cognitive-behavioral strategies. However, in individuals with Panic Disorder With Agoraphobia, the avoidant behavior is also an important target of treatment. Various cognitive-behavioral approaches that involve exposure to feared situations may be especially helpful. This type of therapy involves encouraging the patient to deliberately seek out situations that provoke panic and anxiety symptoms in order to become desensitized through frequent repetition.

Summary

Panic Disorder can be distinguished from other disorders in which panic attacks occur by the requirement that at least some of the panic attacks be unexpected. Many of the symptoms of a panic attack are related to hyperventilation, and helping patients understand this often greatly reduces their concern about the condition. Although it is still a subject of some controversy, most experts believe that the occurrence of panic attacks usually precedes and causes the agoraphobia.

The toughest differential in evaluating panic attacks is how to diagnose those individuals whose disorder began with unexpected panic attacks but who now have panic attacks only in specific predictable situations (e.g., as in Specific or Social Phobia). Although this remains controversial, it is probably better to diagnose the symptoms based on the individual's current presentation rather than on remote history.

Phobias

Specific Phobia

❖   Case Study: A Resident Doctor With a Phobia[1]

Dr. B is a 32-year-old medical resident who is currently training in a large teaching hospital. He has a history of several years of extreme discomfort at the thought of doing a therapeutic removal of a fingernail or toenail for a patient. He first heard descriptions of this procedure while he was doing his undergraduate work in preparation for medical school. He recalls feeling nauseated, faint, and disgusted at the thought of doing this, although he had no similar squeamishness about the thought of performing other procedures. He states that he would rather "take a cockroach out of a kid's ear" than take a fingernail off.

Dr. B was an active child who frequently had minor accidents requiring visits to his family doctor. He had a series of sprains and broken bones and recalls a finger getting smashed in a door when he was about 6 years old. He remembers the finger becoming swollen and bruised and the fingernail eventually coming off as the finger healed. Although he does not remember ever being extremely upset during his visits to the doctor, he does recall

1. Thanks to Suzanne M. Sutherland, M.D., of the Psychiatry Department of Duke University Medical Center for supplying this case.

seeing his mother turn pale and look sick whenever he had to get a shot or stitches. He was always willing to try things with his buddies and describes a self-induced fainting spell when he was 13 years old. He purposely hyperventilated and then stood up quickly and did a Valsalva maneuver. He passed out for about 10 seconds and remembers being very scared as he regained consciousness. He was aware that the voices of his friends seemed abnormal and their faces were distorted and blurry, and he had a sense of unreality and a brief feeling of terror.

During medical school, Dr. B successfully avoided doing a nail removal procedure but as a fourth-year student was forced to observe the procedure. He stood as far back as possible in the examination room and watched the physician remove a toenail. He began to feel sick, became sweaty, noticed his heart beginning to race, and then started to feel faint and weak. He had to sit down to avoid fainting. He explains that "nails are supposed to be there" and that he cannot stop thinking of the "excruciating pain" that might be experienced if the patient were not totally anesthetized.

During the first 2 years of his family medicine residency, Dr. B became known for his willingness to do surgical procedures. He often volunteered to help fellow residents and seemed to enjoy tasks such as setting bones, realigning joints, and even incision and drainage of cysts and boils and stitching acute lacerations. None of his colleagues were aware that he had never removed a nail—a procedure that was commonly done in this general practice. During an evening clinic when he was the only doctor available, a young girl was brought in and needed a nail removed. Unable to perform the procedure himself, he called a fellow resident at home and persuaded her to come in and help him. She agreed on the condition that he see a therapist to deal with the problem.

DSM-IV-TR Diagnosis

Axis I: 300.29   Specific Phobia, Blood-Injection-Injury Type
Axis II: V71.09   No diagnosis
Axis III: None
Axis IV: Residency at major medical center
Axis V: GAF = 75 (current at time of presentation to psychologist);
              90 (highest level in past year)

DSM-IV-TR diagnostic criteria for 300.29 Specific Phobia

A. Marked and persistent fear that is excessive or unreasonable, cued by the presence or anticipation of a specific object or situation (e.g., flying, heights, animals, receiving an injection, seeing blood).

B. Exposure to the phobic stimulus almost invariably provokes an immediate anxiety response, which may take the form of a situationally bound or situationally predisposed Panic Attack. **Note:** In children, the anxiety may be expressed by crying, tantrums, freezing, or clinging.

C. The person recognizes that the fear is excessive or unreasonable. **Note:** In children, this feature may be absent.

D. The phobic situation(s) is avoided or else is endured with intense anxiety or distress.

E. The avoidance, anxious anticipation, or distress in the feared situation(s) interferes significantly with the person's normal routine, occupational (or academic) functioning, or social activities or relationships, or there is marked distress about having the phobia.

F. In individuals under age 18 years, the duration is at least 6 months.

G. The anxiety, Panic Attacks, or phobic avoidance associated with the specific object or situation are not better accounted for by another mental disorder, such as Obsessive-Compulsive Disorder (e.g., fear of dirt in someone with an obsession about contamination), Posttraumatic Stress Disorder (e.g., avoidance of stimuli associated with a severe stressor), Separation Anxiety Disorder (e.g., avoidance of school), Social Phobia (e.g., avoidance of social situations because of fear of embarrassment), Panic Disorder With Agoraphobia, or Agoraphobia Without History of Panic Disorder.

Specify type:
Animal Type
Natural Environment Type (e.g., heights, storms, water)
Blood-Injection-Injury Type
Situational Type (e.g., airplanes, elevators, enclosed places)
Other Type (e.g., fear of choking, vomiting, or contracting an illness; in children, fear of loud sounds or costumed characters)

Guidelines for Differential Diagnosis of Specific Phobia

Specific Phobia must be differentiated from normal and realistic fears of dangerous situations that are not excessive or unreasonable. The important distinction between everyday fears and Specific Phobia is that the latter must cause significant impairment or distress. To make this determination, the clinician needs to take into account the individual patient's situation. For example, a person who has a specific phobia of crossing bridges but lives in an area where there are no bridges to cross would not be considered to have impairment or distress because of the phobia, and a diagnosis of Specific Phobia would not be warranted. If this same individual were forced to move to an area where he or she had to cross a long bridge every day to go to work or run errands and could not function normally because of constant fear of crossing this bridge (e.g., driving an extra 10 miles to avoid crossing the bridge), then the diagnosis would be applicable. Dr. B's phobic dread of performing a nail removal would not be impairing to the average person but creates a definite professional problem for a physician who must regularly perform surgical procedures.

In contrast to the unexpected panic attacks that characterize Panic Disorder, the exposure to the phobic stimulus in Specific Phobia almost invariably provokes an immediate anxiety response. Dr. B becomes nauseated and faint at the thought of performing a nail removal, and he nearly fainted when forced to observe the procedure during medical school. The Blood-Injection-Injury type of Specific Phobia differs from the other types because it is characterized by a slowed rather than elevated heart rate, which is responsible for the fainting that commonly complicates this condition. This slowing of heart rate results from a vasovagal reflex that is excessively well developed in these individuals.

Treatment Planning for Specific Phobia

A common treatment for Specific Phobias is systematic desensitization. Dr. B is seen at the psychology clinic, and a behavioral program using a technique of graduated exposure is devised. Over the next 2 months, he asks fellow clinicians whether he can be present for all nail removals in the clinic. By the end of the 2 months, after watching several procedures and becoming gradually more actively involved, Dr. B is able to perform a nail removal successfully on his own, with only some mild anxiety.

Summary

Phobic fears usually have their onset in early childhood. One way of understanding the types of situations feared in many Specific Phobias is that they represent built-in evolutionary adaptive mechanisms that have gone haywire. Such fears (e.g., of heights; animals; dark, closed spaces; lightning) are very common and are actually adaptive in many cases. They would be considered Specific Phobias only when they cause impairment or distress.

Social Phobia

❖   Case Study: A Woman With No Life of Her Own

Ms. R is a 34-year-old unmarried woman who comes in for evaluation because she is having difficulty coping since her mother's death 3 months earlier. She has always lived at home and, since her father's death 20 years
earlier, she and her widowed mother have been especially close. Ms. R has
always been very shy and fearful of being judged harshly, ridiculed, or embarrassed in social relationships. For this reason, she has depended on her
mother to handle her affairs for her and arrange her social life. Her mother
always took care of all the household business, dealt with repairmen,
helped Ms. R choose her clothing, and planned her vacations. Ms. R doesn't
date and is usually too shy to go out to parties or on blind dates that her
mother's friends try to arrange for her. She has never had any kind of romantic relationship. Ms. R has one close friend whom she has known since
grade school and whom she describes as being very much like her. On weekends, they shop at used book stores and see movies. Except for this one
friend, Ms. R's social life until her mother's death centered around her
mother's friends, who came over regularly for card parties.

   Ms. R attended the local community college and majored in library science. After graduation she took a job at the public library that was arranged
through one of her mother's friends. She says that she is very unhappy with
her current position but can't face the ordeal of going through interviews to
obtain another job.

DSM-IV-TR Diagnosis

Axis I: 300.23   Social Phobia, Generalized Type
             V62.82   Bereavement
Axis II: 301.82   Avoidant Personality Disorder
             301.6   Dependent Personality Disorder
Axis III: 535.50   Gastritis, recurrent
Axis IV: Mother's recent death
Axis V: GAF = 60 (current); 70 (highest level in past year)

DSM-IV-TR diagnostic criteria for 300.23 Social Phobia

A. A marked and persistent fear of one or more social or performance situations in which the person is exposed to unfamiliar people or to possible scrutiny by others. The individual fears that he or she will act in a way (or show anxiety symptoms) that will be humiliating or embarrassing. **Note:** In children, there must be evidence of the capacity for age-appropriate social relationships with familiar people and the anxiety must occur in peer settings, not just in interactions with adults.

B. Exposure to the feared social situation almost invariably provokes anxiety, which may take the form of a situationally bound or situationally predisposed Panic Attack. **Note:** In children, the anxiety may be expressed by crying, tantrums, freezing, or shrinking from social situations with unfamiliar people.

C. The person recognizes that the fear is excessive or unreasonable.
    Note: In children, this feature may be absent.

D. The feared social or performance situations are avoided or else are endured with intense anxiety or distress.

E. The avoidance, anxious anticipation, or distress in the feared social or performance situation(s) interferes significantly with the person's normal routine, occupational (academic) functioning, or social activities or relationships, or there is marked distress about having the phobia.

F. In individuals under age 18 years, the duration is at least 6 months.

G. The fear or avoidance is not due to the direct physiological effects of a substance (e.g., a drug of abuse, a medication) or a general medical condition and is not better accounted for by another mental disorder (e.g., Panic Disorder With or Without Agoraphobia, Separation Anxiety Disorder, Body Dysmorphic Disorder, a Pervasive Developmental Disorder, or Schizoid Personality Disorder).

H. If a general medical condition or another mental disorder is present, the fear in Criterion A is unrelated to it, e.g., the fear is not of Stuttering, trembling in Parkinson's disease, or exhibiting abnormal eating behavior in Anorexia Nervosa or Bulimia Nervosa.

Specify if:

Generalized: if the fears include most social situations (also consider the additional diagnosis of Avoidant Personality Disorder)

Guidelines for Differential Diagnosis of Social Phobia

The social anxiety in Social Phobia must be distinguished from the normal and often adaptive anxiety that most individuals feel when called upon to perform before others or to spend time with new people. Whereas a normal level of anxiety may spur people to try to do their best and make the most favorable impression possible, Social Phobia generally causes people to experience extreme anxiety and distress in such situations and, in many cases, to avoid social situations entirely. When the anxiety has reached this stage, it usually causes the person sufficient distress or interferes enough with normal functioning to be considered pathological. Ms. R has always been a shy and retiring person who has avoided social exposure. Her problems have escalated since her mother's death because she has been forced to deal with many social situations she was able to avoid before, and she now feels extremely lonely and isolated.

Ms. R would be diagnosed with Social Phobia, Generalized, because her fears include almost all social situations. Because her social fears had an early onset and have had a life-long persistent course, she would also be considered to have Avoidant Personality Disorder. In fact, the Generalized Type of Social Phobia usually has an early onset and chronic course that make it indistinguishable from Avoidant Personality Disorder. If Ms. R had only circumscribed performance fears in particular situations (e.g., giving a speech in front of a group), then the Generalized type would not apply.

It can sometimes be difficult to distinguish Panic Disorder With Agoraphobia from Social Phobia in individuals whose social fears are associated with panic attacks. For example, if an individual has an unexpected first panic attack while giving a lecture and then begins to avoid situations in which it is necessary to speak before groups, would this be considered Social Phobia (because the person is anxious and avoids a specific social situation) or Panic Disorder (because the initial attacks were unexpected)? Only by considering the course of the disorder is it possible to determine which diagnosis would best describe the situation. If the individual continues to avoid giving lectures but does not have panic attacks or avoidance associated with other situations, then Social Phobia would probably best describe the situation. If the person begins to have panic attacks in other situations and becomes more generally avoidant, then Panic Disorder With Agoraphobia should be considered.

Treatment Planning for Social Phobia

The treatment of Social Phobia varies dramatically based on which subtype is present. The performance subtype, characterized by fears of situations such as speaking in public, eating in public, or using public rest rooms, responds well to some combination of education, reassurance, rehearsal, systematic desensitization, and treatment with beta-blockers that prevent blushing and trembling. Beta-blockers are ineffective in treating the Generalized Type of

Social Phobia, but fortunately monoamine oxidase inhibitors and selective serotonin reuptake inhibitors are helpful, as is cognitive-behavior therapy with an emphasis on exposure and cognitive restructuring.

Summary

Social Phobia is a diagnostic category that very clearly illustrates the lack of clarity in the boundary between Axis I disorders and Axis II Personality Disorders because the Generalized Type of Social Phobia is often indistinguishable from Avoidant Personality Disorder. In planning the treatment of Social Phobia, the clinician must be especially careful to consider which subtype of the disorder is present because, as indicated above, these have very different treatment implications.

Obsessive-Compulsive Disorder

❖ Case Study: A Schoolteacher's "Habits"
      Affect Her Career and Her Marriage[2]

Ms. A is a 30-year-old elementary schoolteacher with a 5-year history of repetitively checking report card grades; retracing her driving route; and having persistent thoughts about harm coming to her parents, excessive concern about her health, and difficulty grocery shopping alone.

Ms. A first developed checking behaviors during high school, when she would repeatedly check that the stove and her curling iron were turned off before going out of the house. She reports that her checking rituals grew progressively worse during college and, at that time, she began rereading pages in books over and over before exams.

During the past 5 years, Ms. A has experienced further escalation of her symptoms. She often spends 3–4 hours a day engaged in checking behaviors. She spends at least an hour going back and forth between her curling iron, the stove, and the front door. After she is finally convinced that everything is as it should be, the thought comes to her that she should check it all again because, if she doesn't, the house may burn down or a burglar may get in. She often retraces her driving path for fear that she has run over someone or something. Report card time is a nightmare for Ms. A because she repetitively checks and rechecks for hours the grades she has recorded.

---

2. Thanks to Tana A. Grady, M.D., of the Psychiatry Department of Duke University Medical Center for supplying this case.

She reports an association between obsessional thoughts about harm coming to her parents and her behaviors. For instance, she feels that she must call her mother every day both in the morning and evening, no matter how inconvenient this may be. She says that she is obsessed with the thought that if she misses a phone call to check up on her, her mother may have a stroke and die and it will be her fault for failing to call.

In the context of discussing this in the clinician's office, Ms. A can admit that this fear is unrealistic; however, she says that it is almost impossible for her not to make these daily calls without becoming excessively anxious and scared. Ms. A also has certain ritual prayers that she spends a lot of time saying each day, beginning over again whenever she makes the smallest error. She says these prayers ensure that her parents will enjoy continued good health. Again, in the office environment, she can admit that if she should not say these prayers one day, it would not be likely to affect her parents' health. However, she also says that it makes her feel miserable, frightened, and guilty if she tries to omit them from her routine. The patient also has numerous obsessional thoughts and much anxiety about her health, which are not relieved by the checking behaviors.

In addition to these obsessional thoughts and compulsive rituals, Ms. A describes intermittent "blue" feelings but denies any persistent mood disturbance or any neurovegetative signs or symptoms of a Mood Disorder. She does not have a history of any Eating Disorder problems or of motor tics or a Tic Disorder.

Over the past 5 years, Ms. A has become increasingly isolated because of her checking behaviors and obsessional thoughts. She will not go grocery shopping alone because she is terrified that she will do something to "embarrass" herself if she is out alone. Therefore, she will go to shopping malls or grocery stores only when she is with her husband or a friend. Her social isolation and need to be with her husband when she goes out have resulted in increased marital tension. In addition to her tendency to keep herself isolated, the patient is beginning to have doubts about whether she wants a child. Her ambivalence about a possible pregnancy is also contributing to the marital conflict.

Ms. A comes in for her first psychiatric evaluation in response to her husband's urging. He read about new research and clinical programs concerning Obsessive-Compulsive Disorder and encouraged her to come in for assessment and possible treatment. This is a difficult task for Ms. A because she had a negative experience when she first brought these symptoms to the attention of her gynecologist. The patient says she felt humiliated by that interview and was therefore unwilling to seek further treatment until her husband's request.

Her past medical history is unremarkable with the exception of mild mood swings before the onset of menses. She denies any history of head trauma or central nervous system infection. Her family history is notable for superstitions, hoarding behaviors, and extreme meticulousness in her mother and maternal grandmother. There is also a positive family history of motor tics in the patient's father and two paternal uncles. Ms. A has no history of Alcohol or Other Substance Abuse.

On initial evaluation, the patient's mental status exam is notable for increased motor movements, a dysthymic/anxious affect, and intermittent tearfulness. There is no abnormality of thought process or thought content.

DSM-IV-TR Diagnosis

Axis I: 300.3   Obsessive-Compulsive Disorder
             300.23   Possible Social Phobia
Axis II: V71.09   No diagnosis
Axis III: None
Axis IV: Potential breakup of marriage
Axis V: GAF = 55 (current); 75 (highest level in past year)

DSM-IV-TR diagnostic criteria for
300.3 Obsessive-Compulsive Disorder

A. Either obsessions or compulsions:

Obsessions as defined by (1), (2), (3), and (4):

(1) recurrent and persistent thoughts, impulses, or images that are experienced, at some time during the disturbance, as intrusive and inappropriate and that cause marked anxiety or distress

(2) the thoughts, impulses, or images are not simply excessive worries about real-life problems

(3) the person attempts to ignore or suppress such thoughts, impulses, or images, or to neutralize them with some other thought or action

(4) the person recognizes that the obsessional thoughts, impulses, or images are a product of his or her own mind (not imposed from without as in thought insertion)

Compulsions as defined by (1) and (2):

(1) repetitive behaviors (e.g., hand washing, ordering, checking) or mental acts (e.g., praying, counting, repeating words silently) that the person feels driven to perform in response to an obsession, or according to rules that must be applied rigidly

(continued)

DSM-IV-TR diagnostic criteria for
300.3 Obsessive-Compulsive Disorder *(continued)*

(2)   the behaviors or mental acts are aimed at preventing or reducing distress or preventing some dreaded event or situation; however, these behaviors or mental acts either are not connected in a realistic way with what they are designed to neutralize or prevent or are clearly excessive

B.   At some point during the course of the disorder, the person has recognized that the obsessions or compulsions are excessive or unreasonable.   **Note:** This does not apply to children.

C.   The obsessions or compulsions cause marked distress, are time consuming (take more than 1 hour a day), or significantly interfere with the person's normal routine, occupational (or academic) functioning, or usual social activities or relationships.

D.   If another Axis I disorder is present, the content of the obsessions or compulsions is not restricted to it (e.g., preoccupation with food in the presence of an Eating Disorder; hair pulling in the presence of Trichotillomania; concern with appearance in the presence of Body Dysmorphic Disorder; preoccupation with drugs in the presence of a Substance Use Disorder; preoccupation with having a serious illness in the presence of Hypochondriasis; preoccupation with sexual urges or fantasies in the presence of a Paraphilia; or guilty ruminations in the presence of Major Depressive Disorder).

E.   The disturbance is not due to the direct physiological effects of a substance (e.g., a drug of abuse, a medication) or a general medical condition.

Specify if:

With Poor Insight: if, for most of the time during the current episode, the person does not recognize that the obsessions and compulsions are excessive or unreasonable

Guidelines for Differential Diagnosis of Obsessive-Compulsive Disorder

Many people are a little obsessive-compulsive, and it is often a good thing for them and for the people around them. The diagnosis of Obsessive-Compulsive Disorder is reserved for those whose lives are disrupted by their symptoms. In its severe form, Obsessive-Compulsive Disorder can be among the most impairing of the mental disorders.

The DSM-IV-TR criteria describe an obsession as a recurrent, persistent, intrusive, and inappropriate thought that causes marked anxiety and distress and is not simply excessive worry about real-life problems. The person with an obsession attempts to suppress or neutralize the obsession while recognizing that it is a product of his or her own mind. Compulsions are defined as repetitive behaviors or mental acts that the individual feels driven to perform to reduce the distress caused by the obsession or to avert a catastrophe about which he or she is obsessed. However, the relationship between these compulsive behaviors and what they are designed to prevent is not realistic. More than 90% of those with Obsessive-Compulsive Disorder have both obsessions and compulsions; however, a small minority appear to have only obsessions or compulsions.

Most clinicians have been trained to think of obsessions as thoughts and compulsions as actions, but these definitions differ from those of DSM-IV (and DSM-IV-TR), which are based on a functional distinction that has greater treatment implications. Obsessions are thoughts, impulses, or images that are accompanied by anxiety, whereas compulsions are acts or thoughts that are designed to neutralize the anxiety. For example, it is an obsession when Ms. A has the intrusive thought of causing harm to other people or things. However, it is a cognitive compulsion when she engages in the regular mental repetition of a prayer that must be repeated in exactly the same way every time. Most people who have obsessions also have compulsions. This can be useful in the differential diagnosis between Obsessive-Compulsive Disorder and Generalized Anxiety Disorder or Stereotyped Movement Disorder. It is sometimes difficult to distinguish between an obsession and the excessive worries of Generalized Anxiety Disorder, but the presence of accompanying compulsions helps to clarify the diagnosis. It can sometimes be difficult to distinguish between a compulsion and a complex stereotypy, but the presence of obsessions helps in this differential.

Ms. A's obsessive-compulsive behavior has clearly reached a point where it is interfering significantly with her ability to function normally and is threatening the integrity of her marriage. She spends 3–4 hours a day performing senseless rituals and checking behaviors and is unable to go out alone because of fear that she will encounter a situation that triggers her obsessions and causes her to embarrass herself.

The criteria set for Obsessive-Compulsive Disorder allows the clinician to specify "With Poor Insight" for those situations in which the person has lost the ability to recognize that the obsessions and compulsions are excessive and unreasonable. The degree to which those with this disorder actually believe in the reality of their fears varies among individuals and in a single individual over the course of the disorder. The nature of the beliefs falls on a spectrum from those that the individual can readily admit to being senseless to overvalued ideas (which are held with much more conviction but which the person can admit might be wrong) to delusional beliefs (in which the person is completely convinced of the reality of the beliefs). It is more common for individuals to lose the sense of the unreasonableness of their beliefs later in the course of Obsessive-Compulsive Disorder. Some obsessions and compulsions, particularly those having to do with contamination, may with time and in some people become more ego-syntonic (e.g., "germs do exist and it is good to be clean"). Some individuals with Obsessive-Compulsive Disorder may even come to hold their beliefs with delusional intensity. When this happens, an additional diagnosis of Delusional Disorder is made, even though these two diagnoses are probably very closely related. Ms. A is able to admit, at least in the context of a "safe" office visit, that her beliefs are unrealistic and that the house is unlikely to burn down or her mother to die if she does not perform one of her rituals. Nevertheless, she is unable to tolerate the extreme anxiety and guilt that have followed her few attempts to resist her compulsions. In contrast, a psychotic individual might believe that moving a hand or pointing a finger will result in the death of an individual and would have no insight into the impossibility of this relationship.

Although the word *compulsive* is used broadly in colloquial speech to cover many situations (e.g., "compulsive gambler," "compulsive eater"), in DSM-IV-TR, the term compulsive is used in a specific sense and is distinguished from "impulsive behaviors" (e.g., gambling, fire setting, and sexual behaviors) that the individual performs for purposes of pleasure rather than to reduce anxiety. The distinction between "compulsive" and "impulsive" is admittedly hard to draw, however, in dealing with, for example, a pathological gambler who feels driven to gamble to reduce tension and escape feelings of anxiety.

During the process of developing DSM-IV, there was some discussion about creating a new grouping of disorders that would include those forming a spectrum with Obsessive-Compulsive Disorder (i.e., Tic Disorders, Body Dysmorphic Disorder, Hypochondriasis, and Trichotillomania). This proposal was based on studies that suggest these disorders may be related in course, treatment response, and perhaps etiology. It was, however, decided that not enough was yet known about the pathogenesis of these disorders to conclude that a similar mechanism is acting in all of them and to justify such a radical reorganization of the classification.

Treatment Planning for Obsessive-Compulsive Disorder

This is an area of exciting current research, with many clinical studies being done to compare a variety of cognitive, behavioral, and medication treatments.

The clinician may elect to use psychotherapy, medication, or a combination of the two, depending on patient preference and the severity of the disorder. Patients with mild to moderate levels of severity and impairment may be able to benefit from the cognitive-behavioral approach alone. This consists of various techniques designed to expose the individual to the anxiety that results when the ritual is not performed. Treatment of compulsions is much more effective than treatment of obsessions because it is easier to set up response-prevention situations in which patients are exposed to the anxiety that results when they don't give in to the compulsions. The serotonin-specific medications seem to be particularly effective for Obsessive-Compulsive Disorder and often produce positive results in individuals who have not previously responded to psychotherapy. Combinations of psychotherapy and medication are usually indicated for those with moderate to severe symptoms and impairment.

Summary

It is important to remember that compulsions are not always acts but may also be cognitive (e.g., ritualized patterns of thoughts that the individual feels driven to repeat over and over in order to stave off some feared catastrophe). Most people with this disorder have a pattern of obsessions and compulsions that are clearly related to one another (e.g., an individual with an obsession about germs and contamination is very likely to have a compulsion to repeatedly wash and disinfect his or her hands).

Posttraumatic Stress Disorder

❖   Case Study: The Wreck of a Pretty Strong Man

Mr. R, a burly, full-bearded, 37-year-old Irish fireman, was hospitalized for second- and third-degree burns over a third of his body. During the month he spent on the burn unit, he was the model stoic patient, but a week after discharge, during his first appointment in the surgical clinic, he is tremulous, stammering, and unresponsive to the surgeon's assurances. Deeply concerned, the surgeon pages the burn unit's consultant-liaison psychiatrist and introduces him to Mr. R, who shakes hands and mumbles, "I sort of expected you'd be calling in the shrinks."

Although Mr. R tries to appear confident, he chain-smokes, glances around furtively, squirms in his chair, and at times bursts into tears. When he is able to calm down somewhat, he explains that he cannot stop thinking about how, for the first time in his distinguished career, he entered a burning building alone, in a manner contrary to the safety procedures he was responsible for teaching, and sustained near-fatal burns. He tells the interviewer, "You see before you the wreck of what once was a pretty good man."

His hospitalization was bearable because the staff on the burn unit was very supportive, but he admits now that during that month he was troubled by frequent terrible nightmares about the fire. He did not say anything about them because he thought they would pass. Now that he is home, he admits he is constantly jumpy and nervous and drinks to calm his nerves and to sleep. He feels humiliated about his mistake at the fire and cannot stop replaying it in his mind. His recurrent nightmares, in which he reexperiences the fire over and over again, have worsened since he has been home, and he is having great difficulty going to sleep—perchance to dream. At the invitation of his co-workers, Mr. R recently visited the fire station with great reluctance. When a fire alarm sounded, he "nearly leapt out of what was left of my skin" and began to tremble and sweat. He left hurriedly, pleading illness. He is very ashamed about having to face his co-workers in his present condition—shaky, sweating, and frightened—instead of his usual brash and fearless self. He is scheduled to return to his duties on a part-time basis in 2 weeks but doesn't think he ever will be able to stand going back to the firehouse or going out to fight a fire again. He feels that he is cracking up: He paces the floor; is afraid to leave the house on his own; and frequently feels dizzy, numb, and detached. He says he doesn't feel like himself anymore and does not want to talk to anyone. He also expresses a sense of total helplessness and horror about how he looks. For the first time, he has begun to wonder whether life is worth living.

DSM-IV-TR Diagnosis

Axis I:	309.81	Posttraumatic Stress Disorder
		Rule out Alcohol Abuse or Dependence and Withdrawal
Axis II:	V71.09	No diagnosis
Axis III:	942.00	Status post 35% second- and third-degree burns
Axis IV:	Severe burns, potential loss of job	
Axis V:	GAF = 40 (current); 85 (highest level in past year)	

DSM-IV-TR diagnostic criteria for
309.81 Posttraumatic Stress Disorder

A. The person has been exposed to a traumatic event in which both of the following were present:
   (1) the person experienced, witnessed, or was confronted with an event or events that involved actual or threatened death or serious injury, or a threat to the physical integrity of self or others
   (2) the person's response involved intense fear, helplessness, or horror. **Note:** In children, this may be expressed instead by disorganized or agitated behavior
B. The traumatic event is persistently reexperienced in one (or more) of the following ways:
   (1) recurrent and intrusive distressing recollections of the event, including images, thoughts, or perceptions. **Note:** In young children, repetitive play may occur in which themes or aspects of the trauma are expressed.
   (2) recurrent distressing dreams of the event. **Note:** In children, there may be frightening dreams without recognizable content.
   (3) acting or feeling as if the traumatic event were recurring (includes a sense of reliving the experience, illusions, hallucinations, and dissociative flashback episodes, including those that occur on awakening or when intoxicated). **Note:** In young children, trauma-specific reenactment may occur.
   (4) intense psychological distress at exposure to internal or external cues that symbolize or resemble an aspect of the traumatic event
   (5) physiological reactivity on exposure to internal or external cues that symbolize or resemble an aspect of the traumatic event
C. Persistent avoidance of stimuli associated with the trauma and numbing of general responsiveness (not present before the trauma), as indicated by three (or more) of the following:
   (1) efforts to avoid thoughts, feelings, or conversations associated with the trauma
   (2) efforts to avoid activities, places, or people that arouse recollections of the trauma
   (3) inability to recall an important aspect of the trauma
   (4) markedly diminished interest or participation in significant activities
   (5) feeling of detachment or estrangement from others
   (6) restricted range of affect (e.g., unable to have loving feelings)
   (7) sense of a foreshortened future (e.g., does not expect to have a career, marriage, children, or a normal life span)

(continued)

> ## DSM-IV-TR diagnostic criteria for
> ## 309.81 Posttraumatic Stress Disorder *(continued)*
>
> D. Persistent symptoms of increased arousal (not present before the trauma),
>   as indicated by two (or more) of the following:
>   (1) difficulty falling or staying asleep
>   (2) irritability or outbursts of anger
>   (3) difficulty concentrating
>   (4) hypervigilance
>   (5) exaggerated startle response
> E. Duration of the disturbance (symptoms in Criteria B, C, and D) is more
>   than 1 month.
> F. The disturbance causes clinically significant distress or impairment in so-
>   cial, occupational, or other important areas of functioning.
>
> *Specify* if:
> **Acute:**   if duration of symptoms is less than 3 months
> **Chronic:**   if duration of symptoms is 3 months or more
>
> *Specify* if:
> **With Delayed Onset:**   if onset of symptoms is at least 6 months after the stressor

Guidelines for Differential Diagnosis of
Posttraumatic Stress Disorder

This case of Posttraumatic Stress Disorder is much more clear-cut than most
because of the extreme nature of the stressor (a life-threatening fire) and
the characteristic symptom pattern Mr. R reports (i.e., recurrent, intrusive
recollections of the fire and his mistake; recurrent distressing dreams about
the fire and great difficulty sleeping; an exaggerated startle response and immediate and distressing physical reactions to the sound of a fire alarm; an unwillingness ever to return to the firehouse or firefighting; an unwillingness to
go out, see people, or participate in everyday activities; a feeling of detachment and emotional numbness; and a sense that life isn't worth living).

   In common practice, it may often be difficult to distinguish the symptoms of Posttraumatic Stress Disorder from symptoms that are the result of
Malingering or Factitious Disorder, particularly in settings where secondary
gains can be derived from having such symptoms (e.g., in forensic settings as
mitigating circumstances for a crime or in occupational circumstances in
which a person wants to continue to receive disability benefits). It is therefore

important to evaluate carefully for the full range of symptoms described in criteria B, C, and D that involve both anxious and dissociative symptoms as well as symptoms of increased arousal. The disorder must also cause clinically significant distress or impairment, as it obviously is doing in Mr. R's case. The symptoms must have been present for more than 1 month in order to diagnose Posttraumatic Stress Disorder. A new diagnosis, Acute Stress Disorder, has been included in DSM-IV because it has been found that the development of a characteristic symptom pattern in the first month following a trauma often predicts the subsequent development of Posttraumatic Stress Disorder.

Early diagnosis and treatment intervention may help to mitigate the severity of subsequent symptoms. To diagnose Acute Stress Disorder, the same types of symptoms as in Posttraumatic Stress Disorder must develop within 4 weeks of a traumatic event of the same extreme intensity as is required for Posttraumatic Stress Disorder and must last from 2 days to 4 weeks. If symptoms continue after 4 weeks, the diagnosis is changed to Posttraumatic Stress Disorder. Although he did not report them, Mr. R obviously was having certain symptoms (e.g., the recurrent nightmares) during the first 4 weeks after the fire, but, because of the sheltered environment of the burn unit, his symptoms did not come to light until he was discharged. If Mr. R had reported his nightmares while on the unit and had received a psychiatric consultation, it is likely that other symptoms would have been revealed that would have justified a diagnosis of Acute Stress Disorder at that time.

A diagnosis of Adjustment Disorder may be appropriate when an individual develops distressing symptoms in response to a stressor that does not meet criteria for Posttraumatic Stress Disorder (i.e., the stressor did not involve an event or events that entailed actual or threatened death or serious injury or a threat to the physical integrity of self or others) or when the symptoms don't meet full criteria for Posttraumatic Stress Disorder.

Treatment Planning for Posttraumatic Stress Disorder

Experience with Posttraumatic Stress Disorder in the military has demonstrated that the prevention and treatment of the disorder can be greatly improved by providing immediate, proximate, and expectant care to reduce distress and complications. Prevention is much easier than cure in Posttraumatic Stress Disorder. The major reason why the new diagnosis of Acute Stress Disorder was included in DSM-IV was to allow for early identification and intervention. The psychoeducational approach should involve educating the patient about the likely early symptoms that may be experienced after exposure to an extreme stressor. The occurrence of intrusive thoughts and nightmares, startle reactions, and physiological responses to trigger stimuli becomes less terrifying if the patient understands beforehand that these are expectable reactions and likely to be short-lived.

Once Posttraumatic Stress Disorder is established, there is a considerable risk of it becoming chronic, particularly if secondary gains (such as continuing to stay out of work and receive disability payments) enter the picture. Often there is an interaction between the condition and the secondary gain (e.g., the workplace evokes terror, and the symptoms enable the patient to continue to avoid being exposed to the workplace that would trigger the Posttraumatic Stress Disorder symptoms). Treatment should combine continued psychoeducation, exploring cognitions, behavioral exposure, and, very often, medication. It is very important to foster the expectation that the individual will recover.

Summary

An ounce of prevention is worth a pound of cure. A diagnosis of Acute Stress Disorder made shortly after symptoms develop can be helpful if psychoeducation is provided to help individuals know what kinds of symptoms to expect so that they will understand that these reactions are not unusual and that they shouldn't try to avoid them. Psychoeducation, desensitization, and normalization can help these individuals regain a sense of control over their lives. Antidepressants as well as cognitive-behavior therapy have been found to be effective in treating Posttraumatic Stress Disorder. It is also important to evaluate for both Panic Disorder and Major Depressive Disorder because these frequently co-occur with Posttraumatic Stress Disorder. Alcohol and/or Other Substance Abuse may also develop when Posttraumatic Stress Disorder is untreated.

Generalized Anxiety Disorder

❖ Case Study: A Worrier on the Verge of a Nervous Breakdown[3]

Mr. Y, a 30-year-old married real estate investment company owner, goes to a local outpatient psychiatric clinic saying that he "is on the verge of a nervous breakdown." He reports that he has always been a "worrier" but not to

3. Thanks to Mary Soderstrom, M.D., of the Psychiatry Department of Duke University Medical Center for supplying this case.

the extent that his life was affected in any noticeable way. However, over the past year he has been experiencing a "tweaked" feeling of inner agitation and "stays keyed up" most of the time. Mr. Y has frequently complained of stomach upsets and diarrhea over the past 6 months as well as a decreased ability to concentrate at work. His wife, an attractive and well-educated woman in her mid-20s, accompanies her husband to the clinic and says that he tosses and turns in bed until about 2 or 3 A.M. and frequently gets up to urinate. She goes on to complain that her husband has gotten very irritable in the past 6–8 months and frequently yells at people, even at their 5-year-old daughter.

The oldest and only male in a family of four children, Mr. Y is from an affluent and well-educated family steeped in tradition. His father, grandfather, and several other men in the family attended the same northeastern Ivy League university. Mr. Y felt compelled to continue this tradition, but he was apprehensive that his academic skills were not refined enough, although he was in the 90th percentile of his graduating class. Once he was accepted to this prestigious university, he began to feel the pressure to perform exceedingly well. Despite experiencing tremendous anxiety and tension around exam time, Mr. Y graduated from the university with distinction. While in college, Mr. Y began dating his wife and recalls that he would worry for days about whether he had picked the right restaurant for the date, whether he had selected the right flowers, or whether his car, which had recently undergone a minor repair, would break down on the date. He notes that although he worried a lot about something or other not working right, he never had difficulty asking women out on dates or having them accept. He describes himself as driven and generally on the extroverted side.

Three years before the current evaluation, Mr. Y's parents separated and his real estate investment company came close to bankruptcy. Although he has been successful at gradually rebuilding the company over the ensuing years and "getting his feet back on the ground," he has been unable to suppress his nervousness and tension. At night, he lays awake staring at the ceiling and worrying about routine work issues, what the future holds for him, and how he would support himself and his family if his company went bankrupt. It makes him sick to his stomach to think about losing his business and not having health insurance to cover the allergy shots his daughter needs. Mr. Y went to see an internist and a gastroenterologist, but his exams were normal and his symptoms were thought to be "anxiety related." He calms himself down occasionally with a beer or two but denies any alcohol-related problems. He tried cocaine a couple of times in his early 20s but did not like the feeling and denies using any other street drugs. He feels sad but denies feelings of worthlessness or suicidal thoughts.

DSM-IV-TR Diagnosis

Axis I: 300.02   Generalized Anxiety Disorder
Axis II: V71.09   No diagnosis
Axis III: None
Axis IV: Marital stress, problems on the job
Axis V: GAF = 65

DSM-IV-TR diagnostic criteria for
300.02 Generalized Anxiety Disorder

A. Excessive anxiety and worry (apprehensive expectation), occurring more days than not for at least 6 months, about a number of events or activities (such as work or school performance).
B. The person finds it difficult to control the worry.
C. The anxiety and worry are associated with three (or more) of the following six symptoms (with at least some symptoms present for more days than not for the past 6 months).   Note: Only one item is required in children.
    (1) restlessness or feeling keyed up or on edge
    (2) being easily fatigued
    (3) difficulty concentrating or mind going blank
    (4) irritability
    (5) muscle tension
    (6) sleep disturbance (difficulty falling or staying asleep, or restless unsatisfying sleep)
D. The focus of the anxiety and worry is not confined to features of an Axis I disorder, e.g., the anxiety or worry is not about having a Panic Attack (as in Panic Disorder), being embarrassed in public (as in Social Phobia), being contaminated (as in Obsessive-Compulsive Disorder), being away from home or close relatives (as in Separation Anxiety Disorder), gaining weight (as in Anorexia Nervosa), having multiple physical complaints (as in Somatization Disorder), or having a serious illness (as in Hypochondriasis), and the anxiety and worry do not occur exclusively during Posttraumatic Stress Disorder.
E. The anxiety, worry, or physical symptoms cause clinically significant distress or impairment in social, occupational, or other important areas of functioning.
F. The disturbance is not due to the direct physiological effects of a substance (e.g., a drug of abuse, a medication) or a general medical condition (e.g., hyperthyroidism) and does not occur exclusively during a Mood Disorder, a Psychotic Disorder, or a Pervasive Developmental Disorder.

Guidelines for Differential Diagnosis
of Generalized Anxiety Disorder

Since Generalized Anxiety Disorder was introduced in DSM-III, it has been one of the least successful diagnoses in the manual. With each iteration of the system, the criteria set for this disorder has undergone additional changes in an effort to increase its reliability, clarify its boundaries, reduce heterogeneity, and help to predict treatment response. There has been much controversy concerning whether the emphasis in the criteria should be on cognitive symptoms (such as excessive worry) or on the somatic symptoms of anxiety (such as muscle tension or fatigue). The definition of the disorder given in DSM-IV (and DSM-IV-TR) is yet another attempt to balance these two aspects of the disorder. Those who believe that somatic symptoms are the most important aspect of Generalized Anxiety Disorder feel that the DSM-IV definition places too much emphasis on excessive worry, whereas those who are strongly oriented toward cognitive therapy think that the concept of excessive worry is integral to the definition. It is of interest that both the somatic and cognitive aspects were included under Freud's definition of anxiety neurosis. Mr. Y has been worrying excessively about many everyday issues (e.g., keeping his company going and keeping his health insurance to cover his daughter's allergy shots) and has also been experiencing somatic symptoms such as a feeling of inner agitation and being "keyed up" as well as stomach upsets and diarrhea.

Another concern in developing the DSM-IV criteria was to reduce the overlap with Panic Disorder. A number of symptoms that were more characteristic of Panic Disorder were deleted from the DSM-III-R Generalized Anxiety Disorder criteria set to arrive at the DSM-IV definition. The most important features for the differential diagnosis of the two disorders are the different characteristic symptoms and the very different time course. Panic Disorder is characterized by a crescendo effect, with attacks beginning and ending quickly, whereas Generalized Anxiety Disorder is more a way of life, with the anxiety a pervasive presence in the individual's everyday existence. For example, Mr. Y has tended to be a worrier all his life, agonizing in college over the right restaurant or flowers to choose for a date and over how well he would do in his studies, despite his good performance. If criteria are met for both disorders, however, both can be diagnosed.

Another important differential involves the aches, pains, and worries of everyday life that nearly everyone experiences at one time or another. The E criterion for Generalized Anxiety Disorder, requiring that "the anxiety, worry, or physical symptoms cause clinically significant distress or impairment in social, occupational, or other important areas of functioning," is included precisely to help make this distinction. In addition, the criteria require excessive anxiety and worry that are present more days than not for at least 6 months as well as the presence of at least three somatic symptoms (in adults). These requirements are included to help ensure that Generalized Anxiety Disorder is not over-diagnosed in individuals with everyday worries and problems; however, this is ultimately still a matter of clinical judgment that may be influenced by the evaluator's cultural background and own tendencies toward worry.

Although Mr. Y has been a "worrier" all his life, his worry and somatic symptoms appear to have interfered significantly with his functioning only during the past year. He has been worrying almost constantly about everyday affairs; has frequently had trouble sleeping; has been extremely irritable and yelled at people, including his daughter; has had difficulty concentrating at work; and has experienced somatic symptoms that were severe enough for him to seek evaluation by an internist and a gastroenterologist, who could find no physical cause for his problems. Therefore, a diagnosis of Generalized Anxiety Disorder would seem appropriate for Mr. Y at the time of this evaluation, although his symptoms would not have warranted such a diagnosis when he was younger.

Note that anxiety frequently occurs as an associated feature in many other mental disorders and is also a side effect of certain medications and substances. Generalized Anxiety Disorder would not be diagnosed when the anxiety is part of another mental disorder or is due to the direct physiological effects of a substance or a general medical condition (see criteria D and F).

Treatment Planning for Generalized Anxiety Disorder

The treatment of Generalized Anxiety Disorder is an area that has received relatively little study. Because there may be heterogeneous presentations of this disorder, different treatments may be effective for different types of presentations. The results of the studies that have been done are not particularly satisfying or clear-cut enough to suggest any firm recommendations. A variety of medications have been tried without resounding success. Many individuals do seem to benefit from (and want to take) anxiolytic or antidepressant medications.

A cognitive-behavioral approach that focuses on the target symptom of worry and the avoidance that results from this worry is often helpful. A combination of medication and cognitive therapy may be particularly helpful. Individuals with this disorder also sometimes do well with psychodynamic treatments that try to uncover the underlying unconscious dangers that are concealed under the everyday worries with which the individual is preoccupied.

Summary

Generalized Anxiety Disorder was one of the least reliable diagnoses in DSM-III and DSM-III-R. It is not yet clear whether the changes made in the DSM-IV definition of the disorder will improve its reliability. Partly as a result of the lack of diagnostic clarity, very little systematic research has been done on the treatment for Generalized Anxiety Disorder.

Chapter 7

Somatoform Disorders

The Somatoform Disorders in DSM-IV-TR are grouped together because all of them are characterized by the presence of unexplained physical symptoms or bodily preoccupations. In Somatization Disorder, Undifferentiated Somatoform Disorder, Conversion Disorder, and Pain Disorder, the individual experiences physical symptoms that suggest the presence of a general medical condition, but a medical workup cannot establish an etiological general medical condition that adequately explains the problem. Hypochondriasis is characterized by a preoccupation that one has a serious disease. In Body Dysmorphic Disorder, a person is preoccupied with the belief that he or she has a serious defect in appearance.

Before any of the disorders in this section are diagnosed, the clinician must carefully rule out 1) an underlying but as yet undetected general medical condition that is causing the symptoms; 2) another mental disorder that is responsible for the somatic symptoms (e.g., an Anxiety or Mood Disorder may present with primarily somatic symptoms, especially in primary care treatment settings or in certain cultures in which psychological distress is most commonly expressed through somatic symptoms); or 3) symptoms that are intentionally produced or feigned, as in Malingering or Factitious Disorder.

The disorders in this section include the following:

Somatoform Disorders

300.81   Somatization Disorder
300.82   Undifferentiated Somatoform Disorder
300.11   Conversion Disorder
307.xx   Pain Disorder
300.7   Hypochondriasis
300.7   Body Dysmorphic Disorder
300.82   Somatoform Disorder Not Otherwise Specified

We present cases that illustrate Somatization Disorder, Conversion Disorder, Pain Disorder, and Body Dysmorphic Disorder and discuss the other disorders in the differential diagnostic sections of these case studies.

Somatization Disorder

❖   Case Study: A Young Woman
      With a Multitude of Illnesses[1]

Ms. S, a 26-year-old employed married woman is referred to a psychiatrist by her gynecologist. He reports that she is "off work, depressed, suicidal, stumbling around at home on all kinds of medications, and has no active gynecological disease." He says that he has "had it" with both her and her mother who "have just worn me out, always complaining about something and phoning me day and night." Besides, "they never pay their bills." The patient is a member of a locally prominent but erratic family. She has been divorced once and married for the second time 2 years before this evaluation; she has no children.

Ms. S has difficulty walking into the office, bracing herself on the walls and furniture at times but at other times fully supporting herself. She never actually falls. She relates that this sometimes happens to her without warning. She complains that "I am horribly depressed and just want to end it all. I also want to get off all these medications." She reports that she has had many health problems since she was a young teenager. She has seen literally hundreds of doctors but has never found one who has really helped her. She has been seeing her gynecologist for dysmenorrhea, which she says began virtually at menarche. She describes severe cramping (for which she takes Empirin with codeine) and "gushing blood" for 7 or 8 days each menstrual

---

1. Thanks to Ronald L. Martin, M.D., of the University of Kansas School of Medicine at Wichita for supplying the following cases for Somatization and Conversion Disorders.

period. She also says that her menstrual periods are very irregular. However, she has never been anemic, and extensive gynecological workups have not identified any pathology. She takes Fiorinal for "migraine" headaches (which "last for days"). In fact, she reports that she is having a migraine at the time of the interview, although she does not seem to be bothered by light or noise. She also reports having frequent chest pains that convince her she is about to have a heart attack, but numerous electrocardiograms have been negative. She reports that she has "asthma" for which she was once "resuscitated" and that she gets short of breath when "emotionally excited." Although she says that she suffers from "rheumatoid arthritis" and often has pain in "all of my joints" that makes it very difficult to get out of bed, there is no evidence of joint deformities and she is not under a doctor's care for this condition. She also reports problems with nausea and vomiting, a bloated feeling, and sometimes "going days without being able to keep any food down." However, several gastrointestinal workups have never identified a specific illness and she appears to be well nourished. Her neurological examination was within normal limits.

Ms. S reports that she has been depressed "for years," but that it has been worse in the past "few months" since she began having problems at work. She is a political appointee and feels that people are jealous of her and deliberately harass her. She appears distraught but not really sad. She states that she is depressed "all day, every day," has little or no interest in anything, never feels like eating (but has not lost weight), goes "for days" without sleeping unless she uses a hypnotic drug, has no energy, can't concentrate, is a worthless person, and sometimes contemplates suicide (but does not have any specific plan). She describes her "wonderful" husband of 2 years as her only "bright spot" and says he is "fully supportive in every way." Although she initially maintains that there are absolutely no problems in her marriage, she later admits that she usually has pain during sexual intercourse that has prevented relations for several months at a time.

Ms. S was prescribed an antidepressant by her gynecologist (but only takes it "when I really need it"), a benzodiazepine for insomnia (which she has been taking "full dose" every night "for months"), and another benzodiazepine for anxiety (which she takes "to the limit"). She denies current or past use of alcohol or nonprescribed drugs. Although never previously referred to a psychiatrist for depression, she has taken several antidepressants and sedative hypnotics prescribed by other physicians over the years. She states that the medications only made her feel worse.

Her only previous psychiatric contact was 3 years earlier when she was hospitalized for 4 days for a "psychosis." She recalled that people's faces would "melt away and re-form into monsters." She described it as a "difficult period." She was in the process of a divorce from her first husband after 3 years of marriage. She reports that she was treated with "some horrible drug called Haldol," which she was to have continued after discharge.

She never filled the prescription and her "psychotic" symptoms did not recur.

Ms. S is hospitalized and, for observational purposes, is not started on any psychotropic medications. She never shows any objective signs of sedative hypnotic withdrawal. Although she continues to complain of extreme depression and fatigue, she is observed to be very interactive with other patients on the unit and to be in repeated conflict with the nursing staff regarding procedures and rules. After 2 days of hospitalization, she demands a weekend pass to spend time with her husband. Her mood appears to be labile and very situationally sensitive, markedly fluctuating depending on how well visits from her husband, mother, and employer go.

Review of Ms. S's extensive medical records reveals a history of many physical complaints that have been inconsistently reported. Migraine headaches and asthma were mentioned as diagnostic possibilities, but there was a great deal of disagreement from physician to physician. A diagnosis of rheumatoid arthritis or of another connective tissue disease was not supported by laboratory evaluations.

Discussions with Ms. S's husband yield somewhat contradictory information. He reports that she has not been consistently depressed but seemed to be in good spirits until several days before referral when a confrontation with a co-worker occurred and resulted in the patient being placed at a lower level of responsibility. In terms of their marriage, he reports that they have their "rocky times," but he thinks that they can "work it out."

Subsequent to a weekend rounds visit by a colleague of the initial psychiatrist, Ms. S requests that her care be transferred to him because "he has a better sense of humor." Reporting that she now (4 days postadmission) feels much better, she demands to be discharged. Several weeks later when her new psychiatrist is asked about Ms. S's course under his care, he reports that "Things didn't work out too well" and that he is no longer treating her. He also volunteers that the patient is getting divorced.

DSM-IV-TR Diagnosis

Axis I: 300.81   Somatization Disorder
            296.3   Possible Major Depressive Disorder
            305.40   Possible Sedative, Hypnotic, or Anxiolytic
                     Abuse or
            304.10   Sedative, Hypnotic, or Anxiolytic Dependence
Axis II: V71.09   No diagnosis
Axis III: No specific diagnosis
Axis IV: Conflicts with co-workers and demotion at work
           (V62.81), marital problems (V61.10 Partner Relational
           Problem)
Axis V: GAF = 50 (current); 70 (highest level in past year)

DSM-IV-TR diagnostic criteria for
300.81 Somatization Disorder

A.   A history of many physical complaints beginning before age 30 years that occur over a period of several years and result in treatment being sought or significant impairment in social, occupational, or other important areas of functioning.

B.   Each of the following criteria must have been met, with individual symptoms occurring at any time during the course of the disturbance:

   (1) *four pain symptoms:*   a history of pain related to at least four different sites or functions (e.g., head, abdomen, back, joints, extremities, chest, rectum, during menstruation, during sexual intercourse, or during urination)

   (2) *two gastrointestinal symptoms:*   a history of at least two gastrointestinal symptoms other than pain (e.g., nausea, bloating, vomiting other than during pregnancy, diarrhea, or intolerance of several different foods)

   (3) *one sexual symptom:*   a history of at least one sexual or reproductive symptom other than pain (e.g., sexual indifference, erectile or ejaculatory dysfunction, irregular menses, excessive menstrual bleeding, vomiting throughout pregnancy)

   (4) *one pseudoneurological symptom:*   a history of at least one symptom or deficit suggesting a neurological condition not limited to pain (conversion symptoms such as impaired coordination or balance, paralysis or localized weakness, difficulty swallowing or lump in throat, aphonia, urinary retention, hallucinations, loss of touch or pain sensation, double vision, blindness, deafness, seizures; dissociative symptoms such as amnesia; or loss of consciousness other than fainting)

C.   Either (1) or (2):

   (1) after appropriate investigation, each of the symptoms in Criterion B cannot be fully explained by a known general medical condition or the direct effects of a substance (e.g., a drug of abuse, a medication)

   (2) when there is a related general medical condition, the physical complaints or resulting social or occupational impairment are in excess of what would be expected from the history, physical examination, or laboratory findings

D.   The symptoms are not intentionally produced or feigned (as in Factitious Disorder or Malingering).

Guidelines for Differential Diagnosis of Somatization Disorder

What is especially notable in the case of Ms. S and what characterizes Somatization Disorder generally is a complex medical history, inconsistencies between an individual's subjective complaints and objective findings, and an overall dramatic quality to the complaints. Because of the marked discrepancy between the patient's subjective reports and the objective findings that characterizes Somatization Disorder, it is especially important for the clinician to confirm the history supplied by the patient with information from additional informants and with a review of the patient's medical records. To diagnose Somatization Disorder, the clinician must determine that the symptoms cannot be fully explained by a known general medical condition or the direct effects of a substance or, when a general medical condition is present, that the symptoms are in excess of what would be expected given that condition. Despite repeated workups for her gynecological, gastrointestinal, and joint pain problems, no general medical condition has been found that could fully explain Ms. S's symptoms. Note that certain general medical conditions (e.g., multiple sclerosis, porphyria, systemic lupus erythematosus, hyperparathyroidism) may present with numerous atypical symptoms and an unusual course. The clinician should be careful to rule out such conditions before diagnosing Somatization Disorder.

Ms. S's symptoms clearly met the essential requirement of Somatization Disorder. She had many physical complaints that had occurred over several years, with an onset in early adulthood. Her symptoms also more than fulfilled the specific diagnostic algorithm for Somatization Disorder. She had four pain symptoms (i.e., in the head and joints, during menstruation, and during sexual intercourse), three gastrointestinal symptoms other than pain (i.e., nausea, vomiting, and bloating), two reproductive symptoms other than pain (i.e., excessive menstrual bleeding and menstrual irregularity), and two pseudo-neurological symptoms (i.e., difficulty walking and hallucinations that were not part of a psychosis). Ms. S therefore had three more symptoms than the number required to fulfill criteria for the disorder.

The relationship between hallucinations and Somatization Disorder is very interesting. Perhaps the most important point to remember is that not all "hallucinations" indicate that the individual is psychotic. The hallucinations Ms. S experienced were not typical of those that are usually seen in Schizophrenia and Other Psychotic Disorders. Instead, they were characteristic of the types of hallucinations that may occur in Somatization Disorder because they were visual and not auditory, did not occur in the context of a psychotic disturbance, resolved very quickly, and did not recur when antipsychotics were discontinued. Furthermore, they had a dramatic, "fairy tale" flavor, and Ms. S described them eagerly and dramatically. It is of some interest that suggestible individuals ("with hysteria") were hospitalized by Charcot in 19th century Paris on the neurological wards and consequently presented primarily with conversion neurological symptoms. Today such individuals usually wind up in psychiatric hospitals and may consequently develop conversion psychiatric symptoms, especially the kind of atypical hallucinations described above. Of course, visual hallucinations should always suggest the possibility of substance use or a general medical condition.

Individuals with Somatization Disorder may also have Substance-Related Disorders, and this may have been an issue with Ms. S. Although she denied using alcohol or nonprescribed drugs, Ms. S did have a history of problems related to the use of prescription drugs. However, even if an additional diagnosis of Substance Abuse were warranted, many of Ms. S's physical symptoms were present before her drug use and could not be "fully explained" as the effects of Substance Use. In addition, although Ms. S reported a level of Substance Use that would have been expected to produce withdrawal symptoms when she discontinued use, no such symptoms were seen. This suggested that Ms. S was not using the medications to the extent that she reported and that her reports of drug use were very likely exaggerated. However, because abuse of or dependence on prescribed drugs may often be associated with Somatization Disorder, medications should be used judiciously with such patients.

To diagnose Somatization Disorder, the clinician must distinguish it from Factitious Disorder or Malingering, in which symptoms are intentionally produced or feigned. This is a difficult judgment and must be based on an evaluation of the context in which the symptoms occur. There was no evidence that Ms. S's motivation was an external reward, as in Malingering. She also did not appear to be consciously feigning her symptoms, as in Factitious Disorder, but rather to be actually experiencing them.

Other disorders that should be considered in the differential diagnosis of Somatization Disorder are Panic Disorder, Hypochondriasis, and Major Depressive Disorder. It is particularly important to rule out Panic Disorder because it is so much better understood and more treatable than Somatization Disorder. If an individual's symptoms occur only during panic attacks, the diagnosis of Panic Disorder takes precedence over that of Somatization Disorder. However, if the symptom pattern characteristic of Somatization Disorder occurs independently of the individual's panic attacks, both diagnoses can be made.

The question of whether Ms. S was experiencing Major Depressive Disorder is more complicated and reflects the difficulty in evaluating any symptom presentation offered by an individual with Somatization Disorder. Just as the individual is likely to exaggerate and elaborate on somatic symptoms, he or she may also exaggerate and elaborate on psychiatric symptoms. Ms. S reported an adequate number and duration of depressive symptoms to meet the criteria for Major Depressive Disorder. This is not uncommon for patients with Somatization Disorder, even when they do not really have Major Depressive Disorder, because such patients often eagerly claim psychiatric as well as physical symptoms. It seems likely that Ms. S was exaggerating her depressive symptoms because her husband reported that she did not seem to be consistently depressed and was in good spirits until a few days before her referral. Even if a diagnosis of Major Depressive Disorder were indicated, Ms. S's excessive somatic complaints had occurred recurrently throughout her life and had not been limited to periods of depression; therefore, a diagnosis of Somatization Disorder would still be warranted. The clinician might consider a well-monitored, adequate trial of an antidepressant medication, with low overdose lethality potential, the results of which would have diagnostic significance.

The differential between Somatization Disorder and Hypochondriasis rests on a subtle and perhaps not all that meaningful distinction. An individual with Hypochondriasis is preoccupied with the fear or idea of having a serious disease, whereas the person with Somatization Disorder focuses on the symptoms themselves. Moreover, whereas Somatization Disorder is by definition polysymptomatic in nature, individuals with Hypochondriasis are usually concerned with a more narrow range of possible diseases. Although Ms. S reported that she had a number of serious diseases, such as asthma and rheumatoid arthritis, she did not seem particularly concerned with the implications of these diseases but rather concentrated on the actual symptoms themselves. When a preoccupation with fears of having a serious illness occurs only during Somatization Disorder, an additional diagnosis of Hypochondriasis would not be made.

When an individual has somatoform symptoms that do not meet full criteria for Somatization Disorder, Undifferentiated Somatoform Disorder may be diagnosed if the symptoms have persisted for at least 6 months or Somatoform Disorder Not Otherwise Specified may be diagnosed if the duration is less than 6 months.

Treatment Planning for Somatization Disorder

Because there is no well-established treatment for Somatization Disorder, the most crucial issue is "to do no harm." Harm can be done by being either excessively or insufficiently alert to the possibilities of an underlying general medical cause for a patient's extensive and persistent presentation of symptoms. Many patients receive unnecessary medical tests and treatments that often create a remarkable array of complications. On the other hand, individuals with Somatization Disorder are not protected from developing general medical conditions that may require diagnosis and treatment. Once they are labeled as "crocks," such individuals often receive short shrift even when they present with symptoms that are characteristic of serious general medical illnesses. It is also important to evaluate for comorbid mental disorders that may be treatable, particularly Anxiety, Mood, or Substance-Related Disorders.

The tendency toward somatization is probably best managed through long-term supportive psychotherapy that provides an important sympathetic relationship. The practicalities usually require that sessions be relatively brief in duration and fairly widely spaced. The optimum practitioner is often the primary care physician who can work in tandem with a psychiatric consultant.

Summary

In evaluating persistent somatic symptoms, the essential point is to be neither too skeptical nor too credulous. Perhaps the most frequent mistake in diagnosis is to assume that anyone with hallucinations is psychotic. Some suggestible individuals have developed a propensity to experience "hallucinations" as a result of their contact with psychotic patients during inpatient hospital stays.

Conversion Disorder

❖   Case Study: A Woman With Spells

Ms. R, a 20-year-old single woman employed as a salesclerk, is brought to an emergency room in a large metropolitan area by her boyfriend and several other friends. She complains of "numbness" in the left side of her face and her left arm and shoulder subsequent to an incident at a picnic. The "numbness" consists of having no sensation as well as "weakness" in her left arm and shoulder. Apparently, the left side of her head accidentally struck the ground while she was being playfully carried by several friends. Her friends report that immediately following the incident she seemed "dazed" and was inconsistently unresponsive. Within minutes, she was fully conscious but reported the numbness and so was brought to the emergency room.

Upon examination, Ms. R is somewhat perplexed but rather nonchalant about her symptoms. She is fully cooperative with all examination procedures. There are no pupillary abnormalities, and her blink response is normal. There are no signs of facial weakness. On sensory examination, she acknowledges no sensation in any modality on the entire left side of her face, left shoulder, and left arm, with a sharp boundary running down the middle of her forehead and neck, then angling to her axilla. She is seen to move her left arm in conjunction with undressing, but she supports this arm in her right hand and shows weak force in all movements involving her left arm and shoulder. Deep tendon reflexes are symmetrical and normal strength.

Ms. R reports being in good health and denies any past or present abuse of alcohol or drugs. She describes herself as a "shy and sensitive" person who "never feels self-confident like I should" but always has a few good friends nonetheless. She is a high school graduate from an outlying rural area who maintained "OK" grades (Bs and Cs) in the "easiest classes I could take." She especially disliked science and mathematics. Her father worked as a clerk in a feed store and her mother as a waitress in a truck stop. She moved to the city 2 years after graduation when her parents divorced, a breach that upset her greatly. Shortly after relocating, she was hospitalized for a "spell" after she was found walking in a park not knowing who she was and how, when, or why she had gotten there. Although she regained memory function soon after admission, her recollection of the "spell" was vague. She clearly recalled her hospitalization, reporting that after a "thorough evaluation" (which included several types of "brain wave tests"), no explanation for the spell was given other than that she must have been "very upset." No further evaluation or care was recommended, but she did not return to work for several weeks "in order to recuperate."

Ms. R had no recurrence of this or any other neurological symptoms until the present episode. She has stayed with the same job and reports that "I enjoy the people there now that I know all of them so well." She has had two previous serious romantic relationships, but "they just did not work out." Her current relationship has lasted 8 months, but her boyfriend recently told her that "maybe we should date other people." She was distressed by this, especially because it reminded her of her previous breakups. After admission to the hospital, she continues to manifest the same symptoms; however, all objective evaluations are negative. She is advised that there does not appear to be any neurological damage and that her symptoms should progressively improve and disappear. By the next morning, all symptoms have disappeared except for a feeling of "awkwardness" in her left hand for which no objective cause can be found. She is discharged with a referral for outpatient psychiatric care.

DSM-IV-TR *Diagnosis*

Axis I: 300.11   Conversion Disorder, With Mixed Presentation
                      (both motor and sensory symptoms)
           300.12   Dissociative Amnesia (past episode, resolved)
Axis II: V71.09   No diagnosis, avoidant and dependent personality
                      features, dissociation as a specific defense
                      mechanism
Axis III: None
Axis IV: Impending breakup of relationship with her boyfriend
Axis V: GAF = 60 (current); 85 (highest level in past year)

DSM-IV-TR diagnostic criteria for 300.11 Conversion Disorder

A. One or more symptoms or deficits affecting voluntary motor or sensory function that suggest a neurological or other general medical condition.

B. Psychological factors are judged to be associated with the symptom or deficit because the initiation or exacerbation of the symptom or deficit is preceded by conflicts or other stressors.

C. The symptom or deficit is not intentionally produced or feigned (as in Factitious Disorder or Malingering).

D. The symptom or deficit cannot, after appropriate investigation, be fully explained by a general medical condition, or by the direct effects of a substance, or as a culturally sanctioned behavior or experience.

E. The symptom or deficit causes clinically significant distress or impairment in social, occupational, or other important areas of functioning or warrants medical evaluation.

F. The symptom or deficit is not limited to pain or sexual dysfunction, does not occur exclusively during the course of Somatization Disorder, and is not better accounted for by another mental disorder.

Specify type of symptom or deficit:
With Motor Symptom or Deficit
With Sensory Symptom or Deficit
With Seizures or Convulsions
With Mixed Presentation

Guidelines for Differential Diagnosis of Conversion Disorder

Conversion Disorder appears to be much less common in the United States today than was previously the case and is still the case in other cultures. This may be for reasons suggested in the discussion of Somatization Disorder. Suggestible individuals who once might have presented with physical complaints are now more likely to present with psychiatric complaints that mimic other mental disorders rather than neurological disorders.

Ms. R's symptoms fulfilled the requirements for Conversion Disorder: They involved voluntary motor and sensory deficits and appeared to be related to psychological factors (her distress over her boyfriend's recent suggestion that he and Ms. R see other people). The most important diagnostic question is whether Ms. R's symptoms are caused by an underlying neurological condition. Studies have shown that an appreciable number of individuals originally diagnosed with Conversion Disorder are later found to have a neurological disorder that accounts for their symptoms. Although Ms. R's symptoms suggest a possible neurological injury, this explanation does not seem likely because the symptom patterns did not conform to neuroanatomical pathways but were demarcated by a sharp boundary running down the exact middle of Ms. R's forehead and neck.

Although conversion symptoms tend not to follow known anatomical pathways unless the patient is medically knowledgeable, symptoms of some patients do closely mimic a general medical condition. This usually happens in someone who has a knowledge of medicine (e.g., doctors or nurses) or in someone who actually has the disorder (e.g., the majority of people with conversion seizures also have epilepsy) or knows someone who does. Ms. R showed no evidence of any other general medical condition or Substance Abuse etiology. Although all factors point to Conversion Disorder as an explanation for Ms. R's symptoms, the clinician must take care not to reject the possibility of an underlying neurological illness that is early in its course, atypical in its presentation, or so rare as not to have been considered. Follow-up neurological exams may sometimes be indicated.

The requirement that psychological factors be associated with the conversion symptoms is unique in DSM-IV (and DSM-IV-TR). Unfortunately, it is not particularly helpful in improving the specificity of the diagnosis because psychological factors are associated with the presentation of nearly all medical and mental disorders. Criterion B suggests that it may be helpful in making a diagnosis when the symptoms or deficit begins or grows worse after a conflict or stressor. For example, Ms. R's problem began shortly after her boyfriend told her he didn't want to see as much of her.

Ms. R did not appear to be intentionally producing or feigning the symptoms. She seemed fully cooperative with all examinations. Her symptoms did not bring any obvious external rewards (as one would expect in Malingering), and their prompt resolution would indicate there was no conscious intent to assume the sick role (as in Factitious Disorder). It might be possible that

Ms. R's symptoms could bring increased attention and sympathy from her boyfriend (a secondary gain), but as long as the symptoms are not intentionally produced, Conversion Disorder (not Malingering) would be the appropriate diagnosis.

Whenever anyone presents with conversion symptoms, it is important to ask questions that would evaluate whether the other symptoms of Somatization Disorder are also present. By convention and to avoid artifactual comorbidity, conversion-like symptoms that occur as part of a Pain Disorder, Sexual Disorder, or Somatization Disorder are not diagnosed separately. In Ms. R's case, there is no evidence of Somatization Disorder or any other mental disorder that could account for her symptoms.

Treatment Planning for Conversion Disorder

Conversion Disorder tends to occur in people who can be suggested into (and fortunately also suggested out of) the symptoms. Often the best approach to acute symptoms is to provide a positive expectation and a face-saving way (e.g., physical rehabilitation) for the patient to recover. More chronic presentations may require a physical rehabilitation approach as well as psychotherapy and suggestion. Because these symptoms also often occur in the context of psychosocial stressors, other helpful approaches include environmental manipulation, support, advice, and teaching coping skills. In our experience, insight-oriented therapies are usually not indicated despite the fact that psychological conflicts are involved in the etiology of the conversion symptoms. These individuals usually do not find insight particularly helpful and instead may respond to interpretations by feeling blamed for feigning their symptoms.

Summary

Conversion Disorder is easy to miss and easy to overdiagnose. It is crucial to conduct a sufficiently thorough neurological examination, workup, and follow-up to ensure that the symptoms are not the atypical manifestation of an underlying neurological or other general medical condition (e.g., multiple sclerosis, myasthenia gravis, or idiopathic dystonias). On the other hand, some individuals with Conversion Disorder receive a vast array of expensive and potentially dangerous tests and treatment procedures. Clinical judgment is necessary in deciding how far to pursue neurological causes. Conversion Disorder can also be diagnosed when a neurological condition is present if the symptoms are not fully explained by that condition. This is not an uncommon situation. Finally, and perhaps most important, conversion symptoms now much more often may be "psychiatric" than "neurological," although distinguishing between conversion symptoms and primary psychiatric symptoms is certainly no easy task.

Pain Disorder

❖ Case Study: A Man Who Is in Constant Pain

Mr. B is a 37-year-old man who is first seen for psychiatric evaluation 3 years after injuring his back while moving heavy equipment on his job as a truck driver. Two years earlier he underwent lumbar laminectomy, but the operation was only temporarily successful and Mr. B's incapacitating pain has gradually returned.

During the 3 years since his injury, Mr. B has worked for a total of approximately 8 months, but he has felt unable to work for the 6 months before this psychiatric evaluation. He suffers from severe pain in his lower back that occasionally radiates down his left leg. A myelogram is negative, and a physical examination shows no evidence of nerve root compression.

Mr. B's physicians believe that he has instability of his lumbar spine. Everything Mr. B does makes his pain worse, including sitting, standing, bending, and lifting. He has become increasingly preoccupied with his pain and the unfairness of having his entire life ruined by it and is unable to talk or think about anything else. The only relief he gets is from increasing doses of cocaine. Mr. B feels sad and has some difficulty falling asleep but does not have other depressive symptoms that meet criteria for a Major Depressive Disorder. Nevertheless, he keeps loaded guns at home with the intent of killing himself if his back cannot be fixed.

Mr. B is a ruggedly good-looking bearded man who dresses like a cowboy and curses like a sailor. His appearance and mannerisms all seem intended to convince himself and others of his toughness and manliness. Mr. B sees any expression of emotion, except for anger, as weak or effeminate. He has great difficulty in expressing affection, although he shows evidence of deep attachment to family members. Mr. B even views his superior intellectual skills as weaknesses and in high school hid his impressive academic success from friends because he was sure they would laugh at him.

Before his injury, Mr. B saw himself as independent and self-reliant. He dominated his wife and children and generally viewed women as weak and needing to be taken care of. He was proud of how he supported his family, of the heavy work he did, and of the hundreds of hours of overtime he worked each year. He allowed his wife no freedom and became suspicious and angry if he did not know where she was. Only by having her appear totally dependent on him could his own immense dependency needs be kept hidden.

When Mr. B talks about his present condition, it is in terms of loss, mainly because he cannot do the heavy work in which he has previously taken such pride and cannot engage in physical exercise. He was encouraged by his physicians to learn a new, more sedentary trade but refused. He did take courses to be trained as a computer programmer, and, although he was good at it, he quit after several weeks. He couldn't concentrate and said his pain got worse when he sat for long periods. On one occasion he said, "I might be able to learn to live with the pain, but I couldn't do what I used to do." He is constantly searching for a physician who can return him to his former status.

DSM-IV-TR Diagnosis

Axis I: 307.89   Pain Disorder Associated With Both Psychological
                        Factors and a General Medical Condition, Chronic
             305.60   Cocaine Abuse
Axis II: Dependent personality features
Axis III: 715.9   Postlumbar laminectomy
Axis IV: Loss of job and inability to work in chosen field
Axis V: GAF = 45

DSM-IV-TR diagnostic criteria for Pain Disorder

A. Pain in one or more anatomical sites is the predominant focus of the clinical presentation and is of sufficient severity to warrant clinical attention.

B. The pain causes clinically significant distress or impairment in social, occupational, or other important areas of functioning.

C. Psychological factors are judged to have an important role in the onset, severity, exacerbation, or maintenance of the pain.

D. The symptom or deficit is not intentionally produced or feigned (as in Factitious Disorder or Malingering).

E. The pain is not better accounted for by a Mood, Anxiety, or Psychotic Disorder and does not meet criteria for Dyspareunia.

Code as follows:

307.80   Pain Disorder Associated With Psychological Factors: psychological factors are judged to have the major role in the onset, severity, exacerbation, or maintenance of the pain. (If a general medical condition is present, it does not have a major role in the onset, severity, exacerbation, or maintenance of the pain.) This type of Pain Disorder is not diagnosed if criteria are also met for Somatization Disorder.

(continued)

DSM-IV-TR diagnostic criteria for Pain Disorder *(continued)*

Specify if:
Acute: duration of less than 6 months
Chronic: duration of 6 months or longer
307.89   Pain Disorder Associated With Both Psychological Factors and a General Medical Condition: both psychological factors and a general medical condition are judged to have important roles in the onset, severity, exacerbation, or maintenance of the pain. The associated general medical condition or anatomical site of the pain (see below) is coded on Axis III.

Specify if:
Acute: duration of less than 6 months
Chronic: duration of 6 months or longer

Note: The following is not considered to be a mental disorder and is included here to facilitate differential diagnosis.

Pain Disorder Associated With a General Medical Condition: a general medical condition has a major role in the onset, severity, exacerbation, or maintenance of the pain. (If psychological factors are present, they are not judged to have a major role in the onset, severity, exacerbation, or maintenance of the pain.) The diagnostic code for the pain is selected based on the associated general medical condition if one has been established or on the anatomical location of the pain if the underlying general medical condition is not yet clearly established—for example, low back (724.2), sciatic (724.3), pelvic (625.9), headache (784.0), facial (784.0), chest (786.50), joint (719.4), bone (733.90), abdominal (789.0), breast (611.71), renal (788.0), ear (388.70), eye (379.91), throat (784.1), tooth (525.9), and urinary (788.0).

Guidelines for Differential Diagnosis of Pain Disorder

DSM-IV-TR describes three types of Pain Disorder. The first type is pain that is associated with psychological factors. The second type, pain associated with both psychological factors and a general medical condition, is far more common. In this type of Pain Disorder, the patient has a general medical condition that is expected to be painful, but there are also psychological factors that have an important role in "the onset, severity, exacerbation, or maintenance of the pain." The third type of Pain Disorder, pain associated with a general medical condition, is not a mental disorder because the pain is an expected result of the general medical condition and there are no psychological factors involved in its generation. This third type is included in DSM-IV-TR to facilitate differential diagnosis and because pain associated with a general medical condition (especially when it becomes chronic) is often treated by mental health personnel. When a general medical condition is present in association with the pain, it should be coded on Axis III as shown above.

Mr. B was diagnosed as having the second type of Pain Disorder because his pain appeared to go beyond what would be expected on the basis of the physical findings. Admittedly, this is always a judgment call. Procedures and treatments that could have been expected to produce some relief (e.g., the laminectomy and a back brace) did not produce any significant alleviation and, in fact, everything Mr. B did appeared to make his pain worse. In addition, Mr. B displayed a number of personality features that seemed to suggest an important role of psychological factors in the maintenance of the pain. His previous style of almost compulsive independence made it difficult for him to adjust to the aftermath of his back injury, and his own significant but unacknowledged dependency needs could be expressed only through his concerns about the ongoing pain. Despite this, there was no evidence that Mr. B intentionally produced or feigned the pain he experienced (as would be the case with Malingering or Factitious Disorder).

Because complaints about pain are always part of the presentation of Somatization Disorder, a separate diagnosis of Pain Disorder would not be made when Somatization Disorder is present. A separate diagnosis of Pain Disorder is also not made if the pain is restricted to Dyspareunia. In addition, complaints about pain often characterize Mood, Anxiety, and Psychotic Disorders. When the pain is adequately accounted for by another mental disorder, a separate diagnosis of Pain Disorder is not made. Mr. B's symptoms, however, do not meet criteria for any other disorder that could account for his pain complaints, and Pain Disorder Associated With Both Psychological Factors and a General Medical Condition appears to be the appropriate diagnosis.

Treatment Planning for Pain Disorder

Pain management programs often combine the teaching of techniques for coping with pain and the use of various types of medications (e.g., analgesics, anti-inflammatory agents, and antidepressants). Useful cognitive-behavioral techniques include distraction, stress management, cognitive restructuring, activity pacing, and sleep management. The individual may be asked to keep a diary indicating the activities attempted and the level of pain associated with each. Pain is a very real experience for the patient, and it rarely helps to point out that there may be "psychological" factors involved. Rather than challenging the patient's experience, it is more helpful to enlist the patient's cooperation in developing strategies for dealing with pain.

Summary

The adequate diagnosis and treatment of Pain Disorders represent a major public health challenge. It is extremely difficult, and perhaps often inherently impossible, to tease out with any precision the physical and psychological contributions to a particular pain presentation. Most people with chronic pain are probably best considered to have the combined subtype and will usually require treatments targeted to both the physical and psychological aspects of the disorder.

Body Dysmorphic Disorder

❖ Case Study: The "Ugliness" Problem[2]

Ms. J, a 30-year-old single unemployed woman, presents to a psychiatrist with this chief complaint: "My biggest wish is to be invisible so that no one can see how ugly I am. My biggest fear is that people are laughing at me thinking I'm ugly." In reality, Ms. J is an attractive woman who has been preoccupied with her supposed ugliness since age 12. At that time, she became "obsessed" with her nose, which she thought was too "big and shiny." Before the onset of this concern, Ms. J had been confident, a good student, and socially active. However, as a result of her fixation on her nose, she became socially withdrawn and was unable to concentrate in school; her grades plummeted from As to Ds and Fs.

At age 18, Ms. J dropped out of school because of her concern about her nose. Shortly after this, she took a job she disliked and at that time also became excessively focused on her minimal acne. She frequently picked at her few "blemishes"—sometimes all night long—with tweezers and needles, a behavior she found very difficult to resist. Over the following years, Ms. J developed additional excessive preoccupations with the appearance of her hair, which "wasn't smooth and neat enough"; her breasts, which she thought were too small; her supposedly thin lips; and her supposedly large buttocks. Ms. J thinks about her "defects" nearly all day long and states that "I always have two tapes playing—one saying not to worry and the other saying you're ugly."

---

2. Thanks to Katharine A. Phillips, M.D., of the Body Dysmorphic Clinic at Butler Hospital for supplying this case.

Ms. J frequently checks her supposed defects in mirrors and other re-flecting surfaces, such as windows, car bumpers, and spoons. Before she can leave her house, she asks her family members "at least 30 times" whether she looks OK, but she cannot be reassured by their responses. She also combs her hair excessively and attempts to camouflage her supposed de-fects with clothing, posture, and elaborate makeup that takes several hours a day to apply. Despite her efforts to hide her "ugliness," Ms. J thinks that others are probably taking special notice of her, staring at her or laughing at her behind her back. She sometimes drives through red lights because she is "unable to tolerate people looking at me." On one occasion when she was stuck in a traffic jam, Ms. J became so anxious over her belief that other drivers were staring at her nose, skin, and hair that she fled her car and left it in the middle of the highway.

Ms. J thinks that her view of her appearance and her belief that others are ridiculing her are probably accurate. However, she is able to acknowl-edge that she has "a small amount of doubt" about her beliefs, noting that it is possible—although unlikely—that she has a distorted view of her defects. Nonetheless, Ms. J occasionally briefly feels "100%" convinced that she is hideously ugly and is "completely certain" that others are taking special no-tice of her, as happened when she abandoned her car. At these times, she firmly believes that the neighbors are staring at her through binoculars, and she hides where she thinks they cannot see her.

As a result of her preoccupation with her appearance, Ms. J has been able to work only briefly and intermittently. She became increasingly so-cially isolated and avoided dating and other social interactions. As her con-cern intensified, Ms. J began to go out only at night when she could not be seen. Finally, after more than a decade of symptoms, Ms. J stopped working altogether and went on disability. She also became completely housebound, even hiding when relatives came to visit. As she explains, "I didn't leave my house because I didn't want people to see how ugly I was." Although Ms. J relies on her family members to buy her clothes, food, and other necessi-ties, she is unable to tell them about her concerns about her appearance be-cause she is too embarrassed. She has become increasingly depressed, with poor sleep, appetite, and energy, and has suicidal ideation. As a result of her social isolation and her feelings of hopelessness about her appearance, Ms. J has made two suicide attempts and has been hospitalized on several occa-sions.

Before she became housebound, Ms. J received antibiotics from sev-eral dermatologists, but this did not alleviate her concerns about her ap-pearance. She was refused a rhinoplasty by a plastic surgeon she consulted. Ms. J also sought outpatient psychiatric treatment but was never able to discuss her preoccupations with her therapist because she was too embar-rassed to do so.

DSM-IV-TR Diagnosis

Axis I: 300.7   Body Dysmorphic Disorder
            296.33   Major Depressive Disorder, Recurrent,
                       Severe Without Psychotic Features
Axis II: V71.09   No diagnosis
Axis III: None
Axis IV: Lack of employment, social isolation, financial problems
Axis V: GAF = 32 (current); 35 (highest level in past year)

DSM-IV-TR diagnostic criteria for 300.7 Body Dysmorphic Disorder

A. Preoccupation with an imagined defect in appearance. If a slight physical anomaly is present, the person's concern is markedly excessive.
B. The preoccupation causes clinically significant distress or impairment in social, occupational, or other important areas of functioning.
C. The preoccupation is not better accounted for by another mental disorder (e.g., dissatisfaction with body shape and size in Anorexia Nervosa).

Guidelines for Differential Diagnosis of Body Dysmorphic Disorder

The first important differential diagnostic concern is to distinguish the symptoms of Body Dysmorphic Disorder from normal concern about appearance. Most people have at least some reservations about how they look. Criterion B was added in DSM-IV to address this issue by requiring significant impairment or distress. However, the level of preoccupation and associated distress and impairment that can occur in Body Dysmorphic Disorder spans a wide spectrum. At the severe end, as in Ms. J's case, the difference between Body Dysmorphic Disorder and normal concern with appearance is clear. However, milder cases of the disorder blur into everyday concerns about physical appearance. It is likely that Body Dysmorphic Disorder is especially underrecognized and underdiagnosed in the nonpsychiatric settings (e.g., plastic surgery or dermatology) in which these patients often seek treatment.

Another important differential is between Body Dysmorphic Disorder and Obsessive-Compulsive Disorder. Similarities between the two disorders include the obsessional nature of the preoccupations and the presence of ritualistic behaviors, but in Body Dysmorphic Disorder individuals tend to have poorer insight and a higher prevalence of ideas of reference. Whenever an individual's preoccupations center primarily on appearance, the appropriate diagnosis would be Body Dysmorphic Disorder.

Major Depressive Disorder often co-occurs with Body Dysmorphic Disorder, and both can be diagnosed when both are present. However, a separate diagnosis of Body Dysmorphic Disorder is not warranted unless, as was the case with Ms. J, the preoccupation with physical appearance antedates the depression.

Patients with Body Dysmorphic Disorder are sometimes misdiagnosed with Social Phobia because social anxiety and isolation commonly occur as a result of their excessive concerns with appearance. Patients like Ms. J may be reluctant to volunteer their body dysmorphic concerns or may minimize them because of embarrassment. If the clinician elicits concerns that involve appearance and meet criteria for Body Dysmorphic Disorder, this is the appropriate diagnosis and an additional diagnosis of Social Phobia should not be given.

Only Anorexia Nervosa is diagnosed if the person's body image problems are limited to a concern about size and weight. Although Ms. J was concerned that her buttocks were too large, she was not preoccupied with overall "fatness" and did not have other features of an Eating Disorder.

In the process of developing DSM-IV, an interesting issue arose concerning how to handle a preoccupation with appearance that reaches delusional proportions. Three options were considered: 1) adding a delusional subtype for Body Dysmorphic Disorder; 2) requiring a diagnosis of Delusional Disorder, Somatic Type, when the beliefs were delusional in nature; or 3) allowing both diagnoses to be made when appropriate. Pending more data, the third choice was accepted, although this should not be taken to mean that two separate pathogenetic processes are at work.

The beliefs in Body Dysmorphic Disorder occur on a continuum and may vary in a single individual over time. At one end of the continuum are non-pathological concerns about appearance that would not warrant a diagnosis; at the other end lie delusions about appearance, with overvalued ideas falling somewhere in the middle. It is difficult to determine whether Ms. J's usual beliefs about her appearance are delusional or not. After much questioning, her insight appears to be poor and her thinking would probably best be considered to consist of overvalued ideas, making a diagnosis of Body Dysmorphic Disorder alone appropriate.

Treatment Planning for
Body Dysmorphic Disorder

Little systematic investigation of the treatment of Body Dysmorphic Disorder has been done, and no controlled treatment studies have been completed. The treatment data that are available were obtained retrospectively or from open studies. Attempts to reassure those with this disorder that their defect is minimal or doesn't exist are usually not effective. It does appear that serotonin reuptake inhibitors are most likely to be effective in the treatment of Body Dysmorphic Disorder. Adequate treatment often requires a relatively long duration and a higher dose of serotonin reuptake inhibitors than is typically needed for depression. Cognitive-behavioral strategies (e.g., exposure therapy, response prevention, self-esteem building, modification of distorted thinking, and instruction in coping strategies) may also be useful, especially when combined with pharmacotherapy.

Summary

Body Dysmorphic Disorder lies on a continuum that includes normal concerns about appearance at one end and somatic delusions at the other. Although most people don't like at least some aspect of their appearance, the diagnosis of Body Dysmorphic Disorder is reserved for those who have major impairment or distress because of their dissatisfaction. There is some controversy about where to draw the boundary between the excessive somatic concerns of Body Dysmorphic Disorder and the somatic delusions of Delusional Disorder.

Chapter 8

Factitious Disorders

Factitious Disorder is probably the most underdiagnosed condition in psychiatry. It is not in the nature or training of most clinicians to doubt the veracity of the symptoms patients present to us. For the most part, this credulity is usually for the best because it would be very difficult to treat patients empathetically if one were always questioning their motivations and truthfulness. In some settings, such as forensic and Department of Veterans Affairs (VA) settings and some state facilities, the challenge is to avoid becoming cynical. But in most settings the relative innocence of mental health practitioners may lead them to be taken in by individuals for whom hospitalization or some other form of care is an end in itself. Factitious Disorder With Predominantly Physical Signs and Symptoms (i.e., Munchausen syndrome) has been much more commonly and colorfully described in those who present with the "symptoms" of a general medical condition. Although it is likely that Factitious Disorder With Predominantly Psychological Signs and Symptoms is far more prevalent, it is usually missed and is much more difficult to establish.

DSM-III-R listed two separate Factitious Disorders: "With Physical Symptoms" and "With Psychological Symptoms." Those presentations that were a mixture of these two types of symptoms were listed as "Factitious Disorder Not Otherwise Specified." For the sake of simplicity and to capture the common situation in which both psychological and physical symptoms are present, DSM-IV (and DSM-IV-TR) provides a single criteria set for Factitious Disorder, with subtypes that are coded on the basis of the nature of the presentation:

Factitious Disorders

300.xx	Factitious Disorder
.16	With Predominantly Psychological Signs and Symptoms
.19	With Predominantly Physical Signs and Symptoms
.19	With Combined Psychological and Physical Signs and Symptoms
300.19	Factitious Disorder Not Otherwise Specified

A category 300.19 Factitious Disorder Not Otherwise Specified is also included to allow clinicians to note presentations that are factitious in nature but do not meet the criteria for Factitious Disorder. Factitious disorder by proxy is a proposed new category that describes individuals who intentionally produce or feign physical or psychological symptoms, or both, in a person who is under their care (usually a child) for the purpose of indirectly assuming the sick role. Factitious disorder by proxy was not included in DSM-IV because it has not been well studied and might be used to exonerate someone who is engaged in child abuse; however, it is considered an example of Factitious Disorder Not Otherwise Specified and a research criteria set is included in the DSM-IV (and DSM-IV-TR) appendix for proposed categories needing further study.

❖   Case Study: The Voices Will Make Me Do It

Ms. R is a 35-year-old unemployed single mother whose chief complaint is that a voice is commanding her to kill herself. She has a history of 18 previous psychiatric hospitalizations for a variety of frequently changing symptom presentations. Her diagnoses over the years have included Schizophrenia, Bipolar Disorder With Psychotic Features, Major Depression With Psychotic Features, Schizoaffective Disorder, Posttraumatic Stress Disorder, Panic Disorder, Anorexia Nervosa, Multiple Personality Disorder, and Borderline Personality Disorder. She also frequently engages in self-destructive behavior such as cutting her wrists, head banging, and abusing prescription opiate analgesics and alcohol.

Ms. R lives with her parents and her 10-year-old son in a very tense situation. Her parents constantly fight and are threatening to separate after 40 years of marriage. Shortly before Ms. R was admitted, they began making plans to go away for a week to see whether they could resolve their difficulties. Ms. R's son has learning difficulties in school, has frequently been truant, and has conduct problems. Ms. R is frightened that her ex-husband may try to take him away from her because of inadequate mothering. Her lesbian lover, with whom she has been having an affair for the previous 6 months, is also threatening to break up their relationship. Although she has been both physically and emotionally abused by this woman, Ms. R refuses to give up the affair.

Ms. R's medical history includes a congenital heart defect that required several reconstructive surgeries during her preschool years and repeated hospitalizations at ages 10, 13, 17, and 21 because of endocarditis. Her psychosocial history is notable for several years of sexual abuse by her brother. A mental status examination reveals no prominent mania or depression and no psychotic symptoms other than the auditory hallucination; her cognition is intact.

Ms. R is admitted to the inpatient unit, where her command hallucinations seem to disappear almost immediately. Unfortunately, the patient's initial response to the inpatient milieu also includes a marked behavioral regression with childlike speech and mannerisms, dependence on staff members for help in meeting basic needs, and increased self-destructive acts that require restraint. The staff reacts with covert anger toward Ms. R, who appears to them to be behaving in this way to force them to keep her in the hospital. Her parents interpret this behavior as the patient's selfish attempt to prevent them from leaving on vacation.

It becomes clear that the patient's numerous medical and psychiatric hospitalizations have nearly all been in response to threatened separations. The hospital structure, familiar to her from numerous childhood illnesses, serves to contain the sense of panic and disorganization that she feels when she is about to be abandoned. Once the hospital staff members understand this relationship, they are able to prepare Ms. R gradually for discharge through planned, stepwise decreases in structure. She is given off-unit privileges, first with other people and then alone, and short and then longer passes. She also begins attending outpatient sessions before her discharge. On the day before her planned discharge, the patient's "command hallucinations" return; however, she is able to see that this is no more than her way of indicating that she is afraid to go home.

DSM-IV-TR Diagnosis

Axis I:	300.16	Factitious Disorder With Predominantly Psychological Signs and Symptoms
Axis II:	V71.09	No diagnosis
Axis III:	746.9	Congenital heart defect, history of numerous surgeries and endocarditis
Axis IV:	Parents' proposed separation	
Axis V:	GAF = 30 (on admission); 50 (on outpatient follow-up)	

> ## DSM-IV-TR diagnostic criteria for Factitious Disorder
>
> A. Intentional production or feigning of physical or psychological signs or symptoms.
> B. The motivation for the behavior is to assume the sick role.
> C. External incentives for the behavior (such as economic gain, avoiding legal responsibility, or improving physical well-being, as in Malingering) are absent.
>
> Code based on type:
> 300.16 With Predominantly Psychological Signs and Symptoms: if psychological signs and symptoms predominate in the clinical presentation
> 300.19 With Predominantly Physical Signs and Symptoms: if physical signs and symptoms predominate in the clinical presentation
> 300.19 With Combined Psychological and Physical Signs and Symptoms: if both psychological and physical signs and symptoms are present but neither predominates in the clinical presentation

Guidelines for Differential Diagnosis of Factitious Disorder

Factitious Disorder requires a conscious feigning of symptoms. It must be distinguished from V65.2 Malingering, which is listed in DSM-IV-TR as a problem, not a disorder, in the section on Other Conditions That May Be a Focus of Clinical Attention. In both Factitious Disorder and Malingering, the symptoms are intentionally produced or feigned; the difference between these diagnoses is in the motivation. The goal of Factitious Disorder is to assume the sick role in order to receive care, whereas the gains from Malingering are more external and practical (e.g., escaping responsibilities or duties, avoiding prison, and obtaining financial compensation or drugs). Some factors that may make Malingering more likely are presentation in a legal context (e.g., referral by an attorney), failure to cooperate with evaluation or treatment (whereas those with Factitious Disorder tend to eagerly seek treatment), and symptoms that meet criteria for Antisocial Personality Disorder.

Clinicians tend not to think of Factitious Disorder With Predominantly Psychological Signs and Symptoms nearly often enough. Many psychiatric patients become dependent on the treatment system and feign symptoms to get increased help from it.

The first clues that Factitious Disorder might be a concern in Ms. R's case are the frequency of her hospitalizations and the variety of different psychiatric diagnoses she has received over time. When patients are hospitalized frequently, it may reflect the seriousness of their condition or their noncompliance with treatment. But sometimes it results from their use of the hospital to elicit care and to avoid unpleasant situations or seemingly daunting responsibilities. In such situations, it is useful to investigate reasons why the patient might feign symptoms to gain hospitalization or to remain in the hospital. This must be done gently but firmly. Clinicians are often reluctant to confront patients about the possibility that they may be exaggerating or making up symptoms, particularly because it often leads to angry outbursts or requests for another doctor. However, thorough questioning about the nature of the symptoms and pointing out ways in which they are implausible and atypical may at times allow patients to acknowledge that they may have been exaggerating. They may then go on to express their needs in a more direct way. Very atypical presentations, especially ones that conform to popular ideas of the disorder, also suggest the possibility that the symptoms could be feigned.

Treatment Planning for Factitious Disorder

Prevention of Factitious Disorder requires avoiding unnecessary hospitalizations, keeping hospital stays as short as possible, and providing dependency gratification in other ways. There is no specific treatment for Factitious Disorder. The main management goal is to avoid encouraging regressive dependency. This requires careful evaluation before admission to the hospital, shorter rather than longer hospital stays, and provision of support in less intensive outpatient environments. However, it is important to recognize that a determined and self-destructive patient always holds the upper hand. What seems like an unnecessary hospitalization may be unavoidable if the clinician believes that the patient will "raise the ante" with suicide attempts.

Summary

Unfortunately, it is easy both to overlook Factitious Disorder and to overdiagnose it. It is difficult for clinicians not to believe their patients, and Factitious Disorder is probably most often underdiagnosed in psychiatric settings. Psychiatric patients can become addicted to hospitals and may feign symptoms to obtain rehospitalization more often than clinicians realize. On the other hand, as noted above, in settings such as prisons and VA and state hospitals, feigning is sufficiently common that clinicians may become unduly skeptical and overdiagnose Factitious Disorder, attributing to conscious feigning what is in fact primary psychopathology. The most commonly feigned psychiatric symptoms these days are command hallucinations, Posttraumatic Stress Disorder, and Dissociative Identity Disorder, but these styles change with time and with what is current on the television talk shows.

Chapter 9

Dissociative Disorders

D SM-IV-TR defines the essential feature of the Dissociative Disorders as "disruption in the usually integrated functions of consciousness, memory, identity, or perception." This section includes the following disorders:

Dissociative Disorders

300.12 Dissociative Amnesia
300.13 Dissociative Fugue
300.14 Dissociative Identity Disorder (formerly Multiple Personality Disorder)
300.6   Depersonalization Disorder
300.15 Dissociative Disorder Not Otherwise Specified

It should be noted that dissociative symptoms are also associated with several disorders that are included in other sections (e.g., Acute Stress Disorder, Posttraumatic Stress Disorder, and Somatization Disorder). A separate Dissociative Disorder diagnosis would not be made if the dissociative symptoms occurred exclusively in the course of another disorder.

The clinician should be especially careful in evaluating dissociative symptoms in individuals from unfamiliar cultural backgrounds. Dissociative states are commonly accepted as part of religious or social experiences in many cultures. When dissociation does not cause significant distress or impairment, it should not be considered pathological and would not warrant the diagnosis of a mental disorder.

Dissociative Identity Disorder

❖ Case Study: Would-Be Multiple Personality Disorder

Ms. M is a 26-year-old single woman who is hospitalized because of a suicide attempt. She has a long history of psychiatric care. Upon evaluation, she appears to have the symptoms of a typical borderline personality. She feels a great deal of self-hate and confusion about her identity, does not get along with others, feels that she never fits in, and has a hard time making friends. At the same time, Ms. M is highly intelligent and creative and has published poetry in several magazines. Her relationships are extremely intense and passionate, and she often frightens herself and those around her with her unbridled emotions.

Ms. M first intentionally cut herself when she was 15 because she had no date for the junior prom. She has mutilated herself several hundred times over the course of intervening years. She has also used drugs of abuse, including LSD, PCP, and cocaine, fairly intensively since her late teens. She has made two previous serious suicide attempts by overdose, one of which required intubation and a 2-week hospitalization. She has been hospitalized on at least 10 occasions for suicide attempts or ideation or self-mutilation, with stays ranging from 3 days to 3 months. She has received a number of different psychiatric diagnoses, including Borderline Personality Disorder and Bipolar Disorder. None of the treatments she has received have been effective.

During a hospitalization about a year and a half before this admission, Ms. M encountered another patient with Multiple Personality Disorder and decided that this diagnosis might also account for her symptoms. She voraciously devoured books and articles, in the popular press and in psychiatric literature, about Multiple Personality Disorder. She began therapy with a clinician who was reported to be an expert in the area, and after several weeks he was able to identify three personalities: Jane, quiet and subdued; Alice, very aggressive; and Delores, sexually seductive. Ms. M became more and more preoccupied with discovering aspects of her various personalities, and, by year's end, she and the therapist had identified 12 separate personalities. Through the memories retained by one of her personalities, Ms. M discovered that she had been sexually abused by her father as a young child and possibly by her uncle, although she is less sure of this. During the course of the next year, an additional 55 personalities emerged. She attributes her most recent suicide attempt to one of the personalities who was trying to kill only herself but could not avoid potentially harming all the others.

DSM-IV-TR Diagnosis

Axis I:	300.14	Possible Dissociative Identity Disorder
Axis II:	301.83	Borderline Personality Disorder
Axis III:	None	
Axis IV:	None	
Axis V:	GAF = 40	

DSM-IV-TR diagnostic criteria for 300.14 Dissociative Identity Disorder

A. The presence of two or more distinct identities or personality states (each with its own relatively enduring pattern of perceiving, relating to, and thinking about the environment and self).
B. At least two of these identities or personality states recurrently take control of the person's behavior.
C. Inability to recall important personal information that is too extensive to be explained by ordinary forgetfulness.
D. The disturbance is not due to the direct physiological effects of a substance (e.g., blackouts or chaotic behavior during Alcohol Intoxication) or a general medical condition (e.g., complex partial seizures). **Note:** In children, the symptoms are not attributable to imaginary playmates or other fantasy play.

Guidelines for Differential Diagnosis of Dissociative Identity Disorder

The name of this condition was changed from Multiple Personality Disorder to Dissociative Identity Disorder in DSM-IV to more accurately describe the symptoms, which involve disturbances in identity and memory rather than a Personality Disorder. Multiple Personality Disorder was first included in the official psychiatric classification in DSM-III. Since its introduction, there has been a marked increase in the diagnosis of this disorder in the United States—an increase that can be interpreted in two ways. Some clinicians believe that Dissociative Identity Disorder was previously often missed or misdiagnosed as a Psychotic or Bipolar Disorder. These clinicians believe that the current greater awareness of the diagnosis (and of the etiological role of childhood sexual abuse) among mental health professionals has resulted in earlier and more appropriate identification of the disorder. Many other clinicians, however, believe that this disorder is currently being vastly overdiagnosed (or even iatrogenically induced) in individuals who are highly suggestible. These clinicians are particularly concerned that attempts to identify and communicate with previously unrecognized "alters" may encourage dissociation rather than cure it.

Lately, it seems that many patients one encounters proclaim that their problems are due to a Multiple Personality Disorder. This "epidemic" likely is the result of the wide media attention this disorder has received and of the iatrogenic efforts of poorly trained or overzealous therapists.

Patients also learn new symptoms from other patients. Ms. M is clearly an unhappy and creative woman searching for some explanation for her interpersonal difficulties, low esteem, and shaky sense of identity. She first "discovered" herself as a "multiple" after meeting someone else in the hospital who had made the same discovery. She was quick to adopt this currently highly popular metaphor that her psychological conflicts are accounted for by a war between "her multiple personalities."

Treatment Planning for Dissociative Identity Disorder

The most important consideration is to do no harm. Although problems can be created when therapists are callously cynical and refuse to believe their patients' subjective experience, it can also be unhelpful for therapists to wittingly or unwittingly suggest a further compartmentalization in the identities of those who are already on shaky ground. Before Dissociative Identity Disorder became the world's most popular diagnosis, it was relatively uncommon and patients who did present with this disorder reported only a handful of personalities. Now Dissociative Identity Disorder appears to be ubiquitous, and the average number of personalities reported per patient has skyrocketed to 20 and is still growing.

It seems most likely that the development of Dissociative Identity Disorder in Ms. M represents an attempt on her part, in collaboration with her therapist, to make some sense of her very chaotic experiences. However, it is likely this may do more harm than good. By labeling each aspect of Ms. M's ambivalent personality with a different name and by attributing independent powers to each, the therapist is encouraging the disintegration rather than the integration of her personality.

Summary

Throughout the history of psychiatric classification, there has been a succession of fad diagnoses. One of us is very familiar with a long-term inpatient unit that clearly illustrates this problem. When he trained there 25 years ago, nearly all the patients were diagnosed as having "pseudoneurotic schizophrenia." Several years later, there was a change in unit leadership and the prevailing diagnosis became "Borderline Personality Disorder." A few years later, the wheel turned a bit more and most of the patients seemed to have "atypical depressions." It should be no surprise that the unit is now filled with patients with "Multiple Personality Disorder" and/or "Posttraumatic Stress Disorder." We expect that soon most of them will have a diagnosis of "Adult Attention-Deficit Disorder." In fact, the patients treated on this unit have remained remarkably similar over the years—only the diagnostic labels have changed.

Chapter 10

Sexual and Gender Identity Disorders

The Sexual and Gender Identity Disorders section of DSM-IV-TR includes Sexual Dysfunctions, Paraphilias, and Gender Identity Disorders.

Sexual Dysfunctions are characterized by disturbances in sexual desire or functioning that cause marked distress or interpersonal difficulty. The following Sexual Dysfunctions are included in this section:

Sexual Dysfunctions

302.71	Hypoactive Sexual Desire Disorder
302.79	Sexual Aversion Disorder
302.72	Female Sexual Arousal Disorder
302.72	Male Erectile Disorder
302.73	Female Orgasmic Disorder
302.74	Male Orgasmic Disorder
302.75	Premature Ejaculation
302.76	Dyspareunia
306.51	Vaginismus
—.–	Sexual Dysfunction Due to a General Medical Condition
—.–	Substance-Induced Sexual Dysfunction
302.70	Sexual Dysfunction Not Otherwise Specified

Paraphilias refer to disorders that involve unusual sexual preferences that cause clinically significant distress or impairment (or, for some of the paraphilias, marked distress or interpersonal difficulty) or involve children or nonconsenting adults. The following Paraphilias are included in DSM-IV-TR:

Paraphilias

302.4   Exhibitionism
302.81   Fetishism
302.89   Frotteurism
302.2   Pedophilia
302.83   Sexual Masochism
302.84   Sexual Sadism
302.3   Transvestic Fetishism
302.82   Voyeurism
302.9   Paraphilia Not Otherwise Specified

Gender Identity Disorders are characterized by strong and persistent cross-gender identification and a marked discomfort with one's own sex. The Gender Identity Disorders are coded as follows:

Gender Identity Disorders

302.6   Gender Identity Disorder in Children
302.85   Gender Identity Disorder in Adolescents or Adults
302.6   Gender Identity Disorder Not Otherwise Specified

Finally, 302.9 Sexual Disorder Not Otherwise Specified is included for coding a sexual disturbance that does not meet criteria for a specific Sexual Disorder and is neither a Sexual Dysfunction nor a Paraphilia.

We present cases illustrating Female Orgasmic Disorder/Hypoactive Sexual Desire Disorder, Male Erectile Disorder, and Transvestic Fetishism.

Female Orgasmic Disorder/
Hypoactive Sexual Desire Disorder

❖ Case Study: We Live Like Brother and Sister

Ms. G is a very beautiful 28-year-old schoolteacher who presents for consultation because her husband is dissatisfied with their sex life and has insisted that she seek therapy. They have been married for 6 years and for most of that time have had sex approximately once a week, but without passion. Ms. G tends to avoid sexual encounters with her husband by going to sleep early or late or saying she is tired or feels sick. Matters have recently deteriorated to the point where the couple makes love less than once a month and only at Mr. G's insistence.

Ms. G comes from a rigidly proper and religious family. When she was 7 years old, she was surprised and "mortified" when her 13-year-old brother began to regularly expose his penis to her and touch her genitals. Ms. G hated these experiences and knew they were sinful. She tried to confess them to her mother and at church but could not because she was so ashamed of them and because her brother threatened to hurt her if she told. Intermittent sexual contact with her brother continued for about a year and ended only when he was sent away to boarding school because he was having other behavioral troubles as well.

Ms. G was slow to enter puberty and did not date until age 18. Her future husband was the boy next door. Initially, she felt surprised that anyone would find her attractive and was taken aback by his attentions, but soon they became inseparable. He is still her best friend and, as she puts it, "We live like brother and sister."

Even at the height of their sexual activity, Ms. G never experienced an orgasm. She regards this as a major failure in her life and as proof that she is lacking in true femininity. Although Ms. G tries very hard to have an orgasm whenever the couple has sex, she is unable to and feels even more inferior and disappointed in herself. She also tries very hard to fake an orgasm for her husband's benefit but apparently is unconvincing.

Ms. G is very self-conscious about her body and does not let her husband see her undressed except in very dim light. She is also shy about looking at him. In her view, intercourse is meant to be done quickly and to focus on genital contact, not on other kinds of touching or looking.

Although Ms. G has had fleeting sexual feelings toward other men, she finds these sensations horrible and demeaning and reveals them only with great embarrassment. She has never masturbated and believes that to do so would prove that she is sexually inadequate.

DSM-IV-TR Diagnosis

Axis I: 302.73   Female Orgasmic Disorder, Lifelong Type,
                        Generalized Type, Due to Psychological
                        Factors

             302.71   Hypoactive Sexual Desire Disorder, Lifelong Type,
                        Generalized Type, Due to Psychological
                        Factors

Axis II: V71.09   No diagnosis (based on two interviews)
Axis III: None
Axis IV: Marital stress
Axis V: GAF = 70 (current)

DSM-IV-TR diagnostic criteria for 302.73 Female Orgasmic Disorder

A. Persistent or recurrent delay in, or absence of, orgasm following a normal sexual excitement phase. Women exhibit wide variability in the type or intensity of stimulation that triggers orgasm. The diagnosis of Female Orgasmic Disorder should be based on the clinician's judgment that the woman's orgasmic capacity is less than would be reasonable for her age, sexual experience, and the adequacy of sexual stimulation she receives.
B. The disturbance causes marked distress or interpersonal difficulty.
C. The orgasmic dysfunction is not better accounted for by another Axis I disorder (except another Sexual Dysfunction) and is not due exclusively to the direct physiological effects of a substance (e.g., a drug of abuse, a medication) or a general medical condition.

Specify type:
Lifelong Type
Acquired Type

Specify type:
Generalized Type
Situational Type

Specify:
Due to Psychological Factors
Due to Combined Factors

DSM-IV-TR diagnostic criteria for
302.71 Hypoactive Sexual Desire Disorder

A. Persistently or recurrently deficient (or absent) sexual fantasies and desire for sexual activity. The judgment of deficiency or absence is made by the clinician, taking into account factors that affect sexual functioning, such as age and the context of the person's life.
B. The disturbance causes marked distress or interpersonal difficulty.
C. The sexual dysfunction is not better accounted for by another Axis I disorder (except another Sexual Dysfunction) and is not due exclusively to the direct physiological effects of a substance (e.g., a drug of abuse, a medication) or a general medical condition.

Specify type:
Lifelong Type
Acquired Type

Specify type:
Generalized Type
Situational Type

Specify:
Due to Psychological Factors
Due to Combined Factors

Male Erectile Disorder

❖   Case Study: A Stud Gone Limp

Mr. X is a 46-year-old printer whose chief complaint is impotence. He comes in at the urging of his wife, age 48, who does not accompany him to the interview. The couple has been married for 25 years and has two children.

Mr. X's erectile difficulties began about 6 years ago. At that time, he was laid off from a valued job he had held for 15 years because the company he was working for merged with another business. His wife supported the family while he was unemployed. He was able to find another excellent position after being unemployed for a year. Before that time, he had an active and successful sex life with his wife and with numerous other partners.

At first, Mr. X experienced only occasional episodes of erectile failure, but within a year he was having great difficulty having intercourse with any partner on any occasion. He states that he has rarely been able to have intercourse with his wife during the past 5 years because he usually cannot attain an erection. The patient nevertheless still has a strong desire for sex and feels frustrated and defeated by his impotence. He is able to achieve full erections when he masturbates, however, and his orgasms have remained pleasurable. Mr. X occasionally wakes up in the morning with a firm erection and sometimes becomes erect while driving his car, "when I'm not thinking about anything."

Mr. X says that his wife has become increasingly critical of his lack of sexual performance over the past year and recently threatened to leave him if he did not seek help. Before the onset of the problem, the couple had intercourse two or three times a week. Over the past year, Mr. X has increasingly avoided all sexual contact with his wife and with other partners because of his inability to achieve an erection.

An analysis of Mr. X's sexual experiences and functioning reveals that in the past he would become spontaneously erect merely by being in the presence of a sexually available and attractive partner. He could also be aroused by briefly fondling and caressing a woman. He did not require manual or oral stimulation to attain an erection ("I didn't need that"), which he could then maintain as long as he liked. He was very proud of his former erectile capability and "staying power," and he and his wife had both been satisfied with their former sexual pattern.

Since his problem began, Mr. X has been entering sexual situations with intense anxiety, anticipating sexual failure. He will fondle his wife for a few moments and, if he fails to attain an immediate erection, becomes agitated and leaves the bed. His wife makes no attempt to stimulate his genitals.

Three years ago the patient was found to be mildly hypertensive. He has been taking propranolol 30 mg/day since that time. He has suffered from chronic low back pain on and off for many years; there are no signs or symptoms of any other medical illness. The patient has never experienced any major psychiatric signs or symptoms, and he has never required psychiatric treatment.

Ms. X is the dominant force in the marriage, with Mr. X playing the role of "bad boy" while she is "momma." This relationship used to work well for both of them, and both were satisfied with the arrangement; however, Mr. X's current sexual problem seems to have disrupted the previous equilibrium of their relationship and to have evoked ambivalence in both spouses. Although Ms. X was often angered by Mr. X's infidelities earlier in their marriage, she never threatened to leave him until recently. Ms. X also feels that her husband's sexual failures mean she is no longer attractive.

DSM-IV-TR Diagnosis

Axis I:	302.72	Male Erectile Disorder, Acquired Type, Situational Type, Due to Psychological Factors
	V61.10	Partner Relational Problem
Axis II:	V71.09	No diagnosis
Axis III:	401.9	Hypertension
	724.2	Low back pain
Axis IV:	Recent unemployment, dependency on wife	
Axis V:	GAF = 70	

DSM-IV-TR diagnostic criteria for 302.72 Male Erectile Disorder

A. Persistent or recurrent inability to attain, or to maintain until completion of the sexual activity, an adequate erection.
B. The disturbance causes marked distress or interpersonal difficulty.
C. The erectile dysfunction is not better accounted for by another Axis I disorder (other than a Sexual Dysfunction) and is not due exclusively to the direct physiological effects of a substance (e.g., a drug of abuse, a medication) or a general medical condition.

Specify type:
Lifelong Type
Acquired Type

Specify type:
Generalized Type
Situational Type

Specify:
Due to Psychological Factors
Due to Combined Factors

Guidelines for Differential Diagnosis of the Sexual Dysfunctions

The first differential to consider in diagnosing a Sexual Dysfunction is normality. There are no generally accepted guidelines for what should be considered "normal" sexual functioning. Before diagnosing a Sexual Dysfunction, the clinician must take into account the person's age and level of experience; the mores prevalent in the person's cultural and religious background; the adequacy of the sexual stimulation; and, most important, the degree to which the sexual problem is causing the person distress or inter-personal difficulty. Not everyone has to be passionately sexual. If Ms. G were not distressed by her sexual problem and felt satisfied with her mar-riage as it is, a diagnosis of Sexual Dysfunction would not be warranted, especially if her partner were also satisfied with their "brother-sister ar-rangement." Often the differential diagnosis is between a Sexual Dysfunc-tion in one individual and a diagnosis of V61.1 Partner Relational Problem in the couple.

Once it is decided that the Sexual Dysfunction is clinically significant enough to warrant a diagnosis, the next step is to determine the etiology of the disturbance. Sexual problems can result from psychological factors, the ef-fects of a general medical condition, medication side effects, Substance Abuse, or a combination of these factors. If the Sexual Dysfunction is judged to be completely accounted for by a general medical condition (e.g., a neuro-logical or endocrine condition), then Sexual Dysfunction Due to a General Medical Condition is diagnosed and coded according to the predominant type of dysfunction present. If the Sexual Dysfunction is judged to be completely accounted for by a medication side effect or Substance Abuse, then Substance-Induced Sexual Dysfunction is diagnosed and coded according to the type of substance involved, with a specifier indicating the predominant type of dys-function present. When the Sexual Dysfunction is judged to be the result of exclusively psychological factors or, as is often the case, a combination of psy-chological factors and the effects of a general medical condition and/or a sub-stance, then the specific type of Sexual Dysfunction is diagnosed and the appropriate subtype, "Due to Psychological Factors" or "Due to Combined Factors," is noted.

The four phases of sexual response are 1) sexual desire, 2) sexual excite-ment, 3) orgasm, and 4) resolution. Although Sexual Dysfunctions are orga-nized according to the stage of sexual response in which they occur, it is important to remember that individuals often have related problems that oc-cur in more than one phase (e.g., an Arousal Disorder and an Orgasmic Disor-der) that are really different facets of a single problem. This appears to be the case for Ms. G, who is diagnosed with both Hypoactive Sexual Desire Disor-der and Female Orgasmic Disorder. These problems are clearly related to each other. Ms. G's embarrassed attitude toward sex and lack of sexual desire contribute to her inability to have an orgasm, making her even more eager to avoid sexual contact with her husband.

Additional specifiers can be noted to indicate whether the Sexual Dysfunc-tion is the Lifelong or Acquired Type and whether the dysfunction is the General-ized or Situational Type. In the first case we presented, Ms. G's sexual problems appear to have been lifelong and generalized; in the second case, Mr. X 's sexual problems are recently acquired and related to specific situations. The first consideration in evaluating Mr. X's symptoms is whether a medication, a general medical condition, or Substance Use could be causing the erectile problem. However, a physiological factor is ruled out because Mr. X gets a full erection while masturbating or upon awakening. In equivocal cases, laboratory testing may be necessary to confirm and quantify the level of the impairment.

Treatment Planning for Sexual Dysfunctions

The first issue in planning treatment for Ms. G is to evaluate her motivation to participate in a therapy aimed at changing her sexual functioning and the degree to which she wants to work toward a more satisfying sexual relationship with her husband. For individuals who are motivated to participate, the simplest and most straightforward treatment is a cognitive-behavior sex therapy that often includes both partners. Such therapy usually involves teaching the couple about sex, giving them homework exercises that involve giving each other pleasure (e.g., taking showers together, massages, and petting), and generally giving them permission to enjoy themselves. If this approach does not work or if the patient is not motivated, a psychodynamic approach may be indicated. This would entail exploring Ms. G's sexual fears and wishes, relating them to early sexual experiences in the family, and targeting her guilt over her experiences with her brother.

A combination of both methods may be helpful, with the cognitive-behavior therapy focusing on the here and now by teaching Ms. G about her sexuality and helping her to feel free to take pleasure in her sexual relationship with her husband and the psychodynamic therapy focusing on an exploration of her unconscious wishes and fears.

Often a sexual problem is clearly related to other problems in a relationship, and it is difficult to determine which came first. Relationship issues must be addressed to achieve the motivation and goodwill needed for sexual therapy to succeed. For example, Ms. X has felt a long-standing anger about her husband's infidelities, and Mr. X's loss of sexual function has affected the previous roles he and his wife played in the marriage. To treat Mr. X's sexual problems, the therapist will probably need to focus on the couple's relational problems and on Mr. X's loss of self-esteem related to performance anxiety. The presumption is that Mr. X is in the midst of a vicious cycle in which he suffers from high performance expectations that are accompanied by a fear of failure, which has become a self-fulfilling prophecy. Mr. X's sexual failures appear to be due to this performance anxiety and low self-esteem, with each subsequent failure increasing his anxiety and thus making future failures even more likely and further eroding his self-esteem. It is probable that this pattern first developed during the period when Mr. X was out of work and his wife was supporting him, but the problem took on a life of its own and continued even after Mr. X obtained another good job. It would be most helpful for this couple to work together. Both the cognitive-behavioral and the psychodynamic approaches described above can be useful in treating couples as well as individuals. For Mr. X, the psychodynamic approach would focus on the degree to which his self-esteem is invested in his sexual prowess.

Of course, the major change in the treatment of sexual dysfunction over the last decade has been the introduction of sildenafil (Viagra), which is able to improve erectile dysfunction of various etiologies (physical, psychological, medication-induced) in many cases. For some individuals, sildenafil treatment alone appears to be sufficient. Other patients may require a combination of sildenafil and psychotherapy.

Summary

It is very hard to judge what constitutes the "right" amount of sexual potency, adequate sexual performance, or enough sexual desire, given the wide variability among individuals and the degree to which these factors may depend on the vicissitudes of relational matchups and on the cultural norms of the group to which the individual belongs. Clinicians should be careful to follow the judgment of the patient or couple rather than imposing their own values in making this evaluation.

Currently, the most commonly encountered causes of orgasmic difficulties are probably medications (especially the selective serotonin reuptake inhibitors and antihypertensives) and Substance Use, and it is important to rule these out first. Sexual Dysfunctions, especially in older individuals, may also be related to physical problems or hormonal changes. Because the sexual response cycle is continuous, it is not surprising that individuals who have problems at one stage often have problems at other stages. Finally, it is always important to determine whether another mental disorder is present that might account for the Sexual Dysfunction (e.g., Major Depressive Disorder).

Transvestic Fetishism

❖   Case Study: The Secret Cross-Dresser

Mr. L, a 43-year-old accountant, seeks psychiatric consultation after his wife's discovery that he secretly wears women's clothes. He states that he has episodically cross-dressed since adolescence but has kept this behavior secret from his wife during the 3 years of their marriage. When his wife finally discovered this practice, she demanded that he seek psychiatric help or she would leave him.

Mr. L recalls that he first cross-dressed by wearing his mother's undergarments when he was age 7. When he was an adolescent, his cross-dressing increased in frequency and usually was accompanied by sexual excitement and masturbation. Mr. L would secretly purchase women's clothes but would periodically become ashamed of the cross-dressing and would throw them away. In times of stress, however, the urge to cross-dress would recur and he would then go out and buy women's clothing again.

Mr. L was raised in a strict middle-class family. His hardworking father was a stern disciplinarian who was feared by Mr. L's mother, to whom the patient was very close. Mr. L has two siblings who have no unusual sexual practices as far as he knows. As an adolescent, Mr. L was interested in athletics and played two varsity sports in high school and college. He entered the military following college and was awarded various citations for bravery during the Vietnam conflict. He rarely dated and had minimal sexual experience before marriage.

Mr. L met his future wife when she came in for financial assistance. He was attracted by her gentleness and because she made him feel more secure. Mr. L describes his marriage as stable but notes that his wife complains that he is too self-absorbed and not sufficiently interested in her sexually. He goes on to explain that he is usually quiet at home and does not make many domestic decisions, leaving these to his wife. The patient denies any marital infidelity and does not feel there is any problem in the couple's sexual life, which consists of intercourse once a week.

Cross-dressing provides Mr. L with extreme sexual excitement, much more than does actual sex with a woman. The patient describes the pressure to cross-dress fetishistically as "overpowering" and "preoccupying." Because his work requires frequent overnight travel, the patient often cross-dresses in hotel rooms and masturbates but has never appeared in women's garments in public. He views his behavior as a "quirk" in his development and is only slightly embarrassed by it. Mr. L is tall and appears very masculine. He has no homoerotic fantasies and has never had any homosexual experiences, nor is he gender-dysphoric. He has occasionally wondered whether he would be happier as a woman but has never considered sexual reassignment and, in fact, the thought scares him.

Mr. L describes himself as a quiet, moody individual. He is very upset at his wife's reaction to his cross-dressing because this behavior is very important to him. He is not sure what he wants from a psychiatric consultation except to assuage his wife's anger; he does not want to give up his cross-dressing.

On mental status examination, the patient gives his history fluently without any evidence of major psychopathological phenomena. He shows no guilt or anxiety concerning his sexual behavior. He has no vegetative symptoms or any thoughts of self-harm or autocastration. His mood is unremarkable, and his sensorium is intact.

DSM-IV-TR Diagnosis

Axis I: 302.3   Transvestic Fetishism
Axis II: Deferred
Axis III: None
Axis IV: Discovery of cross-dressing by wife
Axis V: GAF = 50 (current); 65 (highest level in past year)

DSM-IV-TR diagnostic criteria for 302.3 Transvestic Fetishism

A. Over a period of at least 6 months, in a heterosexual male, recurrent, intense sexually arousing fantasies, sexual urges, or behaviors involving cross-dressing.

B. The fantasies, sexual urges, or behaviors cause clinically significant distress or impairment in social, occupational, or other important areas of functioning.

Specify if:
With Gender Dysphoria: if the person has persistent discomfort with gender role or identity

---

Guidelines for Differential Diagnosis of Transvestic Fetishism

In DSM-IV-TR, Paraphilia refers to a sexual deviation or perversion. Paraphilias are characterized by recurrent, intense sexually arousing fantasies, urges, or behaviors that involve 1) nonhuman objects, 2) the suffering or humiliation of oneself or one's partner, or 3) children or other nonconsenting individuals.

Some individuals can achieve arousal only through paraphiliac fantasies or stimuli, whereas others can also function sexually in other situations (e.g., Mr. L has a sexual relationship with his wife, although he achieves the most sexual satisfaction through his cross-dressing). Note that with the exception of Sexual Masochism, the Paraphilias occur almost exclusively in males. Although DSM-IV-TR lists eight separate types of Paraphilias, they would perhaps have been better described by a single diagnosis with subtypes because the criteria for each type of Paraphilia are very similar.

The main differential for Transvestic Fetishism is with fantasies and behaviors that form a part of "normal" sexual functioning and do not cause clinically significant distress or impairment in social, occupational, or other important areas of functioning. Mr. L's wife was shocked to discover his cross-dressing and has threatened to divorce him if he does not seek treatment. Mr. L's cross-dressing is therefore clearly having a deleterious effect on his relationship with his wife and a diagnosis of Transvestic Fetishism would be warranted.

Some paraphiliac behaviors are by their very nature problematic, because they involve a nonconsenting individual (e.g., Exhibitionism, Frotteurism, and Voyeurism) or a child (Pedophilia), and the individual with these behaviors can be arrested and incarcerated. It is very important to note that an individual who is diagnosed as having a Paraphilia is in no way absolved of criminal responsibility for the behavior.

Treatment Planning for Paraphilias

The treatment of Paraphilias has considerable forensic and public health significance. It has received very little systematic study. Although a variety of cognitive-behavioral, psychodynamic, hormonal, and medication treatments have been reported, mostly in case study format, the optimal treatment and outcome are not well established. There is a wide consensus, however, that the more severe forms of Paraphilia are persistent and resistant to treatment.

Chapter 11

Eating Disorders

E ating Disorders are included in two sections of DSM-IV-TR. Those that are first identified in infancy or very early childhood (i.e., Pica, Rumination Disorder, and Feeding Disorder) are included in the section on Disorders Usually First Diagnosed in Infancy, Childhood, or Adolescence. Although Anorexia Nervosa and Bulimia Nervosa were also included in this section in DSM-III-R, it was decided in DSM-IV to create a separate section for Eating Disorders because of their importance and because they are often first diagnosed after adolescence. The DSM-IV (and DSM-IV-TR) classification for the Eating Disorders section includes the following disorders:

Eating Disorders

307.1   Anorexia Nervosa
         Specify type: Restricting Type; Binge-Eating/Purging Type
307.51   Bulimia Nervosa
         Specify type: Purging Type/Nonpurging Type
307.50   Eating Disorder Not Otherwise Specified

In DSM-III-R, individuals would receive concurrent diagnoses of both Bulimia Nervosa and Anorexia Nervosa if their body image problems and loss of weight were also accompanied by purging behavior. This led to an artifactual overlap in which individuals who really had only one Eating Disorder nevertheless received two diagnoses. The diagnostic algorithm was revised in DSM-IV so that the diagnosis is either Anorexia Nervosa, Binge-Eating/Purging Type, if the patient is markedly underweight, or Bulimia Nervosa, if the patient is normal weight or overweight. The following two cases will illustrate this distinction.

Anorexia Nervosa

❖ Case Study: The Very Thin Ballet Student[1]

Ms. R is a very thin 19-year-old single ballet student who comes in at the insistence of her parents for a consultation concerning her eating behavior. The patient and her family report that Ms. R has had a lifelong interest in ballet. She began to attend classes at age 5, was recognized by her teachers as having impressive talent by age 8, and, since age 14, has been a member of a national ballet company. The patient has had clear difficulties with eating since age 15 when, for reasons that she is unable to explain, she began to induce vomiting after what she felt was overeating. The vomiting was preceded by many years of persistent dieting begun with the encouragement of her ballet teacher. Over the past 3 years, Ms. R's binges have occurred once a day in the evening and have been routinely followed by self-induced vomiting. The binges consist of dozens of rice cakes or, more rarely, a half gallon of ice cream. Ms. R consumes this food late at night, after her parents have gone to bed. For some time, Ms. R's parents have been suspicious that their daughter has a problem with her eating, but she consistently denied difficulties until about a month before this consultation.

Ms. R reached her full height of 5'8" at age 15. Her highest weight was 120 pounds at age 16, which she describes as being "fat." For the past 3 years, her weight has been reasonably stable at between 100 and 104 pounds. She exercises regularly as part of her profession, and she denies the use of laxatives, diuretics, or diet pills as methods of weight control. Except when she is binge eating, she avoids the consumption of high-fat foods and sweets. Since age 15, she has been a strict vegetarian and consumes no meat or eggs and little cheese. For the past 3 or 4 years, Ms. R has been uncomfortable eating in front of other people and goes to great lengths to avoid such situations. This places great limitations on her social life. Ms. R had two spontaneous menstrual periods at age 16 when her weight was about

1. Thanks to B. Timothy Walsh, M.D., of the New York State Psychiatric Institute for supplying these cases.

120 pounds, but she has not menstruated since.

After completing high school, Ms. R became a full-time member of the ballet company. Ballet classes and rehearsals occupy her for about 4 hours a day, and she spends most of the rest of her time reading. She finds historical novels particularly interesting.

Ms. R's parents describe her as being a serious and able student, although they are concerned about her social isolation. She has few close girlfriends and has never dated or had any sexual experiences.

During the interview, the patient is embarrassed and somewhat guarded in describing her eating behavior and chooses her words carefully. She reports some concern about her inability to control her overeating but thinks she has no particular problems otherwise. Her demeanor is serious and humorless, but she does not seem depressed. There is no evidence of a formal thought disorder.

DSM-IV-TR Diagnosis

Axis I: 307.1   Anorexia Nervosa, Binge-Eating/Purging Type
Axis II: 301.82   Avoidant Personality Disorder
Axis III: 626.0   Amenorrhea
Axis IV: None
Axis V: GAF = 65

DSM-IV-TR diagnostic criteria for 307.1 Anorexia Nervosa

A. Refusal to maintain body weight at or above a minimally normal weight for age and height (e.g., weight loss leading to maintenance of body weight less than 85% of that expected; or failure to make expected weight gain during period of growth, leading to body weight less than 85% of that expected).

B. Intense fear of gaining weight or becoming fat, even though underweight.

C. Disturbance in the way in which one's body weight or shape is experienced, undue influence of body weight or shape on self-evaluation, or denial of the seriousness of the current low body weight.

D. In postmenarcheal females, amenorrhea, i.e., the absence of at least three consecutive menstrual cycles. (A woman is considered to have amenorrhea if her periods occur only following hormone, e.g., estrogen, administration.)

(continued)

> ## DSM-IV-TR diagnostic criteria for
> ## 307.1 Anorexia Nervosa *(continued)*
>
> ---
>
> *Specify* type:
> **Restricting Type:** during the current episode of Anorexia Nervosa, the person
>   has not regularly engaged in binge-eating or purging behavior (i.e., self-
>   induced vomiting or the misuse of laxatives, diuretics, or enemas)
> **Binge-Eating/Purging Type:** during the current episode of Anorexia Nervosa,
>   the person has regularly engaged in binge-eating or purging behavior (i.e.,
>   self-induced vomiting or the misuse of laxatives, diuretics, or enemas)

Bulimia Nervosa

❖   Case Study: A Young Woman Who Can't Stop Eating

Ms. T is a 28-year-old single insurance policy analyst who presents for consultation regarding her eating problems. She is the third of four children of
a well-to-do Midwestern attorney and his wife, who was a homemaker
while Ms. T was growing up. No one in the family has had a problem with
being overweight, but a premium has always been placed on being strong,
fit, and "in shape." As a child, Ms. T was a good student and an athlete and
developed an interest in figure skating. As a young teenager, she placed well
in local competitions and gradually devoted more time and energy to
training.

At age 15, as she entered her sophomore year of high school, Ms. T
transferred to an all-girls boarding school in the East because her parents
felt this would increase her chances of being admitted to an Ivy League college. She made several friends, did well in her courses, and generally coped
well with the demands of the new school. She continued to pursue her interest in figure skating and began training with a new coach. Although for
the most part supportive and encouraging, the coach did comment on one
occasion that Ms. T might do better competitively if she lost a few pounds.
At this time, Ms. T's weight was 128 pounds, normal for her age and height
of 5'7", and her diet was not unusual. Stung by her coach's remark, Ms. T
embarked on a vigorous program of exercise and dieting. In addition to her
daily skating practices, she went to an aerobics class 6 days a week. She also
eliminated desserts and red meat from her diet. Because of the time-
consuming nature of these activities, she grew distant from the new friends
she had made at school.

During the first year at boarding school, Ms. T's weight dropped from 128 to 100 pounds, and her menstrual periods, which had been regular since age 13, ceased. When she returned home for summer vacation, Ms. T's parents were very concerned by her obvious weight loss and insisted that she see her pediatrician who, in turn, referred her to a psychiatrist. It is not clear what diagnosis was made and, after a few visits, Ms. T refused to continue treatment. During that summer, however, her eating habits began to change. Although Ms. T tried to maintain the dieting program she had begun at school, she found herself struggling to control her appetite and, on several occasions, ate a box of cookies and a pint of ice cream late at night after the rest of the family had gone to bed. When she returned to school, Ms. T continued to intermittently overeat and eventually developed a pattern of dieting during the week and overeating on weekends. Although she continued to skate competitively, she was unable to maintain the vigorous exercise program she had initiated during her first year at boarding school. Her weight gradually rose through the rest of high school to 125 pounds, and her menses resumed after 9 months of amenorrhea.

After she graduated from high school, Ms. T entered a competitive Ivy League college where she majored in history and was a good, but not outstanding, student. Her weight continued to rise, reaching a high of 150 pounds in the fall of her freshman year. When she was home for Christmas that year, she found herself unable to stop eating the holiday cookies and snacks in the house. Greatly distressed at the prospect of gaining more weight, she decided she would induce vomiting after overeating. She did so and thus began a pattern of overeating and then inducing vomiting several times a week that has persisted for the past 10 years. On nights when she knows her roommate will be out, Ms. T typically buys a pint of ice cream and a box of chocolate chip cookies on the way home from work. After arriving home, she consumes the cookies and ice cream and any other leftover desserts in the refrigerator over the course of an hour while she watches TV. She then induces vomiting. Ms. T is very ashamed of this "disgusting habit" and has resolved to stop on numerous occasions; however, she has been unable to do so for more than 2 weeks at any given time. When she is not overeating, Ms. T attempts to diet rigorously. She continues to avoid red meat and desserts and her weight is reasonably stable at 145 pounds. She views her appearance as "gross."

Ms. T has been reasonably successful professionally. Since graduating from college, she has been employed by a large insurance firm and is progressing well in the middle-management ranks. She shares an apartment with a woman whom she views as her best friend but whom she has not told about her eating problem. Ms. T reports that her social life has been impaired by her concern about her eating and her weight. She is self-conscious about both and is reluctant to go to dinner with male friends because she fears that her strict dieting will seem incongruous in light of "how big I am."

DSM-IV-TR Diagnosis

Axis I: 307.51   Bulimia Nervosa, Purging Type
             307.1   Anorexia Nervosa (prior history)
Axis II: V71.09   No diagnosis
Axis III: None
Axis IV: None
Axis V: GAF = 65

DSM-IV-TR diagnostic criteria for 307.51 Bulimia Nervosa

A. Recurrent episodes of binge eating. An episode of binge eating is characterized by both of the following:
    (1) eating, in a discrete period of time (e.g., within any 2-hour period), an amount of food that is definitely larger than most people would eat during a similar period of time and under similar circumstances
    (2) a sense of lack of control over eating during the episode (e.g., a feeling that one cannot stop eating or control what or how much one is eating)
B. Recurrent inappropriate compensatory behavior in order to prevent weight gain, such as self-induced vomiting; misuse of laxatives, diuretics, enemas, or other medications; fasting; or excessive exercise.
C. The binge eating and inappropriate compensatory behaviors both occur, on average, at least twice a week for 3 months.
D. Self-evaluation is unduly influenced by body shape and weight.
E. The disturbance does not occur exclusively during episodes of Anorexia Nervosa.

Specify type:
Purging Type: during the current episode of Bulimia Nervosa, the person has regularly engaged in self-induced vomiting or the misuse of laxatives, diuretics, or enemas
Nonpurging Type: during the current episode of Bulimia Nervosa, the person has used other inappropriate compensatory behaviors, such as fasting or excessive exercise, but has not regularly engaged in self-induced vomiting or the misuse of laxatives, diuretics, or enemas

---

Guidelines for Differential Diagnosis of Eating Disorders

The cases of Ms. R and Ms. T illustrate how to distinguish between the diagnoses of Anorexia Nervosa and Bulimia Nervosa. Ms. R, the ballet dancer, receives a diagnosis of Anorexia Nervosa, Binge-Eating/Purging Type, because her body weight of 100–104 pounds is less than 85% of that expected for someone who is 5'8", and she has been amenorrheic for the past 3 years (since age 16). Ms. R is intensely afraid of becoming fat and has a very seriously distorted view of her own body size, describing herself as "fat" even though she weighs only 100 pounds and everyone around her finds her emaciated. The subtype "Binge-Eating/Purging Type" is applicable here because Ms. R binges on rice cakes or ice cream each evening and then vomits.

Ms. T has a history of Anorexia Nervosa, but her current diagnosis would be Bulimia Nervosa because her weight is now not below that which would be expected for her height of 5'7" and she has regular menstrual periods. She regularly binge eats and then vomits in a pattern that has continued over the past 10 years. She also has a distorted sense of her own body, considering herself to be "gross" at 145 pounds. The subtype "Purging Type" is applied because of Ms. T's regular self-induced vomiting.

It is important to note that the diagnoses of Anorexia Nervosa and Bulimia Nervosa are not fixed for a lifetime and often alternate as a result of weight gains and losses. Ms. R's diagnosis of Anorexia Nervosa would change to Bulimia Nervosa if she were to gain enough weight to be within the normal range or her periods were to resume. On the other hand, Ms. T's symptoms would have been diagnosed as Anorexia Nervosa when she was younger because her weight was very low and she was amenorrheic, even though she also engaged in binge-eating and purging behavior. Her diagnosis changed to Bulimia Nervosa when her weight increased to a normal level and her periods resumed. Although this convention is certainly less than elegant and there may be patients who fall in a borderline area at certain times, it does avoid the problem of describing a single set of symptoms with two separate diagnoses.

It probably would have been better to handle these disorders in the diagnostic system by including a single Eating Disorder with different subtypes depending on a patient's current weight and menstrual status and on the presence of binge-eating and purging behaviors.

Nonetheless, the separate categories of Anorexia Nervosa and Bulimia Nervosa have been maintained in DSM-IV (and in DSM-IV-TR) in part because of their different treatment implications and in part because the DSM-IV Task Force was very conservative in making changes. Moreover, there are many individuals with Anorexia Nervosa who never binge or purge (who would receive the diagnosis Anorexia Nervosa, Restricting Type) and many individuals with Bulimia Nervosa whose weight has never been below normal.

In diagnosing Anorexia Nervosa, it is important to distinguish abnormally low body weight from "normal" thinness, particularly in people who work in professions that require low body weight. Although Ms. R is a dancer and is required to maintain a fairly low weight for this profession, her weight loss has gone far beyond what is required for her dancing and is accompanied by features that are characteristic of an Eating Disorder (e.g., excessive fear of weight gain, a distorted body image, amenorrhea, and binge eating and purging). It is also important to rule out other causes of weight loss (e.g., general medical conditions such as cancer, the effects of other mental disorders such as Major Depressive Disorder, or the effects of poverty or poor nutrition) from weight loss that is due to Anorexia Nervosa.

In diagnosing Bulimia Nervosa, it is important to distinguish a regular pattern of binge eating from behavior that involves generalized overeating (often called "grazing") and from overeating that occurs in a specific context on a special occasion (e.g., a party or holiday celebration). To make this distinction, it is helpful to determine what types of food were eaten (binges most often involve sweet, high-calorie foods), how much was eaten (to qualify for a binge, the amount eaten must be what would be considered excessive for most individuals in that situation), the circumstances in which the binge eating took place, and how often the binge eating occurred. Ms. T's binge eating usually involved cookies and ice cream, she binged when she was alone and unobserved, and she had been doing this regularly (several times a week) for 10 years. She consumed a quantity of food that is clearly excessive in those circumstances to most individuals.

To make the diagnosis of Bulimia Nervosa, the individual must also use "inappropriate compensatory behaviors to prevent weight gain." These behaviors most often involve self-induced vomiting or laxative abuse (in which case, the subtype "Purging Type" is used) or less often may involve fasting or excessive exercise (in which case, the subtype "Nonpurging Type" is used). Ms. T regularly induces vomiting after her binges in a pattern that began when she was a teenager. The vomiting that occurs in Bulimia Nervosa is self-induced and is done for the purpose of avoiding weight gain due to the binge eating. This must be distinguished from vomiting that is caused by a general medical condition or by the use of substances.

Overeating and weight gain may also occur in Major Depressive Disorder With Atypical Features. However, the type of overeating that is associated with depression is not associated with inappropriate compensatory mechanisms or a distorted view of one's body weight or size.

Binge eating may occur as part of the impulsive behavior that is characteristic of Borderline Personality Disorder and is usually not accompanied by inappropriate compensatory mechanisms to avoid weight gain. However, Borderline Personality Disorder and Bulimia Nervosa are often comorbid, and, when criteria for both are met, both should be diagnosed.

Two other disorders that may sometimes be confused with Eating Disorders and may also be comorbid with them are Obsessive-Compulsive Disorder and Body Dysmorphic Disorder. Individuals with Obsessive-Compulsive Disorder may have obsessions or compulsions related to food, but they are not driven by an intense fear of weight gain. Their obsessions and compulsions also include concepts that are unrelated to food or eating (e.g., contamination, hurting someone, or damaging something). Like individuals with Eating Disorders, those with Body Dysmorphic Disorder have a distorted image of their bodies, but this is not related to an intense fear of gaining weight and is not associated with low body weight. If the body image problem is characteristic of Anorexia Nervosa, no separate diagnosis of Body Dysmorphic Disorder is necessary. In some cases, however, both diagnoses may be present, for example, an individual who meets criteria for Anorexia Nervosa who also has a pathological preoccupation with the idea that her nose is ugly and misshapen.

Individuals who binge eat without using compensatory mechanisms to avoid weight gain may warrant a diagnosis of Eating Disorder Not Otherwise Specified if their behavior involves impairment or distress. Binge-eating disorder is a proposed diagnosis to describe this situation. As might be expected, these individuals tend to be overweight. Binge-eating disorder is listed as an example of Eating Disorder Not Otherwise Specified with research criteria included in the appendix for "Criteria Sets and Axes Provided for Further Study."

Treatment Planning for Eating Disorders

Both Anorexia Nervosa and Bulimia Nervosa can involve serious medical complications, particularly Anorexia Nervosa. Complications associated with Anorexia Nervosa include constipation, abdominal pain, cold intolerance, lethargy, excess energy, significant hypotension, hypothermia, dry skin, and bradycardia. Some individuals develop lanugo, a fine downy body hair on their trunks; peripheral edema; skin yellowing; hypertrophy of the salivary glands; and (rarely) petechiae. In addition, individuals with Anorexia Nervosa sometimes exhibit laboratory abnormalities and several general medical conditions: normochromic normocytic anemia, impaired renal function, cardiovascular problems, dental problems, and osteoporosis. The long-term mortality of individuals with severe presentations of Anorexia Nervosa who are admitted to university hospitals is more than 10%. Death most commonly results from starvation, multiple organ failure, electrolyte imbalance, or suicide.

Complications associated with Bulimia Nervosa include significant loss of dental enamel due to recurrent vomiting; increased number of dental cavities; enlargement of the salivary glands; and, rarely, potentially fatal problems, including esophageal tears, gastric rupture, and cardiac arrhythmias.

Fortunately, both of these conditions can usually be treated successfully if intervention is timely. The treatment usually consists of some combination of cognitive-behavior therapy and medication.

Summary

Although Anorexia Nervosa and Bulimia Nervosa are listed as separate diagnoses in DSM-IV-TR, they are often different aspects of a single Eating Disorder. Individuals with Eating Disorders are often remarkably embarrassed about their pattern of binge eating and purging, so the clinician should ask specifically about eating patterns, particularly in any relatively young woman who presents with depressive symptoms.

Chapter 12

Sleep Disorders

The Sleep Disorders section in DSM-IV-TR is organized according to presumed etiology and is divided into four groupings: Primary Sleep Disorders, Sleep Disorders Related to Another Mental Disorder, Sleep Disorder Due to a General Medical Condition, and Substance-Induced Sleep Disorder. The Primary Sleep Disorders include the Dyssomnias and the Parasomnias.

The Dyssomnias are characterized by a disturbance in the amount, quality, or timing of sleep and include the following disorders:

Dyssomnias

307.42 Primary Insomnia
307.44 Primary Hypersomnia
347   Narcolepsy
780.59 Breathing-Related Sleep Disorder
307.45 Circadian Rhythm Sleep Disorder
307.47 Dyssomnia Not Otherwise Specified

The Parasomnias are characterized by abnormal behavioral or physiological events associated with sleep and include the following disorders:

Parasomnias

307.47   Nightmare Disorder
307.46   Sleep Terror Disorder
307.46   Sleepwalking Disorder
307.47   Parasomnia Not Otherwise Specified

Sleep Disorder Related to Another Mental Disorder involves a prominent sleep disturbance that results from a diagnosable mental disorder and is severe enough to warrant independent clinical attention. This category includes the following:

Sleep Disorders Related to Another Mental Disorder

307.42   Insomnia Related to Another Mental Disorder
307.44   Hypersomnia Related to Another Mental Disorder

Sleep Disorders may also result from the direct physiological effects of a general medical condition or a substance or a medication. Such disorders would be diagnosed as Sleep Disorder Due to a General Medical Condition or Substance-Induced Sleep Disorder.

In this section, we present one case illustrating Primary Hypersomnia and one case illustrating Insomnia Related to Another Mental Disorder.

Primary Hypersomnia

❖   Case Study: A Man Who Is Always Tired

Mr. P is a 52-year-old man referred for evaluation of excessive daytime sleepiness. He reports a long-standing problem with sleepiness going back to early childhood that has worsened over the past several years. He falls asleep in almost any low-stimulation situation (e.g., meetings at work, talking to customers, doing paperwork, watching television or a movie, or attending church). On several occasions, he has fallen asleep while driving and once had a serious accident as a result. His sleep episodes are typically brief, lasting only a few minutes, and are more likely to occur in the afternoon or evening hours. When he falls asleep during the day, he does not find the sleep particularly refreshing and does not recall dreaming. Mr. P falls asleep three to five times on most days. Upon careful questioning, he denies episodes of muscle weakness with intense emotion, sleep-related hallucinations, or paralysis.

Mr. P regularly goes to bed at about 10:30 P.M., falls asleep almost immediately, and awakens at 7 A.M. He typically has one or two brief awakenings during the night. He works 12-hour shifts as the manager of a discount store but works only during daylight hours. His wife does note some snoring, although this has never been excessively loud and is reduced when he rolls over on his side. She has never observed any breathing pauses during sleep. Mr. P does occasionally awaken at night feeling that he is choking or gasping for air. In the morning, he has difficulty awakening, and if he does not get out of bed immediately, he will fall back to sleep for a prolonged period.

His current medications include a nonsteroidal anti-inflammatory drug and a lipid-lowering drug. He drinks only decaffeinated coffee and cola and does not smoke. His medical history includes a tonsillectomy at age 12 and a minor head injury with a brief loss of consciousness at age 12 or 13, but no hospitalization and no cognitive sequelae. Currently, he has an elevated cholesterol level and essential hypertension. He sustained a "whiplash" injury after his car was struck by another, and he subsequently developed arthritis in his neck.

Although Mr. P currently denies significant depressive symptoms, he did have an episode of Major Depressive Disorder 1 year ago. This occurred in association with marital difficulties and was resolved following marital counseling. Symptoms of major depression at that time included low mood, frequent crying, anxiety, a decrease in appetite, disturbed nocturnal sleep, decreased energy, and anhedonia. The family history is also positive for Major Depressive Disorder and alcoholism in Mr. P's father.

Mr. P is a high school graduate who has been married for 25 years and has two children. He is the manager of a discount store and describes himself as a "workaholic." He reports no particular financial concerns and is pleased that he and his wife have largely resolved their problems.

Mr. P is a well-dressed and neatly groomed man who is not overweight and appears his stated age. On mental status exam, he is awake, alert, and oriented, although he does yawn on several occasions. He does not display any acute distress. When the interviewer leaves the office for several minutes, Mr. P is observed to be asleep when she returns. He does not appear depressed and denies any symptoms consistent with psychosis or cognitive impairment.

When Mr. P is referred for nocturnal polysomnography and a Multiple Sleep Latency Test, nocturnal testing shows a sleep latency of 4 minutes, a sleep duration of 8 hours, and a sleep efficiency (time asleep/time in bed) of 98%. He has six very brief arousals, normal non-rapid eye movement

(NREM) sleep stage distribution, normal rapid eye movement (REM) sleep latency, and 25% REM sleep. Mr. P has no evidence of oxyhemoglobin desaturation but does have 20 hypopnea events during the night. The apnea/hypopnea is 2.5 events per hour of sleep, which is not elevated. During the Multiple Sleep Latency Test, Mr. P falls asleep in each of five nap opportunities with a mean sleep latency of 7.1 minutes. REM sleep is not observed in any of these naps.

DSM-IV-TR Diagnosis

Axis I: 307.44   Primary Hypersomnia
            296.26   Major Depressive Disorder, Single Episode,
                       In Full Remission
Axis II: V71.09   No diagnosis
Axis III: 401.9   Hypercholesterolemia
            715.90   Osteoarthritis
            401.9   Essential hypertension
Axis IV: Marital difficulties (resolved)
Axis V: GAF = 75 (current); 65 (highest level in past year)

DSM-IV-TR diagnostic criteria for
307.44 Primary Hypersomnia

A. The predominant complaint is excessive sleepiness for at least 1 month (or less if recurrent) as evidenced by either prolonged sleep episodes or daytime sleep episodes that occur almost daily.
B. The excessive sleepiness causes clinically significant distress or impairment in social, occupational, or other important areas of functioning.
C. The excessive sleepiness is not better accounted for by insomnia and does not occur exclusively during the course of another Sleep Disorder (e.g., Narcolepsy, Breathing-Related Sleep Disorder, Circadian Rhythm Sleep Disorder, or a Parasomnia) and cannot be accounted for by an inadequate amount of sleep.
D. The disturbance does not occur exclusively during the course of another mental disorder.
E. The disturbance is not due to the direct physiological effects of a substance (e.g., a drug of abuse, a medication) or a general medical condition.

Specify if:
Recurrent: if there are periods of excessive sleepiness that last at least 3 days occurring several times a year for at least 2 years

Guidelines for Differential Diagnosis
of Primary Hypersomnia

Mr. P's long-standing problem with daytime sleepiness, despite an adequate nighttime sleep duration and the absence of accessory symptoms of Narcolepsy or objective findings of sleep apnea, makes Primary Hypersomnia the most likely diagnosis. Although insufficient sleep is probably the most common cause of daytime sleepiness in the general population, Mr. P is getting enough sleep as evidenced by his history and polysomnography test results. Obstructive sleep apnea syndrome is the next most common cause of daytime sleepiness in middle-aged men. Although his wife does report some snoring, she has not observed apneic pauses during sleep. Although Mr. P's systemic hypertension could also raise concern about obstructive sleep apnea, he is not obese. Objective testing does not reveal a significant number of apneic pauses during sleep or any evidence for oxyhemoglobin desaturation.

Narcolepsy is a neurological disorder that can cause daytime sleepiness. Although patients with Narcolepsy typically report brief episodes of sleep during the day, most patients with Narcolepsy report that their naps are refreshing, which is not the case with Mr. P. In addition, most patients with Narcolepsy have disturbed nighttime sleep. The hallmark of Narcolepsy is the presence of accessory symptoms such as cataplexy, sleep-related hallucinations, and sleep paralysis, none of which are present in Mr. P's case.

A Sleep Disorder Due to a Head Injury can be a cause for daytime sleepiness. However, Mr. P's head injuries (i.e., being hit with a rock at age 12 and sustaining a whiplash injury in adulthood) did not produce any other measurable neuropsychological deficits, nor did they appreciably alter the course of his hypersomnia. There is no evidence that Substance Use or Abuse is contributing to Mr. P's hypersomnia.

Hypersomnia Related to Another Mental Disorder is also a consideration, given Mr. P's history of Major Depressive Disorder. However, his sleepiness clearly did not occur exclusively during the course of this disorder and in fact had been present for decades before the Major Depressive Episode. Furthermore, Mr. P's depression tended to cause insomnia rather than a worsening of his hypersomnia.

Other Primary Sleep Disorders are unlikely. There is no evidence of an altered sleep-wake schedule that would suggest Circadian Rhythm Sleep Disorder, nor is there evidence of a subjective or objective difficulty with nighttime sleep that would suggest Primary Insomnia.

Treatment Planning for Primary Hypersomnia

Both behavioral and pharmacological measures can be used to treat Primary Hypersomnia. Patients are well advised to obtain an adequate amount of nighttime sleep to prevent a worsening of symptoms caused by sleep deprivation. Some patients may benefit from a brief daytime nap, although many patients with Primary Hypersomnia report feeling worse after such a nap. Avoiding low-stimulation situations or ensuring that someone else is with the patient at these times can help to prevent accidents. Avoiding substances such as alcohol and caffeine can also maximize the patient's degree of alertness.

Pharmacological treatments include the typical stimulant medications, the most commonly prescribed being methylphenidate, dextroamphetamine, and pemoline. Ritalin 5 mg bid was prescribed for Mr. P, which resulted in a noticeable decrease in his daytime sleepiness and dozing. He also reported no worsening and some improvement in his nocturnal sleep on this regimen.

Insomnia Related to Another Mental Disorder

❖   Case Study: An Anxious Woman
Who Has Trouble Sleeping

Ms. D is a 36-year-old woman who complains of chronic insomnia. Although she has had sleep problems intermittently since her college years, she has developed more persistent problems over the past year and a half. This worsening coincided with several stresses, including a move to a new house, a change of jobs for her husband, her own decision to quit working, and her elderly and ill father's moving in with her family. She claims that she does not sleep at all some nights and is concerned that her sleeplessness will impair her ability to take care of her children and otherwise function during the day. She has been prescribed alprazolam and has used diphenhydramine and alcohol to help with her sleep problems, but the insomnia has always quickly returned upon discontinuation of each of these. In addition, she was treated by a psychologist with visualization and progressive relaxation techniques, but this resulted in only partial relief.

Ms. D often falls asleep on the couch in the family room while watching television at night. She then wakes up, takes an alprazolam tablet, and goes back to bed at about 1:30 A.M. She gets out of bed at approximately 8 A.M. She acknowledges feeling physically and mentally tense about her sleep difficulty and notes that sometimes she clenches her jaw, grips her hands, or feels panicky at night. She also notes an increased heart rate and sweating on occasion at night but denies depersonalization or parasthesias. She denies other unusual behavior during sleep and daytime sleepiness, and she only rarely takes a daytime nap.

Upon further questioning, Ms. D reveals that, although her sleep problem is the biggest difficulty she is having at the moment, it is only one of many symptoms that have been bothering her. She says that she can't stop herself from "worrying about everything": the health and safety of her family, their financial situation, the security of her husband's job, the possibility that their old oil furnace may explode, the state of the tires on the family car, the quality of her children's schools, filling out her tax forms, and so on. She constantly ruminates on these concerns and suffers from somatic tension manifested by tenseness in her neck, shoulder, and jaw muscles; digestive troubles; and general jumpiness. She denies abrupt episodes of panic but says that she does have intermittent episodes of severe anxiety that are characterized by palpitations, sweating, increased muscle tension, difficulty breathing, and a fear that she is losing her mind. She is meticulous about her work and appearance, but denies the presence of specific repeated intrusive thoughts or ritualistic behavior.

Ms. D had one episode of Major Depressive Disorder 8 years earlier that was characterized by low mood, insomnia, decreased appetite and weight loss, poor concentration, and decreased enjoyment and interest, but no suicidal ideation. She saw a minister, and eventually these symptoms resolved. Ms. D has a strong family history of insomnia, depression, and anxiety, and one of her sisters is currently being treated with an antidepressant medication. At the time of this evaluation, Ms. D reports great interest and enthusiasm for her daily activities, although her energy is adversely affected by her sleep disturbance.

Ms. D denies current Alcohol or Other Substance Abuse. She takes alprazolam .75 mg q.h.s. and drinks two cups of caffeinated coffee per day and approximately three alcoholic drinks per month. Her only current medical problem is endometriosis.

Ms. D has been married for 10 years and has two children, ages 4 and 2. She worked as a dietitian but resigned after the birth of the second child to raise her family. She says that she has some marital stress because her husband works long hours and she communicates poorly with him.

On mental status examination, Ms. D is awake, alert, and oriented and does not appear sleepy. She states that she feels anxious and nervous but denies depression. Her cognitive functions are well within normal limits. There is no evidence of psychotic symptoms or of clear-cut obsessions or compulsions. Her speech is normal in rate and rhythm but tends to include detailed answers to all questions.

DSM-IV-TR Diagnosis

Axis I: 307.42   Insomnia Related to Generalized Anxiety Disorder
             300.02   Generalized Anxiety Disorder
Axis II: Obsessive-compulsive personality traits
Axis III: 617.9   Endometriosis
Axis IV: Marital stress, moving to a new house, father's illness
Axis V: GAF = 65 (current); 75 (highest level in past year)

DSM-IV-TR diagnostic criteria for
307.42 Insomnia Related to . . .
[Indicate the Axis I or Axis II disorder]

A. The predominant complaint is difficulty initiating or maintaining sleep, or nonrestorative sleep, for at least 1 month that is associated with daytime fatigue or impaired daytime functioning.
B. The sleep disturbance (or daytime sequelae) causes clinically significant distress or impairment in social, occupational, or other important areas of functioning.
C. The insomnia is judged to be related to another Axis I or Axis II disorder (e.g., Major Depressive Disorder, Generalized Anxiety Disorder, Adjustment Disorder With Anxiety), but is sufficiently severe to warrant independent clinical attention.
D. The disturbance is not better accounted for by another Sleep Disorder (e.g., Narcolepsy, Breathing-Related Sleep Disorder, a Parasomnia).
E. The disturbance is not due to the direct physiological effects of a substance (e.g., a drug of abuse, a medication) or a general medical condition.

Guidelines for Differential Diagnosis of a Sleep Disorder Related to Another Mental Disorder

A number of etiological factors may be involved in sleep problems, and all should be considered before making a diagnosis. The first question is why the sleep problems associated with Generalized Anxiety Disorder should receive a separate diagnosis. The inclusion of Sleep Disorder Related to Another Mental Disorder in DSM-IV (and DSM-IV-TR) is an exception to the manual's general practice of not giving separate diagnoses for individual symptoms that form part of a diagnostic syndrome. This exception was made for consistency with DSM-III-R and with the International Classification of Sleep Disorders and to facilitate the differential diagnosis of insomnia and hypersomnia. A diagnosis of Insomnia or Hypersomnia Related to Another Mental Disorder should be given only in those fairly unusual situations in which the sleep problem is the patient's main complaint and is severe enough to warrant separate clinical attention. It can be argued that Ms. D's insomnia does warrant a separate diagnosis and clinical attention because it is her major concern at the moment, even though it does appear to be related to the Generalized Anxiety Disorder. However, we would also have been comfortable diagnosing Generalized Anxiety Disorder alone and treating the sleep problems as one of the associated symptoms of that disorder.

The next differential diagnosis to be considered is Primary Insomnia, the criteria for which indicate that the disorder does not occur exclusively during the course of another mental disorder. Many patients with Primary Insomnia have anxious overconcern about their sleep, but this anxiety does not carry over to other areas of their life. Ms. D, however, is not only anxious about sleep-related matters but also has pervasive anxiety about many other areas of her life. If her insomnia had been present before she developed anxiety problems or persisted when she no longer had anxiety symptoms, then the diagnosis would most likely be Primary Insomnia.

Other Primary Sleep Disorders are equally unlikely. As in most patients with chronic insomnia, Ms. D does not report daytime sleepiness, excluding a diagnosis of Primary Hypersomnia or Narcolepsy. Her sleep hours are not shifted relative to societal norms or her own need for wakeful function, excluding a Circadian Rhythm Sleep Disorder. The absence of unusual behavior during sleep rules out a Parasomnia.

The next differential to be considered is whether Ms. D's sleep problems are due to the direct physiological effects of a substance or general medical condition. Ms. D's use of alcohol, alprazolam, and caffeine do not appear to be significant enough to be causing her sleep problems, but the only way to determine this for sure is for her to discontinue all these substances. Although Ms. D has endometriosis, she does not appear to have any symptoms that are severe enough to be interfering with her sleep.

Like many patients with chronic insomnia disorders, Ms. D has developed behavioral patterns that may be incompatible with good sleep. These include sleeping on the couch in the evening, going to bed late, and spending an excessive amount of time tossing and turning in bed. In addition, she has used alcohol and over-the-counter agents, as well as prescription medication, in an attempt to control her sleep disturbance, which is also typical of patients with chronic insomnia. Patients with Primary Insomnia as well as Insomnia Related to Another Mental Disorder may note a worsening of symptoms at times of psychosocial stress.

Treatment Planning for a Sleep Disorder
Related to Another Mental Disorder

Both behavioral and pharmacological measures can be useful in treating insomnia. However, when the insomnia is not primary but is due to other causes, the clinician should first address the etiological problem that is causing the sleep disturbance. For example, if the insomnia is due to a general medical condition, the clinician should first treat symptoms such as pain that may be causing the sleep problems. One important aspect of treatment would be to try to undo the possible impact that Ms. D's current Substance Use might be having. It could be helpful for her to stop drinking caffeinated coffee and to withdraw slowly from alprazolam, perhaps switching to a more long-acting benzodiazepine if this is necessary for the treatment of the Generalized Anxiety Disorder or to help her withdraw from the alprazolam. It would probably be helpful for Ms. D to stop using all medications for a period, if possible, because the use of sleep medications is ideally limited to fairly short periods of time. Having established that Ms. D's insomnia is related to Generalized Anxiety Disorder, the clinician should try to treat both the anxiety symptoms and the insomnia. See p. 188 for a discussion of "Treatment Planning for Generalized Anxiety Disorder."

Behavioral measures would include restriction of time in bed to approximate more nearly the patient's actual ability to sleep. In addition, a regular period of relaxation to "unwind" in the evening would be advisable. Regular daily exercise and a regular time for going to bed and awakening would further help to reinforce a normal sleep-wake routine. Further training in relaxation techniques, such as progressive muscular relaxation, may help to diminish the patient's cognitive and somatic symptoms of anxiety at bedtime.

Pharmacological measures could include either benzodiazepine or antidepressant medication. Ms. D was switched from alprazolam to a longer acting benzodiazepine, clonazepam. The dose was lowered to a total of 0.25 mg/night. When she continued to exhibit daytime anxiety symptoms and overconcern about sleeplessness, a trial of sertraline was instituted. At a dose of 50 mg/day, Ms. D noted a dramatic improvement in her daytime and nighttime worrying, became much less focused on her difficulty with sleep, had an easier time tolerating everyday stresses, and reported a general decrease in all anxiety symptoms.

Summary

Sleep Disorders are very commonly encountered in clinical practice. The essence of the evaluation is to determine whether a defined etiology (i.e., another mental disorder, a general medical condition, medication or Substance

Use, or a combination of these) is causing the sleep problem or whether the disturbance is a Primary Sleep Disorder. This is the one area in psychiatry in which we have very sensitive and specific laboratory tests that are remarkably useful in diagnosis. The major problem in using these tests on a routine basis is that they are expensive and not always accessible. For the most part, diagnosis can be made on clinical grounds, with the sleep laboratory serving as a backup for the more confusing or difficult to treat conditions.

Chapter 13

Impulse-Control Disorders Not Elsewhere Classified

I mpulsive behaviors that can be harmful to oneself or others are a feature of a number of mental disorders classified in other sections of DSM-IV-TR (e.g., Substance-Related Disorders, Borderline and Antisocial Personality Disorders, Conduct Disorder, and Bipolar Disorder). The section titled "Impulse-Control Disorders Not Elsewhere Classified" is reserved for those disorders that involve impulse control that is not part of the presentation of another mental disorder. The disorders in this section are characterized by a sensation of increased tension or arousal before giving in to the impulse, followed by a feeling of pleasure or relief afterward.

The following disorders are included in this section of DSM-IV-TR:

Impulse-Control Disorders Not Elsewhere Classified

312.34 Intermittent Explosive Disorder
312.32 Kleptomania
312.33 Pyromania
312.31 Pathological Gambling
312.39 Trichotillomania
312.30 Impulse-Control Disorder Not Otherwise Specified

We discuss one case illustrating Intermittent Explosive Disorder and one case illustrating Pathological Gambling.

Intermittent Explosive Disorder

❖   Case Study: A Man Who Blows Up

Mr. P is a 46-year-old plumber who comes for consultation at the insistence of his wife, an extremely attractive 32-year-old waitress, because she is terrified of his temper outbursts. Mr. P and his wife have been fairly happily married for 4 years and have even been contemplating having children. Mr. P is crazy about his pretty young wife, but he is preoccupied with getting older and fears that he is losing his powers and will not be able to keep her affections. He often feels as if his wife is taking him for granted, and he is very jealous of the men with whom she comes into contact at work. Mr. P would like her to change jobs, even though she makes more money as a waitress in the expensive restaurant where she works than she is likely to make doing anything else.

Mr. P's wife reports that their marriage has been reasonably happy despite occasional fights and that there are no grounds for Mr. P's jealousy but says that "if he keeps blowing up like he has been, I will have to leave him." She says that every once in a while Mr. P completely loses control and "becomes a different person." On one occasion, he began breaking up the furniture in the apartment when she got home a little late and he was convinced she was with another man. On another occasion, he tore up most of her wardrobe because he said she dressed too provocatively. His wife says that it is hopeless for her to try to reason or interfere with Mr. P during these episodes because he goes blindly on with his destructive behavior despite anything she does or says. Ms. P is especially concerned because these episodes seem to be occurring more often. Mr. P remembers everything he has done during these episodes and feels a tremendous sense of remorse and disbelief that he could be so carried away but says that when these "spells" come over him, he "just sees red." Neither Mr. P nor his wife drink alcohol or use any other drugs, and no medical problems were found during Mr. P's annual physical 3 months before this evaluation.

DSM-IV-TR Diagnosis

Axis I: 312.34   Intermittent Explosive Disorder
Axis II: V71.09   No diagnosis
Axis III: None
Axis IV: Marital difficulties
Axis V: GAF = 55 (current); 65 (highest level in past year)

DSM-IV-TR diagnostic criteria for
312.34 Intermittent Explosive Disorder

A. Several discrete episodes of failure to resist aggressive impulses that result in serious assaultive acts or destruction of property.
B. The degree of aggressiveness expressed during the episodes is grossly out of proportion to any precipitating psychosocial stressors.
C. The aggressive episodes are not better accounted for by another mental disorder (e.g., Antisocial Personality Disorder, Borderline Personality Disorder, a Psychotic Disorder, a Manic Episode, Conduct Disorder, or Attention-Deficit/Hyperactivity Disorder) and are not due to the direct physiological effects of a substance (e.g., a drug of abuse, a medication) or a general medical condition (e.g., head trauma, Alzheimer's disease).

Guidelines for Differential Diagnosis of Intermittent Explosive Disorder

Intermittent Explosive Disorder is one of the least well-described and studied disorders in DSM-IV. The nosology of aggression has never been well established, and the DSM-IV-TR criteria for this disorder are not really much of an improvement over those in DSM-III-R. One change from DSM-III-R to DSM-IV is to allow the presence of impulsive behavior between episodes of Intermittent Explosive Disorder. This change was made because the DSM-III-R construct was so narrowly defined as to be almost nonexistent because it excluded "any generalized impulsiveness or aggressiveness" between episodes.

Before making a diagnosis of Intermittent Explosive Disorder, the clinician must rule out all other possible causes of the aggressive impulses. The first differential is with aggressive behavior that does not indicate the presence of a mental disorder but is the result of irresponsibility, thrill seeking, lack of conscience, or a desire for gain.

It is also important to determine the role of substances or a general medical condition in the etiology of the symptoms because Intermittent Explosive Disorder would not be diagnosed if the behavior is the result of the direct effects of a substance of abuse (e.g., alcohol, PCP, or cocaine), a medication, or a general medical condition. Aggressive behavior that is the direct physiological result of a head trauma would be diagnosed as Personality Change Due to a General Medical Condition, Aggressive Type. Aggressive behavior can be associated with delirium or dementia, in which case no separate diagnosis would be made. Intermittent Explosive Disorder would also not be diagnosed if the aggressive episodes are better accounted for by one of the several disorders with which such episodes may be associated, such as Antisocial Personality Disorder, Conduct Disorder, or Bipolar Disorder. Finally, the clinician should be alert to the possibility that a person may be Malingering, especially in forensic settings where someone may be trying to evade responsibility for his or her actions. Mr. P does not use any substances of abuse, is not taking any medications, does not appear to have any general medical problems that might be responsible for his outbursts, and does not have the symptoms of any other mental disorder; therefore, the appropriate diagnosis appears to be Intermittent Explosive Disorder.

Treatment Planning for Intermittent Explosive Disorder

There is a paucity of studies specifically addressing the treatment of Intermittent Explosive Disorder. Any treatment recommendations must be extrapolated from more generic studies of medication and cognitive-behavioral treatments of aggression and violence. There is some indication that a variety of different medications (e.g., beta-blockers, anticonvulsants, or mood stabilizers) may be useful, but this is by no means definitively established.

Pathological Gambling

❖   Case Study: A Lawyer Who Has
       Gotten in Way Over His Head[1]

Mr. A is a 59-year-old attorney who is referred for psychiatric evaluation by his lawyer. For the past 15 years, he has been taking the money that his clients have given to him to invest for them and using it to gamble. This practice began when an intended investment was not available. Mr. A was afraid to risk disappointing the client, so he paid the client regular "interest payments" out of his own pocket. Mr. A says that he sometimes actually paid clients more money than they would have gotten had the investments been made. Mr. A has been able to keep this deception secret until recently.

     Mr. A has been gambling regularly since he was 10 years old. He was first introduced to it by his father, who loved sports betting, going to the

---

1. Thanks to Richard Rosenthal, M.D., of Beverly Hills, California, for supplying this case.

racetrack, and playing the stock market. He shared these interests with his two sons, frequently taking them to ball games and having friends over to watch or listen to games and wager on them. He took his sons to the track at a young age and taught them to handicap. These were exciting times for Mr. A. It undoubtedly added to the experience that their father was a successful gambler who made most of his money in the stock market and was later successful in real estate speculation.

By the time he was 15, Mr. A was going to the track on his own and betting as much as $50 a race. He was also playing cards and shooting baskets for money. When he entered college at age 17, he felt socially unprepared, anxious, and overwhelmed. Instead of going to classes, he usually spent all day at the track and, by the end of the first semester, had to drop out. He was subsequently able to complete his college education elsewhere, however, and went on to graduate from law school.

What attracts Mr. A to gambling is the excitement of the competition and the immediate feedback. Unlike the practice of law, where cases tend to drag out over months or even years, when he gambles, Mr. A quickly learns whether he is right or wrong and knows where he stands. Mr. A's games of choice are horse racing, casino gambling (blackjack), bridge, backgammon, golf, and the stock market.

Until shortly before this referral, Mr. A believed himself to be a skillful and winning gambler. During the course of this evaluation, however, he realizes that as early as the late 1970s he was regularly overdrawn at the bank, owed money to the casinos, and had significant financial problems. Although he keeps records of his winnings and losses for tax purposes, his memory of his losses is poor. As Mr. A got deeper and deeper into debt, he continued to underestimate his losses and was convinced that he could win all the money back. When he recently realized that he was not going to be able to do this, he became anxious and then seriously depressed.

It becomes clear that the two previous periods when Mr. A's gambling escalated also occurred when he was under increased stress. The first was during college. The second period was in response to the death of his father and the breakup of his first marriage. During that period, he felt lost and alone and sought solace at the track. He also bought two hotels in a state that he expected would soon legalize casino gambling. When this did not happen, he poured large amounts of money into his "investment" before finally selling at a big loss. Mr. A lost $300,000 a year at a time when his best annual income was $100,000.

During the past 3 years, Mr. A has increased his gambling in an unavailing attempt to escape his ever-increasing debts. Unfortunately, his "chasing" buried him even further. Before he saw an attorney to turn himself in for embezzling from his clients, he contemplated suicide daily because he felt that he had betrayed everybody and that if he killed himself his second wife would at least have the insurance money.

When he first comes for consultation, Mr. A has still not told his wife about the extent of his gambling losses or the legal difficulties he faces because he is afraid of what her reaction will be. In fact, his secrecy and his desperate chasing were an all-out effort to repay the money and undo the problems before she could find out.

The mental status exam reveals a guilt-ridden and severely depressed man. He cries frequently during the session and appears overwhelmed by the enormity of what he has done. His thoughts center on self-disgust and anger at himself. He repeatedly says, "I can't believe I could do such a thing. I can't believe I did this." He has difficulty concentrating, impaired functioning, multiple somatic complaints, insomnia, and a loss of appetite.

Although Mr. A's intelligence is superior, he demonstrates poor judgment and minimal insight and at times appears naive. He has always lived in fear of not living up to the expectations of others, beginning with his father. Although Mr. A presents himself during the interview as someone who acts independently and does not need to ask others for help, his passivity during the interview is notable and his dependency on his wife and others is obvious.

DSM-IV-TR Diagnosis

Axis I: 312.31   Pathological Gambling
             296.23   Major Depressive Disorder, Single Episode,
                       Severe Without Psychotic Features
Axis II: V71.09   No diagnosis
Axis III: None
Axis IV: Overwhelming debts, legal problems because of embezzlement
Axis V: GAF = 45 (current); 35 (past year)

DSM-IV-TR diagnostic criteria for
312.31 Pathological Gambling

A. Persistent and recurrent maladaptive gambling behavior as indicated by five (or more) of the following:
    (1) is preoccupied with gambling (e.g., preoccupied with reliving past gambling experiences, handicapping or planning the next venture, or thinking of ways to get money with which to gamble)
    (2) needs to gamble with increasing amounts of money in order to achieve the desired excitement

(continued)

DSM-IV-TR diagnostic criteria for
312.31 Pathological Gambling *(continued)*

---

(3) has repeated unsuccessful efforts to control, cut back, or stop gambling

(4) is restless or irritable when attempting to cut down or stop gambling

(5) gambles as a way of escaping from problems or of relieving a dysphoric mood (e.g., feelings of helplessness, guilt, anxiety, depression)

(6) after losing money gambling, often returns another day to get even ("chasing" one's losses)

(7) lies to family members, therapist, or others to conceal the extent of involvement with gambling

(8) has committed illegal acts such as forgery, fraud, theft, or embezzlement to finance gambling

(9) has jeopardized or lost a significant relationship, job, or educational or career opportunity because of gambling

(10) relies on others to provide money to relieve a desperate financial situation caused by gambling

B. The gambling behavior is not better accounted for by a Manic Episode.

Guidelines for Differential Diagnosis of Pathological Gambling

In diagnosing Pathological Gambling, the first differential is with recreational gambling. In recreational gambling, individuals are able to stop gambling and do not "chase" their losses over a long period, and the gambling does not cause any major problems for the person or his or her family. Pathological Gambling should also be distinguished from professional gambling, in which the individual carefully monitors risk factors to make a profit. To meet the criteria for Pathological Gambling, the person must exhibit "persistent and maladaptive gambling behavior" that meets at least 5 of the 10 criteria. Such behavior causes dislocations and disturbances in the individual's family and professional life. Although Mr. A had for a long time considered himself to be almost a professional gambler and had believed that he was very successful, this was clearly no more than wishful thinking on his part and his gambling loses have been out of control. Mr. A's behavior appears to meet the majority of the 10 criteria for Pathological Gambling. He is preoccupied with gambling and unable to stop himself despite the growing losses that he continues to chase ever more feverishly. His gambling escalates

in periods of stress (e.g., when he first went away to college and when his father died and his first wife left him), when he uses the excitement of the
wager to forget his troubles. He has concealed his debts and dishonest behavior from his wife. In fact, one of the motivations for his ever more frenzied
chasing has been to avoid having to tell her the truth. Mr. A has embezzled
money from his clients to gamble and by this act has jeopardized his professional career.

During a Manic Episode, individuals may gamble excessively and with
poor judgment in a way that resembles the behavior of a pathological gambler.
If the gambling behavior occurs only during the Manic Episode and appears to
be well accounted for by the Manic Episode, then a separate diagnosis of
Pathological Gambling would not be appropriate. Conversely, if manic-type
symptoms appear only during an individual's Pathological Gambling (which
does happen in the excitement and heat of the moment), this does not by itself indicate the presence of a Manic Episode. Mr. A has a lifelong history of
increasing involvement and problems with gambling and does not show any
evidence of manic behavior that is not related to his gambling; therefore, a diagnosis of Pathological Gambling would be appropriate.

Major Depressive Disorder may co-occur with Pathological Gambling,
especially when the individual is faced with increasing losses and family and
occupational problems because of the losses, as Mr. A was. A 20% prevalence
of attempted suicide has been reported among those being treated for Pathological Gambling, and the clinician should be alert to the need to identify and
treat suicidal ideation in such individuals. In addition, individuals with Antisocial Personality Disorder may have an increased tendency to have problems
with gambling, and both diagnoses may be given when appropriate.

Treatment Planning for Pathological Gambling

Clinicians who treat Pathological Gambling often use cognitive-behavioral
approaches similar to those used for treating Substance Dependence. It is
also very important to evaluate for and treat conditions that are commonly
comorbid, especially substance-related problems and Mood and Anxiety
Disorders.

Summary

The disorders covered in this section represent a heterogeneous grouping of
residual Impulse-Control Disorders that did not fit in very well elsewhere in
the manual. Remember that problems with impulse control are also associated with a number of other disorders in the manual and that a more specific
diagnosis should be made whenever possible.

Chapter 14

Adjustment Disorders

A djustment Disorders describe emotional or behavioral problems that occur as a reaction to a stressor. These problems must cause significant distress or impairment but do not meet criteria for any other specific mental disorder. Adjustment Disorders are coded on the basis of the type of symptoms that predominate as shown below:

Adjustment Disorders

309.0	With Depressed Mood
309.24	With Anxiety
309.28	With Mixed Anxiety and Depressed Mood
309.3	With Disturbance of Conduct
309.4	With Mixed Disturbance of Emotions and Conduct
309.9	Unspecified

Adjustment Disorder With Depressed Mood

❖ Case Study: "An Old Bird With an Empty Nest"

Mrs. A is a 50-year-old woman who comes for consultation because she feels that she has wasted her life and because of a loss of sexual interest. Her recent inability to achieve orgasm has convinced Mrs. A that her sexual life and femininity are things of the past. The patient's symptoms began suddenly 3 weeks ago after an extremely unpleasant argument with her husband of 30 years. The patient's youngest daughter had just left home to begin college, a move that spurred Mrs. A to try to establish greater intimacy in her marriage "since it's really just going to be the two of us from now on." Mrs. A's husband rebuffed her in no uncertain terms, making it clear that he was and would remain totally preoccupied with his business and community activities (he is active in a number of clubs and societies) and had no supply of time or emotion left for her. He told her that he was perfectly satisfied with the way things were as long as she kept the house well and performed the other tasks that she does so well. He told her he thought her efforts to increase their marital satisfaction were "silly and sappy" and that they were too old for "that kind of nonsense." Mrs. A says that, although her husband has never been particularly demonstrative, she never realized he felt that way. Mrs. A says she feels "totally deflated" by her husband's rejection and ridicule and by her loneliness for her youngest daughter to whom she is very close. Mrs. A contemptuously describes herself as "an old bird with an empty nest."

Mrs. A has always been a highly competent, popular, and attractive woman. She is widely regarded as an ideal wife, mother, and friend and has also managed a successful side career as an interior decorator. She grew up in a stern and demanding environment and was expected to be a letter-perfect little lady. She was a hardworking student, a dutiful wife, and a devoted mother but never felt completely satisfied with her performance. She now feels she is trapped in an unhappy and unfulfilling marriage and that she has wasted her life.

Although the patient would like to leave her husband, she does not believe in divorce. She admits that she has recently been thinking of having affairs but is sure that she would not be able to deal with the guilt because she believes they are sinful. When Mrs. A informed her husband that she planned to seek treatment and asked whether he would come with her, he refused, saying that she was the one with a problem, not him, and that he didn't believe in all that "mumbo jumbo" anyway.

Despite her discouragement, Mrs. A continues to function well at work and is not suicidal, and her sleep and appetite are unaffected. She relates well to the therapist and brightens in response to a joke.

DSM-IV-TR Diagnosis

Axis I:	309.0	Adjustment Disorder With Depressed Mood, Acute
Axis II:	No personality disorder, compulsive personality features	
Axis III:	None	
Axis IV:	Marital dissatisfaction, youngest daughter leaving home	
Axis V:	GAF = 65 (current); 85 (highest level in past year)	

Adjustment Disorder With Mixed
Disturbance of Emotions and Conduct

❖ Case Study: A Small Boy With a
Long and Complicated History

Jimmy is a 6-year-old first grader who is brought for consultation by his adoptive parents because of school problems that have been growing steadily worse over the past year. He has been hitting his peers, is excessively active, and gives up easily on school tasks. His adoptive parents are also uncertain about the effects of the death of Jimmy's first adoptive mother when he was age 4 and his father's remarriage a year later. Placement testing performed several months before this consultation showed that Jimmy had difficulty with small motor movements and poor imaginative drawing.

Little is known about Jimmy's biological parents, but there were no noted perinatal or antenatal insults. Jimmy was a "good baby" during his first year, but his first adoptive mother had leukemia and was indulgent and unable to exert discipline. He was cared for intermittently by different au pair girls and developed a strong attachment to his father. Physical affection and indulgence characterized his early years.

Jimmy walked and spoke at 12–14 months but continued to have nocturnal enuresis and daytime soiling until his second adoptive mother took over his care. Before that time, Jimmy had been sleeping with his father, who had taken the path of least resistance with the idea that Jimmy had "gone through enough" and that he deserved coddling because of his mother's recent death. Jimmy did not seem very disturbed when told of her death, although he did ask to see her body, which he was permitted to do.

When the boy's father introduced his future wife to the child, she found him "charming but spoiled" and immediately sensed that his rearing had been "unfair" in its indulgence and lack of social boundaries. Once married to his father, she took a firm disciplinary hand but complained that her husband remained too passive and foolishly indulgent. Although Jimmy's behavior at home has been improving (aside from intermittent angry tantrums), his teachers complain that he does not like school, is picking fights, and is not making much academic progress. Jimmy says that people at school don't like him and that he hates school and doesn't have any friends there. Although he was popular and a leader in nursery school, he now seems angry and negative and often refuses to participate in class activities, games, or parties. He often displays passive resistance and occasionally has outbursts in which he erupts and angrily lashes out at his peers because of minor irritations. By contrast, when his new mother invites children to play with him at home, his play is imaginative and amiable.

Jimmy is a bright-eyed, handsome youngster with two front teeth missing. During the consultation, he appears animated and lively. Although he initially protests against coming into the office without his mother or father, once inside he quickly becomes absorbed in play with a set of toy soldiers. He is well coordinated and agile. Despite previous test results to the contrary, his handling of small toys shows good fine motor coordination and his skill at building barriers with larger blocks is excellent for his age. His neediness is displayed in his insistent inquiries about the other toys in the closet. The content of his play with the toy soldiers involves killing off the therapist's army one by one. As he kills the soldiers, he indicates that they "go to God" and says that it is possible "to revive them back to life again."

When the therapist asks about his mother's death, Jimmy says that she too is with God in heaven but insists that he can make her alive again anytime that he wants to, although it seems clear from his tone that Jimmy only half-believes what he is saying with such insistence. He begins a discussion about his attachment to his father and about his "new mom." He then says that the boys at school don't like him, but he doesn't understand why. He describes a good friend in his neighborhood with whom he plays at home.

When asked to draw a person, Jimmy draws a simple figure consisting of two circles with legs appropriately placed and facial features. His drawing of a boy and girl are similarly rudimentary, with no clear differentiation between the sexes. The Bender Gestalt test for visual-motor assessment shows poor form, impulsivity, poor angulation, and haphazard approach to the task; graphomotor deficits are also observed clinically. Jimmy is right-handed but has poor consistency in distinguishing right from left in others. Jimmy displays an excellent vocabulary and is emotionally expressive with a good range of affects, but he also appears to be preoccupied with needs, aggression, and death. The psychological testing reveals similar preoccupations. A full-scale Wechsler Preschool and Primary Scale of Intelligence shows an IQ of 119 (verbal IQ 116, performance 119). None of the subtest scores are below average.

DSM-IV-TR Diagnosis

Axis I:	309.4	Adjustment Disorder With Mixed Disturbance of Emotions and Conduct, Chronic
	V61.20	Parent-Child Relational Problem
Axis II:	V71.09	No diagnosis
Axis III:	None	
Axis IV:	Death of first adoptive mother, new adoptive mother, inconsistent and overly indulgent parenting, school problems	
Axis V:	GAF = 65	

> ## DSM-IV-TR diagnostic criteria for Adjustment Disorders
>
> A. The development of emotional or behavioral symptoms in response to an identifiable stressor(s) occurring within 3 months of the onset of the stressor(s).
> B. These symptoms or behaviors are clinically significant as evidenced by either of the following:
>   (1) marked distress that is in excess of what would be expected from exposure to the stressor
>   (2) significant impairment in social or occupational (academic) functioning
> C. The stress-related disturbance does not meet the criteria for another specific Axis I disorder and is not merely an exacerbation of a preexisting Axis I or Axis II disorder.
> D. The symptoms do not represent Bereavement.
> E. Once the stressor (or its consequences) has terminated, the symptoms do not persist for more than an additional 6 months.
>
> *Specify* if:
> **Acute:** if the disturbance lasts less than 6 months
> **Chronic:** if the disturbance lasts for 6 months or longer
>
> Adjustment Disorders are coded based on the subtype, which is selected according to the predominant symptoms. The specific stressor(s) can be specified on Axis IV.
> **309.0**   **With Depressed Mood**
> **309.24** **With Anxiety**
> **309.28** **With Mixed Anxiety and Depressed Mood**
> **309.3**   **With Disturbance of Conduct**
> **309.4**   **With Mixed Disturbance of Emotions and Conduct**
> **309.9**   **Unspecified**

Guidelines for Differential Diagnosis of Adjustment Disorders

The first crucial point in making a diagnosis of Adjustment Disorder is ensuring that criteria for a more specific mental disorder are not met. Although Mrs. A has some depressive symptoms, they are relatively mild. If her symptoms met full criteria for a Major Depressive Episode, then that would have been the appropriate diagnosis rather than Adjustment Disorder. Similarly, Jimmy's condition does not meet full criteria for any of the specific Mood Disorders, Oppositional Defiant Disorder, Conduct Disorder, or Attention-Deficit/Hyperactivity Disorder.

A second requirement for a diagnosis of Adjustment Disorder is the presence of an identifiable stressor or stressors that triggered the symptoms. Mrs. A's symptoms began after two upsetting incidents: her youngest daughter's departure for college and her husband's total rejection of her attempts to improve their marriage. Although understandable, Mrs. A's unhappiness and her feeling that she has wasted her life are a source of clinically significant distress that is severe and persistent enough to warrant a diagnosis of Adjustment Disorder. Jimmy lost his first adoptive mother and then had to adjust to a new mother. He was initially coddled and spoiled and is now having to adjust to a more sensible but less indulgent type of discipline. Although he does not report any overt distress about his mother's death or the change in discipline, psychological testing reveals a preoccupation with death. He also has begun having marked difficulties functioning in school since his father's remarriage, in contrast to his previously successful performance in nursery school.

For symptoms to be considered Adjustment Disorder, they must develop within 3 months of the stressor and can persist for no more than 6 months after the stressor (or its consequences) has terminated. This is a change from the DSM-III-R criteria set for Adjustment Disorder, which put an absolute limit of 6 months on the duration of symptoms for Adjustment Disorder. The DSM-III-R time limit was unrealistic because there are many types of stressors (e.g., a chronic general medical condition or a divorce that has long-term financial, emotional, and social effects) that have long-term effects. Basically, DSM-IV allows the symptoms of Adjustment Disorder to persist for as long as the stressors (or their effects) do. For example, because of the ongoing consequences of Jimmy's mother's death, a diagnosis of Adjustment Disorder continues to be appropriate even though his symptoms have persisted for longer than 6 months.

Treatment Planning for Adjustment Disorders

Most individuals with Adjustment Disorder recover on their own with the passage of time and/or the amelioration of the stressor, but, in some cases, the symptoms become chronic or go on to meet the criteria for a another more specific disorder. Treatment should target resolving the specific problem that causes the symptoms or modifying an individual's reaction to the problem. More than in other cases, environmental manipulation may be helpful, and family interventions are particularly likely to be useful and desirable. A statement by the patient that other family members are not willing to join in the consultation should not be taken at face value because a call from the therapist to invite them will often be successful. This is particularly true when it is made clear that only a commitment for consultation is involved, that the therapist and patient will not be "ganging up" against the family member, and that the potential gain for everyone far outstrips the risks.

Although Mr. A spoke negatively to his wife about her treatment, he clearly does depend on her in many ways and wants her to function well. He may be more willing to be involved in her treatment if he comes to recognize that her problems may get more severe and cause him great inconvenience if she is not helped quickly.

Strategies that might be helpful in Jimmy's case include ensuring that his caretaking is good, that discipline is fair and consistent, that time is scheduled for him to be with other relatives, and that all possible attempts are made to maintain a stable and consistent home environment. Psychotherapy and play therapy could also be useful to allow him to grieve for his lost adoptive mother and to teach alternative coping skills for dealing with his ongoing problems at school and with his family.

Summary

There are three common misconceptions in applying the diagnosis of Adjustment Disorder. The first is that the presence of a precipitating stressor is restricted to Adjustment Disorder.

Stress is a factor in the onset or exacerbation of all DSM-IV disorders. Adjustment Disorder is a residual category to be used only when there is a clinically significant maladaptive response to stress that does not meet the criteria set for a more specific disorder. Therefore, before settling on a diagnosis of Adjustment Disorder, it is important to conduct a thorough evaluation to rule out the presence of a more specific condition. The second misconception—that all Adjustment Disorders are mild—arises from the requirement that criteria not be met for a more specific disorder. However, some Adjustment Disorders can be deadly. Particularly in adolescence, suicide attempts or successful suicides may occur in individuals with a diagnosis of Adjustment Disorder. The third misconception is that Adjustment Disorder is brief. Some stressors are long term or have long-term consequences that cause enduring adjustment problems.

Chapter 15

Personality Disorders

"**P**ersonality traits are enduring patterns of perceiving, relating to, and thinking about the environment and oneself that are exhibited in a wide range of social and personal contexts. Only when personality traits are inflexible and maladaptive and cause significant functional impairment or subjective distress do they constitute Personality Disorders" (DSM-IV-TR, p. 686). This is how DSM-IV describes the boundary between normal variations in personality traits that occur in all individuals and Personality Disorders that cause a pattern of long-term impairment. A general criteria set defining a Personality Disorder is given in DSM-IV-TR to specify the features that are common to all Personality Disorders and to help distinguish them from both Axis I disorders and normal personality variants.

DSM-IV-TR general diagnostic criteria for a Personality Disorder

A. An enduring pattern of inner experience and behavior that deviates markedly from the expectations of the individual's culture. This pattern is manifested in two (or more) of the following areas:
(1) cognition (i.e., ways of perceiving and interpreting self, other people, and events)
(2) affectivity (i.e., the range, intensity, lability, and appropriateness of emotional response)

(continued)

DSM-IV-TR general diagnostic criteria for a Personality Disorder *(continued)*

    (3) interpersonal functioning
    (4) impulse control

B. The enduring pattern is inflexible and pervasive across a broad range of personal and social situations.

C. The enduring pattern leads to clinically significant distress or impairment in social, occupational, or other important areas of functioning.

D. The pattern is stable and of long duration and its onset can be traced back at least to adolescence or early adulthood.

E. The enduring pattern is not better accounted for as a manifestation or consequence of another mental disorder.

F. The enduring pattern is not due to the direct physiological effects of a substance (e.g., a drug of abuse, a medication) or a general medical condition (e.g., head trauma).

To be considered a Personality Disorder, the individual's traits must "deviate markedly from the expectations of the individual's culture." To assess the degree of deviation, the clinician must either be familiar with the individual's cultural background or obtain this knowledge from other informants.

The traits and behaviors that define a Personality Disorder may be apparent in how a person perceives and interprets what is going on around him or her (cognition), in the type and intensity of emotional responses (affectivity), in the way the person interacts with other people (interpersonal functioning), and in how the person regulates impulses (impulse control). The pattern of traits and behaviors that constitutes a Personality Disorder must have been apparent no later than early adulthood and must show up in nearly every aspect of an individual's life (i.e., at home, at work, and in social situations). It is important to be sure that the traits and behaviors are not the result of another mental disorder (e.g., a Mood or Anxiety Disorder). Making this distinction is especially complicated in situations where an Axis I disorder, such as Major Depressive Disorder, is also present. Taking a careful history and obtaining information from informants, especially family members, may be helpful in determining whether a preexisting Personality Disorder is present. In some cases, a definite determination cannot be made until the Axis I disorder has remitted. In the case of chronic Axis I disorders, such as Dysthymic Disorder, it may be very difficult and perhaps not very useful to try to make an absolute determination of which features are associated with a Personality Disorder and which are related to an Axis I disorder.

To be considered a disorder, the traits and behaviors must cause distress for the individual or must interfere with how he or she is able to function either socially or occupationally or both. If a person is not distressed or impaired by the traits or behaviors, then a Personality Disorder would not be diagnosed. In some cases, although individuals are not distressed by or dissatisfied with their personality traits, their behavior is so irritating or so disruptive to others that it causes enough social or occupational impairment to be considered a Personality Disorder.

When personality problems develop as a result of a general medical condition, a diagnosis of Personality Change Due to a General Medical Condition is made and the specific condition involved (e.g., head trauma) is specified and listed on Axis III. Unlike Personality Disorders, changes can occur at any age and their onset is associated with the general medical condition causing the problem. The diagnosis of a Personality Disorder can be made in the presence of a Substance-Related Disorder if the Substance Use is judged to be secondary to the Personality Disorder.

Specific Personality Disorders

Criteria sets for 10 specific Personality Disorders are included in DSM-IV-TR. Individuals often meet criteria for more than one Personality Disorder, and all the disorders for which criteria are met should be diagnosed.

Personality Disorders

301.0	Paranoid Personality Disorder
301.20	Schizoid Personality Disorder
301.22	Schizotypal Personality Disorder
301.7	Antisocial Personality Disorder
301.83	Borderline Personality Disorder
301.50	Histrionic Personality Disorder
301.81	Narcissistic Personality Disorder
301.82	Avoidant Personality Disorder
301.6	Dependent Personality Disorder
301.4	Obsessive-Compulsive Personality Disorder
301.9	Personality Disorder Not Otherwise Specified

An additional category, 301.9 Personality Disorder Not Otherwise Specified, is included to allow clinicians to code Personality Disorders that do not meet criteria for any of the specific disorders listed above but that do meet the general criteria for a Personality Disorder. Personality Disorders that might be coded as "Not Otherwise Specified" include those with presentations of features of several different Personality Disorders that do not meet the full criteria for any one of the specific disorders included in this section. Also, if criteria are met for a Personality Disorder that is not included in the formal DSM-IV-TR classification, a Personality Disorder Not Otherwise Specified would be coded. Research criteria sets for two such Personality Disorders, depressive personality disorder and passive-aggressive (negativistic) personality disorder, are included in the DSM-IV-TR appendix for criteria sets provided for further study.

Paranoid Personality Disorder

❖   Case Study: Principal "Queeg"

Mr. Q, a 51-year-old middle school principal, comes in for evaluation at his wife's insistence after a battle with the school board that has put his job in jeopardy. She says that their current marital situation is intolerable and that if he doesn't stop fighting with everyone, she will be forced to leave.

During the initial interview, Mr. Q readily admits that, although he has always been a suspicious person, this characteristic has lately gotten out of hand. Despite this admission, he goes on to describe his feeling that members of the school board are conspiring with his staff and a group of unhappy parents to have him ousted from his position. He feels that the teachers and staff are "keeping him in the dark" and not telling him what is going on in the school so that he will look bad and lose his position. He says that he thinks his wife's insistence on this psychiatric evaluation may actually be part of the school board's plot to oust him, because his wife is good friends with one of the school board members, and Mr. Q suspects she may not be completely loyal to him. He says that the school board administrator told him recently that, since his promotion to principal 2 years ago, he has been driving everyone nuts. Mr. Q insists that he has been trying to do the best job he can and that this statement must stem from jealousy and the school board's determination to get rid of him, "probably because they want to put one of their buddies in the job." When questioned in more detail, Mr. Q does admit, however, that he might possibly be overreacting and that perhaps some aspects of his behavior could have been at fault. Nevertheless, Mr. Q says that he constantly thinks about how he is being mistreated and that this is interfering with his ability to perform his duties at school.

When his wife is interviewed separately, she says that Mr. Q has always had a tendency to be suspicious of others and to keep his feelings and thoughts to himself but that since his promotion to principal these traits had become much worse. She reports that she and Mr. Q have been having frequent fights because she tells him that he is creating his own problems. According to his wife, Mr. Q is constantly irritable and argumentative with her and with his teachers and staff. She is also very concerned about several incidents that have recently occurred at the school. For example, he accused the kitchen staff of deliberately wasting food so that his budget report would look bad. When the head of the kitchen staff showed him figures demonstrating that the cafeteria in his school did as well or better than any of the other cafeterias in the system, Mr. Q accused her of showing him falsified figures. The head of the kitchen staff then complained to the central office and requested a transfer, which was granted. On another occasion, Mr. Q became convinced that the seventh-grade teacher was privately making derogatory reports about him to the school superintendent, who was a personal friend of the teacher. On several occasions he called this teacher into his office and berated him for his "betrayal of trust." Mr. Q refused to accept the teacher's assurances that his relationship with the superintendent was completely social and that he would not have considered discussing Mr. Q behind his back in such a situation. The conflict finally grew so stressful that this teacher also requested a transfer to another school. After this incident, the school board administrator told Mr. Q that if matters continued this way, he would be unable to staff Mr. Q's school.

The recent battle with the school board was the result of Mr. Q's insistence that he had been unfairly passed over for an adequate pay raise. Despite being reassured by the administrator in charge of the budget that no other principal in a comparable position with a similar level of experience had received any larger increase, Mr. Q insisted on presenting his case to a closed session of the school board. Ms. Q's friend on the school board told his wife privately that Mr. Q's behavior and accusations during this meeting were so out of line with what the school board expected from a principal that she was seriously worried about him and concerned that he might lose his job. It was after this conversation that Ms. Q insisted that her husband go for psychiatric evaluation or she would leave him.

Mr. Q's wife says that Mr. Q will not talk to her parents because he is convinced that they think he isn't good enough for their daughter. He believes that they are trying to persuade her to leave him, which Ms. Q says is not true. He also tries to keep his wife and children from having any contact with Ms. Q's parents because, he claims, seeing her parents shows a lack of loyalty and attachment to him.

When the clinician interviews Mr. Q's two children, a 12-year-old girl and a 15-year-old boy, they complain that Mr. Q runs the house like a military base by constantly monitoring every expense, friend, and party. He insists that everyone give him a complete itinerary of where they plan to be at every minute. His daughter attends the school where he is principal, and he constantly grills her about what the other kids are saying about him. Mr. Q's family admits that he is right when he claims that they are keeping things from him. Because of his excessive vigilance, Mr. Q's wife and children have stopped telling him about almost everything; however, this leads to furious outbursts when he catches them in evasions or half-truths.

When asked to describe himself, Mr. Q says he takes pride in being the sort of person who can spot sham and phoniness in others. He discusses at length how he came from a very poor family, how he always had to work against the odds, and how he succeeded in finishing graduate school and achieving his present position despite adverse circumstances and the hindrances of a number of hostile professors and employers.

DSM-IV-TR Diagnosis

Axis I: 309.0   Adjustment Disorder With Depressed Mood
Axis II: 301.0   Paranoid Personality Disorder
Axis III: None
Axis IV: Promotion to principal, marital discord
Axis V: GAF = 50

DSM-IV-TR diagnostic criteria for
301.0 Paranoid Personality Disorder

A. A pervasive distrust and suspiciousness of others such that their motives are interpreted as malevolent, beginning by early adulthood and present in a variety of contexts, as indicated by four (or more) of the following:

   (1) suspects, without sufficient basis, that others are exploiting, harming, or deceiving him or her

   (2) is preoccupied with unjustified doubts about the loyalty or trustworthiness of friends or associates

   (3) is reluctant to confide in others because of unwarranted fear that the information will be used maliciously against him or her

   (4) reads hidden demeaning or threatening meanings into benign remarks or events

   (5) persistently bears grudges, i.e., is unforgiving of insults, injuries, or slights

(continued)

> ## DSM-IV-TR diagnostic criteria for
> ## 301.0 Paranoid Personality Disorder *(continued)*
>
>   (6)   perceives attacks on his or her character or reputation that are not apparent to others and is quick to react angrily or to counterattack
>   (7)   has recurrent suspicions, without justification, regarding fidelity of spouse or sexual partner
>
> B. Does not occur exclusively during the course of Schizophrenia, a Mood Disorder With Psychotic Features, or another Psychotic Disorder and is not due to the direct physiological effects of a general medical condition.
>
> **Note:** If criteria are met prior to the onset of Schizophrenia, add "Premorbid," e.g., "Paranoid Personality Disorder (Premorbid)."

Guidelines for Differential Diagnosis of Paranoid Personality Disorder

Mr. Q is obviously paranoid. However, the first question to be considered is whether there are legitimate grounds for his feelings because there is actually a threatening environment to be paranoid about or whether Mr. Q is bringing the situation to a head because of features within his own personality. Determining the reasonableness of Mr. Q's feelings hinges on the degree to which he meets every new situation with suspicion, regardless of whether the situation is realistically threatening, and whether his paranoid feelings and constant battles with others cause him distress and clinically significant impairment in his ability to function. Making this determination can be difficult in some cases, partly because a certain degree of suspiciousness can be adaptive and also because being paranoid leads to a vicious cycle of self-fulfilling prophecies. When you are paranoid, other people start feeling unable to reveal things to you, thus confirming your feeling that they are concealing things and are in league against you, as has happened with Mr. Q's family. Taking a careful history and including other informants can help to confirm that there has been a long-standing pattern of suspiciousness that is not related to a particular stressor (in which case the only diagnosis would be Adjustment Disorder) and that the feelings and behaviors are severe enough to warrant a diagnosis of Paranoid Personality Disorder, not only paranoid personality traits. In some individuals with paranoid personality traits, an external stressor or the presence of an Axis I disorder such as depression can result in a clinical presentation that cross-sectionally is identical to Paranoid Personality Disorder. However, this presentation differs in terms of premorbid history and has a much better prognosis for recovery once the stressor is reduced or the Axis I condition is successfully treated. For example, an individual with mild suspicious tendencies may develop a Major Depressive Episode during which the paranoid beliefs and fears transiently increase in severity; however, the person will usually return to a normal level of mild suspiciousness once the depression is in remission.

Mr. Q appears to have had a long-standing pattern of suspicion and paranoia that has caused him problems and distress for most of his adult life, justifying a diagnosis of Paranoid Personality Disorder. He describes hostility from professors in graduate school and from former employers. He has always regarded his in-laws as hostile and has tried to sever his wife's connection with them. His behavior to his wife and family has been characterized by suspicion and distrust. An additional diagnosis of Adjustment Disorder With Depressed Mood is warranted because the effects of Mr. Q's promotion to principal have caused his symptoms to intensify. His suspicions have gotten out of hand, and his functional impairment is becoming severe (e.g., he is likely to lose his job).

At times it is difficult to distinguish between Paranoid Personality Disorder and Delusional Disorder, especially because individuals with Paranoid Personality Disorder tend to create hostility in others. For example, Mr. Q's teachers and staff often are really angry with him and the school board really is considering terminating him—his conviction that they are hostile is factual. It is best to have a high threshold before calling such plausible concerns delusions. However, if Mr. Q's suspicious beliefs should become fixed, unshakable, and weighty enough to be considered delusions, both diagnoses could then be given, with "(premorbid)" noted after the Personality Disorder diagnosis.

Treatment Planning for
Paranoid Personality Disorder

There is no specific treatment for Paranoid Personality Disorder. Patients often respond to a supportive and structured psychotherapy. Once rapport is established, it is useful to explore systematically the patient's fears, convictions, and grudges to determine whether alternative explanations are possible and to suggest other strategies for dealing with the people and situations involved. At times, treatments geared toward impaired relationships in the family may be useful in identifying sources of misunderstanding. Patients with milder forms of Paranoid Personality Disorder may have sufficient insight to engage in psychodynamic treatments aimed at understanding the internal conflicts and self-dislike they are projecting onto others. It may help to point out the vicious cycles in which these individuals become embroiled in order to increase their understanding of how their own behavior is contributing to other people's reactions.

For example, the clinician could try to help Mr. Q explore the feelings he and the teachers have about each other to determine whether he can find ways in which he is causing these feelings. It would then be useful to help Mr. Q plan new strategies for dealing with his staff, teachers, and the school board. People with this disorder often respond best to straightforward reality if it can be presented in a way that is not challenging or confronting. The clinician needs to help Mr. Q gain intellectual control of the situation so that Mr. Q can try to retain his position.

Schizoid Personality Disorder

❖ Case Study: A Man Who Prefers to Be Alone

Mr. S is a 38-year-old unmarried laboratory technician who is referred by his employer, a university scientist, because he is having difficulty being a team player on a project. For the past 5 years, Mr. S has been employed in the laboratory working on a project more or less by himself and doing very well at it. The renewal grant that Mr. S's employer recently received, allowing for Mr. S's continued employment, involves a substantial expansion of the project. The scientist therefore hired a number of new employees to work in the lab, and he expected Mr. S to train them. Several of the newly hired people quit within 3 weeks, saying that Mr. S was impossible to learn from and to work with. They complained that he did not provide any guidance and that he was unfriendly and arrogant. When the scientist confronted Mr. S with these charges after the third individual quit, Mr. S was bland and surprised. He said that he was trying to do his best and that he couldn't understand the complaints. He did admit that he was somewhat annoyed at the change in his role and was not really clear about what was expected of him. His employer had previously been pleased with the thoroughness and accuracy of Mr. S's work and was reluctant to lose him, but he realized that the success of his expanded project was in jeopardy if Mr. S was unable to learn to train and work with others. He therefore suggested to Mr. S that he seek some professional help in dealing with his new duties and hence Mr. S came in for evaluation.

During the initial interview, Mr. S describes himself as a loner who has always felt awkward and unhappy when forced into relationships with others. He says that he has always been detached from the rest of his family. When asked to describe his life growing up, it becomes apparent that Mr. S has never had a good friend, was never chosen to be on teams, and never participated in any school activities. Mr. S describes these facts in a de-

tached manner and does not appear at all distressed by them. He says that
he has never dated or had any sexual experiences with others, nor does he
express any desire to do so when asked. His interest in science began with a
chemistry set he received for his 13th birthday, after which he spent long
hours as a teenager conducting solitary experiments. When asked about
how he spends his leisure time, he says that he mostly enjoys playing computer games.

DSM-IV-TR Diagnosis

Axis I: V71.09   No diagnosis
Axis II: 301.20   Schizoid Personality Disorder
Axis III: None
Axis IV: Potential loss of job
Axis V: GAF = 50 (current); 65 (highest level in past year)

DSM-IV-TR diagnostic criteria for
301.20 Schizoid Personality Disorder

A. A pervasive pattern of detachment from social relationships and a restricted range of expression of emotions in interpersonal settings, beginning by early adulthood and present in a variety of contexts, as indicated
by four (or more) of the following:
  (1) neither desires nor enjoys close relationships, including being part of
      a family
  (2) almost always chooses solitary activities
  (3) has little, if any, interest in having sexual experiences with another
      person
  (4) takes pleasure in few, if any, activities
  (5) lacks close friends or confidants other than first-degree relatives
  (6) appears indifferent to the praise or criticism of others
  (7) shows emotional coldness, detachment, or flattened affectivity
B. Does not occur exclusively during the course of Schizophrenia, a Mood
Disorder With Psychotic Features, another Psychotic Disorder, or a Pervasive Developmental Disorder and is not due to the direct physiological effects of a general medical condition.

Note: If criteria are met prior to the onset of Schizophrenia, add "Premorbid,"
e.g., "Schizoid Personality Disorder (Premorbid)."

Guidelines for Differential Diagnosis
of Schizoid Personality Disorder

The concept of Schizoid Personality Disorder belies Aristotle's idea of man as a social animal. These individuals appear to lack that spark of enjoyment or pleasure that characterizes most people's reactions to social intercourse. In diagnosing Schizoid Personality Disorder, the most important differential is with people who are loners but do not have a Personality Disorder. If an individual prefers to be solitary and is not distressed or impaired by this, a diagnosis of Schizoid Personality Disorder would not be appropriate. If Mr. S were able to function successfully at work and feel satisfied with his life, a Personality Disorder diagnosis would not be appropriate. However, because Mr. S's lifelong pattern of avoiding contact with others is causing a problem that places his job in danger, this diagnosis is relevant.

The next important differential in diagnosing Schizoid Personality Disorder is with Avoidant Personality Disorder. In Avoidant Personality Disorder, individuals want to be accepted and avoid social situations because of a fear of being embarrassed or rejected, whereas those with Schizoid Personality Disorder appear uninterested in social involvement, from which they derive little or no pleasure. For example, Mr. S does not appear to be distressed by his isolation, although he has never had a close friend and has never dated.

Individuals with Schizoid Personality Disorder resemble those with Schizotypal Personality Disorder in their lack of interest in social intercourse and their restricted range of emotions, but they do not have the distortions of cognition and perception and the odd or magical beliefs that are characteristic of Schizotypal Personality Disorder. Individuals with Paranoid Personality Disorder may avoid social contact, but this is because they fear that others are hostile or conspiring against them, not because of a lack of interest.

Treatment Planning for
Schizoid Personality Disorder

Individuals such as Mr. S rarely volunteer for (or stay in) therapy, nor is there a specific treatment for this disorder. However, it may be helpful to increase an individual's cognitive awareness of how his or her personality features are causing problems and to encourage certain environmental manipulations. The therapist might explore with Mr. S precisely what needs to be done to meet the new demands of his job. Although Mr. S will undoubtedly always have trouble naturally and easily providing others with information, once he understands how important this is for maintaining his role in the project he may be better able to fulfill the new requirements of his position. In dealing with individuals with this disorder, it is often very important to help them select the right job, because they may do very well in positions that require only minimal interaction with others, as did Mr. S during the 5 years he worked largely alone. If Mr. S's efforts to adjust to his new role prove to be impossible, he might be better served by switching to a position more similar to the one he held previously, which does not require working as part of a team. In addition, education of a patient's family or employer may help them to provide enough space so the patient does not feel interpersonally surrounded.

Schizotypal Personality Disorder

❖   Case Study: Odd Woman Out

Ms. G is a 60-year-old woman who has never been married and lives by herself with 13 cats. Ms. G's appearance is strange, and her behavior is obviously eccentric. Although she has an endearing quality and is likable, anyone who sees her immediately senses that she is "different." Ms. G dresses in a crazy quilt of colors in an eclectic style that favors the 1920s. She has never been able to work, but she lived on an inheritance from her parents until she was in her 40s and since then has been supported by disability payments and welfare. Ms. G was raised in a devout Roman Catholic home and believes that she is destined to receive a visitation from the Virgin Mary, as the children at Lourdes did. She is constantly on the lookout for messages or clues that she believes will reveal to her when and where the visitation will occur. For example, she carefully reviews the most ordinary statements made by individuals (e.g., the checker at the grocery store or the clerk at the post office) to see whether their words have hidden and deeper meanings. Ms. G experiences almost constant feelings of depersonalization and derealization: She says she feels as if she is not connected to herself and as if she is a character in a movie. She is fascinated by the subject of out-of-body experiences and describes frequent episodes of astral travel. Her apartment is filled with signs and refuse she has collected over the years. Despite her odd beliefs, Ms. G is not delusional and is able to acknowledge that she may be mistaken in her beliefs. She often feels that other people are talking about her when she leaves the apartment but acknowledges that this may be because of the unusual way she dresses. For this reason and because she is extremely stilted and shy in social situations, Ms. G generally goes out only at night to avoid talking to others or meeting them in the elevator. She sneaks in and out of her apartment surreptitiously and does her shopping at the 24-hour store at 3 A.M. when hardly anyone is there.

Ms. G had a maternal uncle who was schizophrenic. She has been very shy and retiring since she was a child and says that she was always "odd" and never fit in with her brothers or sisters or fellow students. Although her siblings have suggested at various times over the years that Ms. G seek some sort of psychiatric treatment, she has refused. Ms. G is brought in for evaluation at this time because she was picked up by the police after she took a figure of the Virgin Mary from a religious supply store without paying for it, claiming that she was meant to have it. When the policeman insisted that Ms. G must return the statue, she became argumentative, irritable, and threatened to strike him. At this point she was handcuffed and brought to the emergency room.

Ms. G has four brothers and two sisters. To varying degrees, they have tried to remain in contact with her over the years. She has rejected most of their overtures, however, and is irritated at each one of them for different reasons. She says she feels more comfortable alone. Although in earlier years she used to be invited to family gatherings for holidays, her brothers and sisters have long since abandoned their attempts to get her to participate in these social occasions. For the past 15 years she has lived in almost complete isolation, except for an occasional phone call from one of her brothers or sisters. Her siblings have arranged for her to receive disability and welfare payments, however, and also provide her with hand-me-down clothes.

DSM-IV-TR Diagnosis

Axis I: V71.09   No diagnosis
Axis II: 301.22   Schizotypal Personality Disorder
Axis III: None
Axis IV: Trouble with the law
Axis V: GAF = 45

DSM-IV-TR diagnostic criteria for
301.22 Schizotypal Personality Disorder

A. A pervasive pattern of social and interpersonal deficits marked by acute discomfort with, and reduced capacity for, close relationships as well as by cognitive or perceptual distortions and eccentricities of behavior, beginning by early adulthood and present in a variety of contexts, as indicated by five (or more) of the following:

(continued)

**DSM-IV-TR diagnostic criteria for
301.22 Schizotypal Personality Disorder (continued)**

(1)   ideas of reference (excluding delusions of reference)
(2)   odd beliefs or magical thinking that influences behavior and is in-
      consistent with subcultural norms (e.g., superstitiousness, belief in
      clairvoyance, telepathy, or "sixth sense"; in children and adoles-
      cents, bizarre fantasies or preoccupations)
(3)   unusual perceptual experiences, including bodily illusions
(4)   odd thinking and speech (e.g., vague, circumstantial, metaphorical,
      overelaborate, or stereotyped)
(5)   suspiciousness or paranoid ideation
(6)   inappropriate or constricted affect
(7)   behavior or appearance that is odd, eccentric, or peculiar
(8)   lack of close friends or confidants other than first-degree relatives
(9)   excessive social anxiety that does not diminish with familiarity and
      tends to be associated with paranoid fears rather than negative judg-
      ments about self
B.   Does not occur exclusively during the course of Schizophrenia, a Mood
     Disorder With Psychotic Features, another Psychotic Disorder, or a Perva-
     sive Developmental Disorder.

Note: If criteria are met prior to the onset of Schizophrenia, add "Premorbid,"
e.g., "Schizotypal Personality Disorder (Premorbid)."

Guidelines for Differential Diagnosis of Schizotypal Personality Disorder

In diagnosing Schizotypal Personality Disorder, the clinician must first rule
out the presence of past or present psychotic symptoms that may indicate
Schizophrenia, Delusional Disorder, or a Mood Disorder With Psychotic
Features. Although individuals with Schizotypal Personality Disorder often
cling to very odd and magical beliefs (e.g., Ms. G's expectation of a divine
vision and her belief in astral travel), they do not experience persistent psychotic symptoms such as hallucinations and delusions. They may, however,
experience transient psychotic episodes that remit within minutes to hours
and would not warrant an additional diagnosis. These very brief psychotic
experiences are particularly likely to occur when these individuals are under
stress.

Individuals with Schizotypal Personality Disorder may occasionally develop Schizophrenia, in which case the Schizotypal Personality Disorder would still be noted on Axis II as "premorbid." It can sometimes be difficult to distinguish adults with Schizotypal Personality Disorder from those with the residual symptoms of mild Autistic Disorder or Asperger's Disorder. However, individuals with a Pervasive Developmental Disorder usually have a history of severe social withdrawal and strange behavior from early infancy. Schizotypal Personality Disorder can be distinguished from the other Personality Disorders, especially by the presence of distortions in cognition and perception and odd, eccentric, and magical beliefs. Borderline Personality Disorder and Major Depressive Disorder are very often comorbid with Schizotypal Personality Disorder, although neither of these is a feature of Ms. G's presentation.

Treatment Planning for Schizotypal Personality Disorder

There is no specific treatment for this condition. Low doses of antipsychotic medications have been tried and may be symptomatically helpful; however, many individuals find the side effects unacceptable and compliance tends to be low. It may sometimes be useful to provide these individuals with clarifications of reality to help them understand how their behaviors are not working out very well and to suggest alternative ways to deal with the world. For example, the clinician might try to make Ms. G understand why the store owner and policeman reacted to her shoplifting as they did and to explain the need to avoid this behavior in the future.

Antisocial Personality Disorder

❖   Case Study: A Bad Man

Mr. Y is a 26-year-old man who is transferred from prison to a psychiatric unit as a result of a suicide attempt. Mr. Y has a history of three previous suicide attempts and multiple problems with the law. From information contained in the patient's social services, medical, and legal records, the clinician is able to piece together Mr. Y's history.

Mr. Y's mother was a prostitute and drug addict, and he never knew his father. He had a history of very serious conduct problems from a young age. He began getting into fights with other children almost from the day he began school and was caught torturing animals on a number of occasions when he was in elementary school. When he was 9 years old, Mr. Y threw his baby brother out of the window of their first floor apartment, causing multiple fractures. During his childhood, Mr. Y spent several years in a group home and stayed in many foster homes, but these placements were never successful. He would occasionally stay with his maternal grandmother, who was taking care of up to eight other grandchildren at the same time. Mr. Y began using drugs at age 10.

In early adolescence, Mr. Y joined a gang where he became involved in selling drugs and running numbers. He fathered his first child at the age of 13. Before he was 17, he was arrested on a variety of charges that included theft, possession of illegal drugs, and assault, but, because of his age, he received a series of suspended sentences. He was constantly truant from school and finally dropped out permanently at age 15. At that time, he began living on the street with other friends from his gang who were also engaged in using and selling drugs. At age 17, he was sentenced to 2 years in prison for stabbing someone in a fight in a bar. During this imprisonment, he attempted suicide by hanging himself with an article of clothing. As a result of this, he was transferred to the infirmary for several weeks and did not have to participate in his work detail.

By the time Mr. Y was 23, he had fathered five children, none of whom he sees or supports. When he's not crossed, Mr. Y is a manipulative person who can be charming, funny, and gregarious. When he is on drugs or when he does not get his way, however, he can become coldly furious and ruthlessly destructive.

Mr. Y has been treated for a series of drug overdoses, several of which were intentional. He has been hospitalized in psychiatric facilities on three occasions because of depression and suicide attempts. This is the fourth such hospitalization. Mr. Y's behavior follows a characteristic pattern during these hospitalizations. Initially, he seems to blossom and get better right away and is helpful with staff and patients. Soon, however, Mr. Y begins stirring up trouble on the ward and leading the other patients in revolt concerning smoking privileges, passes, and the need for medication. On one occasion during his most recent hospitalization, he was caught having intercourse with a 60-year-old female patient.

DSM-IV-TR Diagnosis

Axis I: V71.09   No diagnosis
Axis II: 301.7   Antisocial Personality Disorder
Axis III: None
Axis IV: Imprisonment
Axis V: GAF = 40

**DSM-IV-TR diagnostic criteria for
301.7 Antisocial Personality Disorder**

A. There is a pervasive pattern of disregard for and violation of the rights of others occurring since age 15 years, as indicated by three (or more) of the following:

    (1) failure to conform to social norms with respect to lawful behaviors as indicated by repeatedly performing acts that are grounds for arrest

    (2) deceitfulness, as indicated by repeated lying, use of aliases, or conning others for personal profit or pleasure

    (3) impulsivity or failure to plan ahead

    (4) irritability and aggressiveness, as indicated by repeated physical fights or assaults

    (5) reckless disregard for safety of self or others

    (6) consistent irresponsibility, as indicated by repeated failure to sustain consistent work behavior or honor financial obligations

    (7) lack of remorse, as indicated by being indifferent to or rationalizing having hurt, mistreated, or stolen from another

B. The individual is at least age 18 years.

C. There is evidence of Conduct Disorder with onset before age 15 years.

D. The occurrence of antisocial behavior is not exclusively during the course of Schizophrenia or a Manic Episode.

Guidelines for Differential Diagnosis of Antisocial Personality Disorder

The most fundamental question concerning Antisocial Personality Disorder is whether it should be considered a mental disorder and be included in DSM-IV. There are many cogent arguments for not considering Antisocial Personality Disorder a mental disorder, not least of which is that there is no effective treatment and that including the disorder in the manual could conceivably result in people's evading responsibility for their actions. This disorder continues to be included in DSM-IV (and DSM-IV-TR), however, because of a long historical tradition and because the more early onset and severe forms of the disorder are familial, probably with both genetic and cultural transmission.

Antisocial Personality Disorder is comorbid with a number of other psychiatric conditions and is associated with a high suicide rate of 5%–10%. However, not everybody who commits a crime has a Personality Disorder. Most individuals who commit antisocial acts do not have any mental disorder. Some individuals choose a life of crime as a means of earning a living and do not meet the other criteria for Antisocial Personality Disorder (e.g., someone who commits the acts purely for gain such as a professional drug dealer or killer). When evaluating someone who has committed antisocial acts, other diagnoses to consider are Substance-Related or Bipolar Disorders or Schizophrenia.

Antisocial Personality Disorder is not meant to be used to describe individuals who perform isolated antisocial acts. If late-developing or isolated antisocial behaviors become a focus of clinical attention, they can be noted by using "Adult Antisocial Behavior," which is included in the DSM-IV-TR section "Other Conditions That May Be a Focus of Clinical Attention."

Antisocial Personality Disorder is meant to describe a pattern of behavior beginning in early life that would have warranted a diagnosis of Conduct Disorder before the person was 15 years old. If a late adolescent or young adult continues to display disruptive and antisocial behaviors that are not severe enough to meet the criteria for Antisocial Personality Disorder, a diagnosis of Conduct Disorder may be warranted. According to the DSM-IV-TR definition, the diagnosis of Antisocial Personality Disorder cannot be given to anyone under 18 years of age.

Two other important issues in considering the appropriateness of a diagnosis of Antisocial Personality Disorder are the relationship of the behaviors to drugs and to an individual's cultural background. This is in many ways an example of the classic chicken and the egg problem: People with a proclivity for conduct disturbance tend to use drugs early and join gangs; however, people who might otherwise avoid antisocial behavior may become involved in such behavior secondarily because of the consequences of drug use and peer pressure. Because it is often impossible to tease out the role of drugs and peer pressure in the etiology of antisocial behavior, their presence does not preclude this diagnosis. A diagnosis of Antisocial Personality Disorder requires that there be evidence that Conduct Disorder was present and had its onset before the individual was 15 years old. A number of other Personality Disorders may be comorbid with Antisocial Personality Disorder, in particular Borderline, Histrionic, and Narcissistic Personality Disorders.

Treatment Planning for Antisocial Personality Disorder

The only effective treatment for Antisocial Personality Disorder appears to be the passage of time. Those individuals who do not get killed or kill themselves and survive into their 40s tend to mellow out and become less impulsive and predatory. When Substance Abuse is a prominent part of the clinical picture, it provides an important target for intervention. Individuals with this Personality Disorder often also have episodes of depression that may require treatment and suicide risk prevention, especially given the high suicide rate associated with the disorder.

One major problem is where and how treatment should be provided. Individuals with Antisocial Personality Disorder are usually noncompliant with outpatient intervention. Prison rehabilitation programs have not been very effective, and these individuals become wolves among sheep when hospitalized in psychiatric facilities, as seen in the way Mr. Y behaved during his psychiatric hospitalizations. If this discussion of the treatment of Antisocial Personality Disorder sounds pessimistic, it is meant to.

Borderline Personality Disorder

❖   Case Study: A Woman With an Unstable Life

Ms. E is a 25-year-old woman brought to the emergency room by her boyfriend, who has become progressively more alarmed at her complaints, demands, and erratic behavior. Her chief complaint to the staff is "I keep thinking about wanting to kill myself." Ms. E is a competent secretary, has her own apartment, and is self-supporting. She is also attending university classes in the evening because she wants to advance her education and does not "want to stay a secretary all my life."

The current crisis began when her boyfriend, Mr. M, refused to consider her demands for marriage after a 2-year exclusive relationship. Ms. E began to call him at work demanding more and more time, finally threatening to kill herself if he didn't spend every evening with her. Mr. M reported that her demands, phone calls, and escalating threats were becoming intolerable and were making him want to break off the relationship entirely. On the evening Mr. M brought Ms. E to the emergency room, he had told her that he had to go on a business trip and would be away for several days. Ms. E insisted that he was doing this just to get away from her. She became severely agitated and began to talk wildly about killing herself. In the emergency room, Ms. E angrily belittles her boyfriend in front of the staff and accuses him of using and then rejecting her. After physically separating the arguing couple, the staff is able to obtain a history of the progressive development of Ms. E's symptoms.

In response to the stress of the past several months, Ms. E has developed fluctuating depressive moods, a tendency to oversleep (especially sleeping in the evenings and on weekends), and a tendency to binge eat that has resulted in a 20-pound weight gain. Ms. E says she is constantly anxious and has been having increasing difficulty concentrating on her studies. She has continued to work throughout this stressful period, seeking support from those in her office. Attention from Mr. M or her co-workers produces a brightening of her mood that she is able to sustain while they are with her.

Ms. E experiences her most severe symptoms when she is alone. These include prolonged fantasies about killing her boyfriend and a desire to hurt herself. She says that on several occasions she has cut her thighs with razor blades and describes watching herself do this as if from a distance, numb and dead inside and feeling little pain. Ms. E says that at these times she feels fat and unattractive as well as completely unlovable and worthless. At such moments, she calls Mr. M on the phone and threatens to commit suicide unless he comes and keeps her company. Mr. M reports that she has also begun to lose control of her temper. For example, shortly before he brought her to the emergency room, she attacked him with her fists in the midst of an argument.

Ms. E was the youngest of four children and one of two girls. Her parents separated and divorced when she was 3 years old because of her father's alcoholism and physical abuse of his wife and children. A family secret was that Ms. E was sexually abused when she was 10 years old by a brother 5 years her senior.

In adolescence, Ms. E associated with a rebellious group and became involved in drug abuse and early sexuality to fit in. Ms. E said that her mother attributed Ms. E's teenage rebellion to a need to "find a father" and that she thought that Ms. E had gotten "her sexual urges confused with wanting to be loved and cared for." By age 16, Ms. E had already embarked on the pattern of chaotic unstable involvements with men that continues to characterize her adult life.

Her first drug overdose occurred at age 17 in response to a perceived rejection by her boyfriend. A series of intense relationships followed this incident, each of which followed a similar pattern: Ms. E would become progressively more clinging until she gradually alienated her partners. Each rejection was marked by a period of anger and self-abuse, followed quickly by a new and identical relationship. Ms. E's current boyfriend is only the latest in a long series of disappointing partners.

DSM-IV-TR Diagnosis

Axis I:	296.32	Major Depressive Disorder, Moderate, Recurrent, With Atypical Features, Without Full Interepisode Recovery, Without Preexisting Dysthymic Disorder
Axis II:	301.83	Borderline Personality Disorder
Axis III:	None	
Axis IV:	Breakup of relationship with boyfriend	
Axis V:	GAF = 35 (current); 80 (highest level in past year)	

DSM-IV-TR diagnostic criteria for
301.83 Borderline Personality Disorder

A pervasive pattern of instability of interpersonal relationships, self-image, and affects, and marked impulsivity beginning by early adulthood and present in a variety of contexts, as indicated by five (or more) of the following:

(1) frantic efforts to avoid real or imagined abandonment. **Note:** Do not include suicidal or self-mutilating behavior covered in Criterion 5.

(2) a pattern of unstable and intense interpersonal relationships characterized by alternating between extremes of idealization and devaluation

(3) identity disturbance: markedly and persistently unstable self-image or sense of self

(4) impulsivity in at least two areas that are potentially self-damaging (e.g., spending, sex, substance abuse, reckless driving, binge eating). **Note:** Do not include suicidal or self-mutilating behavior covered in Criterion 5.

(5) recurrent suicidal behavior, gestures, or threats, or self-mutilating behavior

(6) affective instability due to a marked reactivity of mood (e.g., intense episodic dysphoria, irritability, or anxiety usually lasting a few hours and only rarely more than a few days)

(7) chronic feelings of emptiness

(8) inappropriate, intense anger or difficulty controlling anger (e.g., frequent displays of temper, constant anger, recurrent physical fights)

(9) transient, stress-related paranoid ideation or severe dissociative symptoms

Guidelines for Differential Diagnosis of
Borderline Personality Disorder

Although Mood Disorders and Borderline Personality Disorder can often occur together (as was the case for Ms. E), they may also be confused with each other. The diagnosis of Borderline Personality Disorder is frequently used inappropriately and pejoratively for individuals who are temporarily irritable, demanding, manipulative, and self-destructive during a Major Depressive Episode. Such behavior does not warrant a diagnosis of Borderline Personality Disorder unless the features have an early onset, a pervasive impact, and a more or less chronic course. In some cases, the patient's "borderline symptoms" disappear as the mood symptoms remit, whereas, in others, both diagnoses are warranted. An individual's response to treatment may be helpful in making the distinction.

The same kinds of issues apply to individuals with Substance-Related Problems who may behave in unstable and impulsive ways when intoxicated with substances but who may behave very differently when off substances. The clinician is faced with the same chicken and egg problem we discussed for Antisocial Personality Disorder: Because Borderline Personality Disorder is often characterized by self-destructive Substance Use, it can be very difficult to establish whether the destructive personality features led to the Substance Use or whether the Substance Use produced the impairment in personality.

Borderline Personality Disorder tends to be comorbid with many Axis I conditions, including Mood Disorders, Substance-Related Disorders, Eating Disorders (especially Bulimia Nervosa), Posttraumatic Stress Disorder, and Attention-Deficit/Hyperactivity Disorder, each of which must be considered in the differential diagnosis. Because completed suicide occurs in 5%–10% of individuals with Borderline Personality Disorder, it is especially important to identify and treat comorbid Mood Disorders when they are present. Borderline Personality Disorder is also often comorbid with other Personality Disorders.

Treatment Planning for
Borderline Personality Disorder

In treating an individual with Borderline Personality Disorder, the clinician must first focus on the target symptoms of depression and Substance Use. After these have been evaluated and treated, several promising treatments that have been developed specifically for Borderline Personality Disorder can be used. These include cognitive-behavior therapy (dialectical behavior therapy), which focuses on particular problems such as interpersonal rejection sensitivity, self-destructive and aggressive behavior, depersonalization, and a tendency to see the world without shades of gray. Long-term psychodynamic therapy, with an emphasis on increasing insight and providing a corrective emotional experience, is also often very helpful. Whatever the treatment chosen, it is important to avoid creating conditions in which regression can take place or that reinforce suicide attempts. Hospitalization can often do as much harm as good and should be avoided or kept brief whenever possible.

Time is on our side in treating Borderline Personality Disorder. A number of studies indicate that the long-term prognosis is surprisingly good because patients seem to mellow out with age.

Histrionic Personality Disorder

❖ Case Study: The "King" Bee

Mr. C is a 45-year-old television actor who presents for consultation after his girlfriend has abruptly walked out. Although Mr. C is very attractive, he is dressed in a fashion that seems suited to a much younger man. He is wearing a tank top, tight jeans, a large medallion, and has longish hair. At the beginning of the interview, he is wildly disconsolate about the loss of his girlfriend, tearing at his hair and declaring that he sees no purpose in going on living. However, his theatrically expressed despair rapidly vanishes as he becomes increasingly interested in the female therapist and begins to make a series of sexually seductive remarks to her.

His recent romantic "tragedy" apparently repeats a pattern that has occurred frequently in Mr. C's life. He falls quickly and deeply in love, soon becomes a "love junkie" who can't stand for his latest girlfriend to spend any time away from him, and then can't tolerate the "cold-turkey" withdrawal of love that seems to follow inevitably from relationships that are too intense and torrid to have any staying power. Whenever a relationship does seem to be leading toward marriage, however, Mr. C loses interest, discovers previously undetected faults in the woman, and breaks off the affair himself. Mr. C has been in serious relationships in which marriage was discussed at least six times, but the woman never turned out to be the "right one."

Mr. C has a "passion" for restaurants but complains that he has a difficult time finding others to accompany him because so few people "share my discriminating tastes." After hearing Mr. C describe his usual behavior in a restaurant, it becomes clear that eating with him must be torture. He mobilizes all the waiters and the maitre d' so that his table becomes a center of activity and attention. Before ordering, Mr. C insists on speaking to the head chef, the dessert chef, and the wine steward; demands detailed descriptions of how each entree is prepared; and usually insists on visiting the kitchen or the wine cellar. Before long, the whole restaurant seems to be involved in his selection of delicacies. Despite all this, few dishes live up to Mr. C's expectations and it is very unusual for him to finish a dinner without sending at least one dish back. Mr. C is equally fussy about women— one is too tall, another too short, one is too talkative, another too quiet, one is too flamboyant, another too mousy; no one is "just right."

Mr. C has been in psychotherapy many times in his life and is aware of the self-defeating and self-destructive nature of his love relationships. He is a very intelligent, well read, and psychologically sophisticated man who can provide a detailed and convincing psychodynamic formulation for his behavior. None of this apparent insight has any perceptible effect on his behavior once he leaves the office, however, a fact he also recognizes and points out with a combination of thoughtfulness, regret, and insouciance.

Mr. C has been very successful in his work but has never fulfilled his early promise. When he was in his 20s, he landed several important roles in serious stage plays. However, he always had a hard time sticking with the parts and with the tremendous commitment of time and energy required. Over the years, he has turned more and more to television work and has had parts in a number of daytime soap operas. Mr. C is as fickle in work as in love, starting each new role with tremendous commitment and initially doing very well but after a few months heading off to do something else. He is much more interested in being liked and admired by his fellow actors and by the production crew, particularly the females, than in actually getting the job done. He also enjoys describing all the important and influential people in his field, such as actors, producers, and directors, with whom he has close relationships, always referring to them on a first-name basis. He reports that he has great difficulty working with other men because they are jealous of him and excessively competitive. Although he has many female friends, he has never had a close male friend.

The youngest, handsomest, and most talented of three brothers, the patient was prized and indulged by both of his parents. They were always convinced that he had a great future and encouraged him to cultivate his good looks and acting skills, happily paying for expensive clothes and acting courses. Mr. C matured early and began his many erotic adventures at the age of 14. Ever since that time, he has experienced his life as an unhappy but exciting melodrama.

In much the same pattern as that seen in his love relationships, Mr. C begins each new psychotherapy relationship with enthusiasm and ends with a feeling of disappointment or rejection. He typically falls in love with his female therapists and has trouble keeping them out of his mind. He feels frustrated when his affection is not reciprocated, even though he has been in therapy often enough to know that it would be inappropriate and unprofessional for such a relationship to develop. Mr. C has never received medication.

DSM-IV-TR Diagnosis

Axis I: V71.09   No diagnosis
Axis II: 301.50   Histrionic Personality Disorder
             301.81   Narcissistic Personality Disorder
Axis III: None
Axis IV: Breakup with current girlfriend
Axis V: GAF = 65

DSM-IV-TR diagnostic criteria for
301.50 Histrionic Personality Disorder

A pervasive pattern of excessive emotionality and attention seeking, beginning by early adulthood and present in a variety of contexts, as indicated by five (or more) of the following:

(1) is uncomfortable in situations in which he or she is not the center of attention

(2) interaction with others is often characterized by inappropriate sexually seductive or provocative behavior

(3) displays rapidly shifting and shallow expression of emotions

(4) consistently uses physical appearance to draw attention to self

(5) has a style of speech that is excessively impressionistic and lacking in detail

(6) shows self-dramatization, theatricality, and exaggerated expression of emotion

(7) is suggestible, i.e., easily influenced by others or circumstances

(8) considers relationships to be more intimate than they actually are

---

Guidelines for Differential Diagnosis of Histrionic Personality Disorder

The main problem in diagnosing Histrionic Personality Disorder is that it is often missed in males. For example, in Tennessee Williams's play, *A Streetcar Named Desire*, most people would immediately notice that Blanche Dubois might be a good candidate for a diagnosis of Histrionic Personality Disorder because of her constant need to be the center of attention, her wildly dramatic utterances, her femme fatale sexual posture, and her insistence on maintaining her fragile southern belle appearance. However, many people would fail to see that the very same diagnosis could easily apply to Stanley Kowalski, who is equally focused on his sexual seductiveness and physical appearance, is self-dramatizing, and is uncomfortable when not the center of attention and object of deference, especially for the women around him. In fact, it is the clash between these two individuals who both need to be the absolute center of their universe that drives the dramatic tension in the play.

Histrionic Personality Disorder often co-occurs with Borderline, Narcissistic, Antisocial, or Dependent Personality Disorders. The main characteristics that help to distinguish individuals with Histrionic Personality Disorder from those with the other Personality Disorders are their flamboyant, overly dramatic quality; their preoccupation with sexual seductiveness and physical appearance; and their willingness to accept whatever role is required (e.g., to be helpless, fragile, dependent) to gain the attention they so desperately desire. Mood, Somatoform, and Anxiety Disorders are the most common comorbid Axis I disorders in individuals with Histrionic Personality Disorder and are particularly likely to develop if the individual has lost or fears losing attention.

Treatment Planning for Histrionic Personality Disorder

In our experience, it is usually not a good idea for a man with Histrionic Personality Disorder to be treated by a female therapist, nor for a female with this disorder to have a male therapist. When treated by a female therapist, the main thing a male patient with this disorder will seek is the female's attention (just as a female patient will seek the attention of a male therapist). However, this outcome is usually not helpful to these patients and often is not analyzable no matter how insightful the patient seems to be on the surface. If the patient can tolerate it, a therapist of the same sex would be a better choice, and group therapy might also be indicated because in this situation the individual will begin to learn to share attention. In deciding how to treat the individual with Histrionic Personality Disorder, the clinician must choose between providing supportive therapy or therapy to help the patient become more aware of and actually change destructive and impairing personality traits. When an Axis III disorder is present and complicates the presentation, it is probably best to provide supportive treatment until the other condition has been treated. For example, a woman with Histrionic Personality Disorder who has recently had a mastectomy because of breast cancer should be complimented on how attractive her hair or dress is.

Narcissistic Personality Disorder

❖   Case Study: A Man With Expectations
      That No One Can Live Up To

Mr. R is a 50-year-old professor of pathology who presents with great surprise because his wife has announced that she wants a divorce. He has always considered her very lucky to be married to him and was amazed when he recently learned that she did not share his high opinion of the marriage and of his performance as a husband. His wife has agreed to give him one more chance if he will go into therapy. He is coming "only to appease her" because he doesn't think there is anything wrong with him. Within the first 15 minutes of the first session, he regales the therapist with his accomplishments: how he was the youngest graduate from his medical school, the prizes he has won, the papers he has published, the big house he owns in the nicest neighborhood in town, the fact that he met John Kennedy once, and the wonderful trips he takes to out-of-the-way and exclusive resorts. He says that he has "given his wife so much and asks for so little," and he cannot understand how she could be dissatisfied.

More detailed questioning by the therapist, however, makes it clear that, despite all his "accomplishments," Mr. R's wife takes care of all mundane details for him. She does all the household work and chores, handles all the finances and correspondence, and makes all the actual travel arrangements for the wonderful trips Mr. R wants to take. Mr. R insists that his house be beautifully furnished and impeccably maintained at all times, and he admits that his wife has always done an admirable job of this but speaks of this as if it was only his due.

In his professional life, Mr. R reports that he can't keep secretaries and that younger colleagues with whom he has worked often leave his department. On one occasion, he overheard someone call him an "insufferable horse's ass." He attributes these problems to jealousy and the fact that these individuals are not talented or hardworking enough to live up to his expectations and keep up with his achievements. He angrily claims that he should have been named chairman of his department because his professional achievements are far superior to those of the person who was chosen. Mr. R insists that he was passed over only because of the jealousy of some of his colleagues in the administration of the medical school and because the current department head exploited certain "connections" to get the job.

In picking a therapist, Mr. R has already rejected the first two whom he visited because they were not "qualified" or "expert" enough. He has finally condescended to meet with the chairman of the psychiatry department but only after being assured that he is considered a well-known authority in the field.

In a subsequent interview with the patient's wife and family, they describe how Mr. R refuses ever to wait in lines because he considers himself too busy and important to waste time. This has often caused his family much embarrassment. When they eat out, Mr. R always insists on having the best table and the most expensive wine on the wine list. He insists that everyone in his family wear only the "right" clothes with the "right" labels. Mr. R's wife is a very attractive woman who was considered a beauty when she was younger. She says that her husband has lately been pressuring her to have a face-lift, to color her hair, and generally to make herself more attractive. Mrs. R's resistance to these suggestions has led to frequent arguments and altercations, ultimately culminating in her request for a divorce. She complains that her husband does not seem to care about her as a person but only as a beautiful object that belongs to him and he can show off. Mr. R's two high school-age children say that they feel they can never please him. Despite doing well in school, being involved in a number of activities, and being well liked by their classmates, they are constantly made to feel that this is not good enough—they should be at the very top of their classes and be the captain of the football team or the homecoming queen. They both express the thought that, even if they should achieve these goals, it would still not be enough to satisfy their father.

When the therapist discusses his family's feelings with Mr. R, he reiterates that he feels that he "asks so little of others, why can't they comply?"

DSM-IV-TR Diagnosis

Axis I: V71.09   No diagnosis
Axis II: 301.81   Narcissistic Personality Disorder
Axis III: None
Axis IV: Marital stress
Axis V: GAF = 55

DSM-IV-TR diagnostic criteria for
301.81 Narcissistic Personality Disorder

A pervasive pattern of grandiosity (in fantasy or behavior), need for admiration, and lack of empathy, beginning by early adulthood and present in a variety of contexts, as indicated by five (or more) of the following:

(1) has a grandiose sense of self-importance (e.g., exaggerates achievements and talents, expects to be recognized as superior without commensurate achievements)
(2) is preoccupied with fantasies of unlimited success, power, brilliance, beauty, or ideal love
(3) believes that he or she is "special" and unique and can only be understood by, or should associate with, other special or high-status people (or institutions)
(4) requires excessive admiration
(5) has a sense of entitlement, i.e., unreasonable expectations of especially favorable treatment or automatic compliance with his or her expectations

(continued)

> ### DSM-IV-TR diagnostic criteria for
> ### 301.81 Narcissistic Personality Disorder *(continued)*
>
> ---
>
> (6) is interpersonally exploitative, i.e., takes advantage of others to achieve his or her own ends
> (7) lacks empathy: is unwilling to recognize or identify with the feelings and needs of others
> (8) is often envious of others or believes that others are envious of him or her
> (9) shows arrogant, haughty behaviors or attitudes

Guidelines for Differential Diagnosis of Narcissistic Personality Disorder

Most people have a little bit of normal narcissism that does not necessarily qualify as a mental disorder. In diagnosing Narcissistic Personality Disorder, the clinician must first distinguish feelings of grandiosity and entitlement that have become pathological and impairing from a normal and expectable degree of pride in one's accomplishments. Although Mr. R sees nothing out of line in his evaluation of his own accomplishments or in his expectations of others, his attitudes and behavior are clearly causing great disruption in his personal life (his wife is asking for a divorce and his children feel they constantly let him down) as well as in his professional role, where he cannot keep secretaries and alienates his associates.

The second major differential to be considered is whether the individual's grandiosity is due to personality functioning or is the result of a Manic or Hypomanic Episode or Substance Use. Although Axis I disorders may also co-occur with Narcissistic Personality Disorder, Narcissistic Personality Disorder should not be diagnosed unless there is a long-standing, pervasive pattern of narcissistic personality traits that causes impairment and can be traced back to early adulthood. The symptoms of a Depressive Disorder may resemble the feelings individuals with Narcissistic Personality Disorder have when criticized or faced with incontrovertible evidence of having failed to achieve the success they feel they deserve. When full criteria for a Major Depressive Episode are met, both diagnoses may be made.

Narcissistic Personality Disorder often overlaps with Histrionic, Borderline, and Antisocial Personality Disorders and, when more than one are present, all should be diagnosed. Despite marked similarities among these disorders, certain features do help to distinguish them. Although Histrionic and Borderline Personality Disorders are also associated with a strong need for the attention of others, the main feature that distinguishes those with Narcissistic Personality Disorder is the grandiose sense of self-importance and entitlement. They desperately need attention but require that the attention they receive be unstintingly admiring in recognition of their superiority. Individuals with Narcissistic Personality Disorder have a fairly stable self-image and do not usually behave in the self-destructive or impulsive ways that characterize those with Borderline Personality Disorder. Individuals with Narcissistic Personality Disorder tend to be exploitative without realizing it, believing that their special qualities and abilities entitle them to special treatment. For example, despite all his wife does for him, Mr. R is convinced that he asks very little from her and can't understand why she won't comply with his every request. Although those with Antisocial Personality Disorder also exploit others and lack empathy for their feelings, they are also characterized by irresponsibility, aggression, impulsivity, deceit, and an early history of severe conduct problems, none of which are typically associated with Narcissistic Personality Disorder.

Treatment Planning for
Narcissistic Personality Disorder

As in treating all Personality Disorders, the clinician must first establish whether the goal of therapy is support or change. Individuals with Narcissistic Personality Disorder often come to treatment only when there has been a narcissistic injury, such as a family problem, job reversal, medical illness, or a growing awareness of the wear and tear of aging. The disappointments associated with such factors cause the individuals to realize that they are not perfect, a fact they find unpalatable. For example, although Mr. R continues to maintain that nothing is wrong with him and that he has no idea why his wife is unhappy, the very fact that she has asked for a divorce and insisted that he come for therapy has obviously struck a severe blow to his self-esteem.

The immediate need is for Mr. R to try to make some fairly rapid changes in his behavior that may enable him to persuade his wife to give the relationship another chance. For this, the supportive approach would probably initially be best. The clinician helps the patient to lick his wounds by finding things to admire in him. Increasing Mr. R's self-esteem will make it easier for him to cope with the disappointments he is experiencing. The therapist might focus on Mr. R's good qualities (e.g., he is caring, concerned, and protective and has been faithful and loyal to his wife). While acknowledging that Mr. R has every reason to feel proud of the wonderful things he has achieved, the therapist can try to show him ways in which his current behavior is creating problems. This could set the stage for the therapist to help Mr. R plan a course of action that might not come naturally to him but that he might be willing to pursue when advised to do so by a clinician whose reputation and status he respects. This plan might include encouraging Mr. R to express admiration and appreciation for his wife's accomplishments as well as her physical attractiveness instead of focusing on his desire for her to "upgrade" her physical appearance. Mr. R could be encouraged to find the positive attributes in his children and offer them praise and encouragement for the many good things they are doing. It might help to encourage Mr. R to see his children's very real successes as yet another source of pride to himself.

To attempt to produce a lasting change in an individual's narcissistic traits usually requires long-term psychotherapy using combined psychodynamic and cognitive approaches. The individual needs to have the corrective emotional experience of being accepted by the therapist despite not being perfect. The establishment of an effective therapeutic alliance is obviously crucial, and it is essential that the patient work with someone he or she can respect. During this type of long-term therapy, the individual can explore the disappointments he or she feels both inside and outside the treatment setting.

Avoidant Personality Disorder

❖ Case Study: A Shy and Beaten Man

Mr. D is a 32-year-old single graduate student who presents for consultation because he feels he is getting nowhere in his work or love life. For several years now, he has been unable to complete his dissertation. Although he has amassed thousands of index cards and hundreds of references, Mr. D finds himself unable to bring the project any nearer to completion. He works as an assistant cashier in a book store and is becoming increasingly convinced that he will be behind a cash register for the rest of his life. This is particularly painful to him because he hates his job and is constantly fearful of making a mistake and being reprimanded by a customer or his boss.

Mr. D is painfully shy. He has great trouble initiating conversations with strangers for fear he will say something stupid. When invited to parties, he usually makes excuses not to go. When he does venture forth, he feels awkward and embarrassed and is sure that he is blushing all the time. He generally becomes so anxious and overwhelmed by these feelings that he leaves before having a chance to talk to anyone. This makes him feel like an idiot and makes him even less willing to accept the next invitation.

Very occasionally, Mr. D has become briefly involved with a woman, generally someone who has been introduced by a mutual acquaintance, but the relationships usually end badly. Women are surprised by his lack of sexual forwardness and find that they have to take the initiative. Mr. D then becomes painfully self-conscious and fearful of performing badly and is often plagued by premature ejaculation.

Mr. D grew up as the eldest of three children in a lower-middle-class family. He was the apple of his mother's eye and always felt that she had very high, perhaps unattainable, expectations for him. His father, on the other hand, is a very pious, humble, and unambitious man whose favorite expressions are "nobody has anything to be proud of" and "self-praise stinks." Despite his resentment toward his father, Mr. D is very attached to both his parents and to the room in which he has lived his entire life. He continues to live at home and spends a great deal of his spare time with his parents.

Mr. D was apparently a fairly aggressive, free-spirited, lusty 5-year-old until his father caught him in the process of stripping the neighbor's little daughter and playing with her vagina. Mr. D had the stuffing beaten out of him and was also subjected to a round of mortification of the soul delivered by the local priest. After months of rigorous training in religion and self-discipline, he lost his spunk and defiance, became increasingly timid, and was proclaimed forgiven for his sins. He has been avoidant and an underachiever ever since.

Mr. D is intelligent and psychologically sophisticated. He volunteers that his self-consciousness and fear of criticism stem from the vigilance with which he felt both parents tracked his behavior. When the consultant asks how this affects his sexual performance, he laughs and says, "It's like always having my father watching." He then recalls a dream in which he is making love to a woman in the backseat of a taxi, but the taxi driver interrupts and takes over the lovemaking. The patient is forced to move to the front seat and watch the sexual proceedings in the rearview mirror. He mentions in passing that the woman is much older and not really very pretty.

During the second session, Mr. D becomes silent and self-conscious in relation to the therapist and consciously withholds a sexual memory. When pressed to investigate what is happening, he notices with surprise that he is already expecting the therapist to be demanding and critical. Mr. D is interested in understanding his behavior and changing it, but he is not sure he can stand the embarrassment of having to reveal all of his thoughts to someone who he is sure must judge what is said to him. This self-consciousness is why he has never appeared previously for treatment, and he is not sure how long he will stay with therapy. He is also concerned that time and energy spent in treatment will distract him from working on his dissertation and that he may be opening a Pandora's box. His financial situation is also very tenuous.

DSM-IV-TR Diagnosis

Axis I: 300.23 Social Phobia, Generalized Type
Axis II: 301.82 Avoidant Personality Disorder, compulsive and dependent personality traits
Axis III: None
Axis IV: Trying to complete dissertation, sexual problems
Axis V: GAF = 60

DSM-IV-TR diagnostic criteria for 301.82 Avoidant Personality Disorder

A pervasive pattern of social inhibition, feelings of inadequacy, and hypersensitivity to negative evaluation, beginning by early adulthood and present in a variety of contexts, as indicated by four (or more) of the following:

(1) avoids occupational activities that involve significant interpersonal contact, because of fears of criticism, disapproval, or rejection
(2) is unwilling to get involved with people unless certain of being liked
(3) shows restraint within intimate relationships because of the fear of being shamed or ridiculed
(4) is preoccupied with being criticized or rejected in social situations
(5) is inhibited in new interpersonal situations because of feelings of inadequacy
(6) views self as socially inept, personally unappealing, or inferior to others
(7) is unusually reluctant to take personal risks or to engage in any new activities because they may prove embarrassing

---

Guidelines for Differential Diagnosis of Avoidant Personality Disorder

Before diagnosing Avoidant Personality Disorder, the clinician should first carefully rule out normal shyness. It is also important to take into account the cultural background of the individual and the situations in which the symptoms appear. Different cultural groups have varying standards for the degree of social forwardness that is considered appropriate in certain situations. Individuals from different backgrounds, and especially those who may have difficulties with a second language, may also be fearful and reluctant to expose themselves to strange or stressful social situations. Shy and socially avoidant behavior in such situations would not be considered evidence of Avoidant Personality Disorder.

Mr. D would clearly meet criteria for Social Phobia, Generalized Type. He is anxious in most social situations and usually responds by leaving without speaking to anyone, even though he knows his fear is excessive and that he is only making things worse for himself by running away. He generally tends to avoid social situations altogether. His social anxiety and fear of being upbraided for a mistake make his job a nightmare for him and make it impossible for him to establish any kind of long-term relationship with a woman. Mr. D also meets criteria for Avoidant Personality Disorder because his social fears, feelings of inadequacy, and hypersensitivity go back to his early childhood and he appears to meet every criterion for this Personality Disorder. Avoidant Personality Disorder, as defined in DSM-IV-TR, is virtually equivalent to generalized Social Phobia. This is perhaps the clearest instance in which the distinctions between Axis I and Axis II become meaningless.

The Personality Disorder that is most often comorbid with Avoidant Personality Disorder is Dependent Personality Disorder because individuals with this disorder become very closely attached to the few people with whom they feel comfortable. Although Mr. D does not appear to meet the full criteria for Dependent Personality Disorder, he does demonstrate some significant dependent traits. He is very attached to his parents, spends much of his time with them, and continues to live at home. From the case history, it is not completely clear why Mr. D has been unable to complete his dissertation. To the degree that this may be related to the fear of being exposed to ridicule during the process of completing and defending the dissertation, the procrastination would be characteristic of Avoidant Personality Disorder. To the degree that it is related to a need for perfection, it would be more closely related to the obsessive-compulsive personality traits that also seem to be present.

Individuals with Avoidant Personality Disorder may be distinguished from those with Schizoid and Schizotypal Personality Disorders, who are also socially isolated but do not seem to feel much, if any, desire for social intercourse. In contrast, individuals with Avoidant Personality Disorder would love to be well liked and socially successful but find it extremely difficult to get involved in social situations or close relationships because they are so afraid of being embarrassed or ridiculed. Note that Schizoid Personality Disorder is rarely diagnosed and that the social isolation encountered in most clinical situations is much more likely to be the result of Avoidant Personality Disorder. Avoidant Personality Disorder may also co-occur with Borderline, Paranoid, Schizoid, or Schizotypal Personality Disorders.

Individuals with Avoidant Personality Disorder are likely to have comorbid Anxiety Disorders (in addition to Social Phobia) and Mood Disorders and may use substances to help reduce their anxiety or dysphoria. The one feature of Mr. D's presentation that is atypical is his lack of avoidance in early childhood. Usually those who later develop Avoidant Personality Disorder show a tendency toward avoidance shortly after birth that may, at least to some degree, reflect a genetically inherited temperament.

Treatment Planning for
Avoidant Personality Disorder

Avoidant Personality Disorder is a frequently encountered problem in outpatient practice. Several techniques work well in individuals with this disorder, especially when they are used in a complementary way. These individuals often benefit from a psychotherapy that combines psychodynamic techniques to help them gain insight into the source of their fears, cognitive techniques to target their false assumptions about the effects of failure, and behavioral desensitization and social skills retraining. Once the therapeutic alliance with such patients is established, it may be possible to design a graded hierarchy of activities to expose them to situations they have previously avoided. Paradoxical injunctions are often used in treating such individuals. For example, the therapist could instruct the individual to perform a task at which he would most likely be expected to fail (e.g., asking a very attractive woman out for a date) as a means of reducing the fear of failure. The behavioral exercises also help to desensitize the patient and to produce material for psychodynamic explorations. Treatment with monoamine oxidase inhibitors may also be helpful, particularly for those patients who also qualify for a diagnosis of Social Phobia.

During the first week of desensitization, Mr. D was assigned the task of chatting with customers at the register. During the second week, he was assigned to go to a lecture and strike up a conversation with someone in the audience. By the third week, he had progressed to the point where he was assigned to try to get a date with one of the customers who he was sure would refuse. Mr. D was told that if he did not ask for the date, he would have to take a tennis lesson instead. Interestingly, Mr. D chose to complete neither the task nor the penalty, but instead went to a lecture at the YMCA and struck up an unexpected conversation with a young woman.

Dependent Personality Disorder

❖   Case Study: Lost at Sea

Mrs. T is a 53-year-old woman with three children in their 20s who comes in at their insistence. A year ago, her husband of 30 years left her for a younger woman. Since then, she has been unable to mobilize herself. She has felt fearful every day and incapable of making decisions about what she should do about any aspect of her life (e.g., whether to continue living in her house, whether to seek a job, how to handle her finances, and even what clothes to buy). She is constantly begging her children for the advice and emotional support that her husband had previously provided. Her children love her and understand her plight but are becoming increasingly annoyed by her inability to stand on her own feet. Friends who had previously been very fond of Mrs. T have also been put off by her constant demands for assistance and have begun to avoid her.

Most of Mrs. T's friends and acquaintances cannot understand why she is so devastated by her husband's desertion. He had been chronically unfaithful, impossible to please, and was always very tight with money. He did, however, make all the important decisions for Mrs. T. He decided how they would spend and invest their money, where they would live, when and where they would go on vacation, when they would eat out and where, what movies they would see, whom they would entertain, where the children would go to school, and even what careers the children should be encouraged to pursue. Mr. T always shopped with her and even helped her choose all her clothes. After he left, Mrs. T collapsed, felt unable to do anything, and lapsed into a helpless funk.

Mrs. T was the only child of a doting mother. Her father died in World War II when she was 3 years old. Her mother was a strong and possessive woman who dressed her, treated her like a fragile doll, and made all her decisions. Mrs. T's mother scheduled her days with a round of lessons and prearranged social activities and also selected her friends for her. The patient continued to live at home during her first 3 years of college. During her third year of college, her mother died suddenly in a car accident.

Mr. T, her mother's lawyer and executor of the will, took charge of handling all Mrs. T's affairs after her mother's death and soon became her adviser and confidant. Mrs. T was relieved when he asked her to marry him because she had quickly become totally dependent on him to fill the void left by her mother's death.

DSM-IV-TR Diagnosis

Axis I: 309.0   Adjustment Disorder With Depressed Mood
Axis II: 301.6   Dependent Personality Disorder
Axis III: None
Axis IV: Marriage breaking up, husband leaving her for younger woman
Axis V: GAF = 60 (current); 70 (highest level in past year)

DSM-IV-TR diagnostic criteria for
301.6 Dependent Personality Disorder

A pervasive and excessive need to be taken care of that leads to submissive and clinging behavior and fears of separation, beginning by early adulthood and present in a variety of contexts, as indicated by five (or more) of the following:

(1) has difficulty making everyday decisions without an excessive amount of advice and reassurance from others

(2) needs others to assume responsibility for most major areas of his or her life

(3) has difficulty expressing disagreement with others because of fear of loss of support or approval. **Note:** Do not include realistic fears of retribution.

(4) has difficulty initiating projects or doing things on his or her own (because of a lack of self-confidence in judgment or abilities rather than a lack of motivation or energy)

(5) goes to excessive lengths to obtain nurturance and support from others, to the point of volunteering to do things that are unpleasant

(6) feels uncomfortable or helpless when alone because of exaggerated fears of being unable to care for himself or herself

(7) urgently seeks another relationship as a source of care and support when a close relationship ends

(8) is unrealistically preoccupied with fears of being left to take care of himself or herself

Guidelines for Differential Diagnosis of Dependent Personality Disorder

The most common error in diagnosing Dependent Personality Disorder is to mistake the state of dependency with the trait of dependency. When faced with medical or psychiatric illness or difficult situations, most individuals regress at least to some degree and become much more dependent. Such situations must be distinguished from Dependent Personality Disorder, which has an early onset and is a lifelong pervasive pattern that causes clinically significant impairment. Dependency may also be adaptive. An interesting question is whether a diagnosis of Dependent Personality Disorder would have been warranted if Mrs. T had never had to fend for herself and was not notably distressed by the price exacted by her husband for his support. This is very much a judgment call. The individual may have adapted and may be functioning well in a situation that only in the eyes of some outside beholder would be considered pathological. In fact, individuals with Dependent Personality Disorder most often come to clinical attention when they either lose the support on which they have depended or the individuals upon whom they are dependent come to find them unbearably burdensome.

This is one of the Personality Disorders that is bedeviled by a criteria set that may be applied in a way that is sex biased. The criteria describe a submissive dependency that is perhaps more common in women but ignore a domineering type of dependency that is more common in men but less likely to be diagnosed as pathological (especially by male therapists). Individuals who display domineering dependency need others to perform many necessary tasks for them and make decisions for them but obtain these services by giving orders to the individuals upon whom they depend. Another issue is the degree to which certain societies and cultures encourage dependent and submissive behaviors, especially in women. When an individual's dependent behavior is the result of cultural values, this would not be considered pathological and would not warrant a diagnosis of Dependent Personality Disorder.

Dependent Personality Disorder is frequently comorbid with other Personality Disorders, in particular Borderline, Avoidant, and Histrionic Personality Disorders. When criteria are met for more than one of these Personality Disorders, all those that are applicable should be diagnosed. Dependent Personality Disorder differs from Borderline Personality Disorder because an individual with Dependent Personality Disorder will usually react to potential abandonment with increasingly desperate clinging and submissiveness, whereas the person with Borderline Personality Disorder becomes enraged, impulsive, demanding, and self-destructive. When individuals with Dependent Personality Disorder find their dependent position threatened, they are prone to develop Anxiety, Mood, or Adjustment Disorders. Mrs. T received an additional diagnosis of Adjustment Disorder With Depressed Mood because she did not meet full criteria for a Major Depressive Episode but had prominent depressive symptoms in response to the continuing stress of being abandoned by her husband and left to fend for herself. These individuals may also express their help-seeking through Hypochondriasis or other somatoform symptoms. It is of interest that individuals with Dependent Personality Disorder frequently gravitate toward those who are controlling, obsessive, and narcissistic and will make all their decisions for them (as Mr. T did for Mrs. T).

Treatment Planning for
Dependent Personality Disorder

Supportive treatment that helps to meet a patient's dependency needs is usually necessary, at least at the beginning of treatment. These individuals are very likely to turn to a therapist for advice, structure, and decision making. If the therapist expects too much too soon in the way of insight and independence, the patient is likely to find the treatment unsupportive and anxiety provoking and experience it as just one more demand to be filled. However, once a therapeutic alliance is established, it may be possible to formally or informally encourage the patient to seek out opportunities to experience increased self-assertion and independence. For example, when Mrs. T first began treatment, the therapist had to take a very supportive and directive role to help her get her affairs in order. Gradually, however, he was able to encourage Mrs. T to find ways to take more responsibility for her own life, beginning with making a number of small and relatively unimportant decisions for herself and then progressing to more important issues.

Cognitive-behavioral approaches (e.g., assertiveness and socials skills training) are often helpful to individuals with Dependent Personality Disorder. Group therapy may be particularly useful if patients can be brought to overcome their fears that this setting will not meet their needs.

Obsessive-Compulsive Personality Disorder

❖   Case Study: In Control

Ms. C, a 41-year-old grocery store manager, comes for an evaluation at the insistence of the regional manager of the chain for which she works. Ms. C has failed to turn in the last four periodic reports on time, and her store has one of the lowest productivity ratings in the chain, even though she usually comes in earlier and stays later than any of the other managers and appears to be busy every minute of the day. Ms. C has frequent battles with her employees and has the highest turnover rate of employees in the chain. When confronted with these problems, she insists that her store is being run "properly" and by the book—unlike the others in the chain, which are maintaining "shoddy" standards.

It is easy to identify the source of difficulty in the store. Ms. C insists that her employees shelve and arrange goods in exquisitely straight lines. She checks, double-checks, triple-checks, and quadruple-checks all her figures, which is why her periodic reports never get in on time. She micromanages every aspect of the store's operation and, consequently, her meat and produce managers are always transferring to other stores. Instead of appreciating Ms. C's constant supervision, her managers find it annoying and time consuming. She is constantly drawing up charts, tables, graphs, and employee directives. She spends much of her time each morning constructing an elaborate to-do list that she never finds time to complete.

Ms. C has been married for 15 years and has two children in their early teens. Her husband is a postal worker. Mr. C reported to the therapist that until Ms. C began working at the store 6 years ago they had lots of marital struggles because of Ms. C's need to oversee and direct every aspect of his life. She had insisted on knowing where he was at every moment and had tried to plan all his leisure time activities. He said that it was a great relief to him when she began to work at the store and became too busy to pay so much attention to his life. Mr. C says that he and the children have a hard time persuading his wife to take a vacation and that it generally does not turn out to be much fun when she does agree to go. Ms. C plans their itinerary and activities minutely and insists that everyone must participate in what she has scheduled. Nothing is allowed to be spontaneous or unplanned, and everyone is expected to spend their time "productively" even when on vacation.

Ms. C comes by her perfectionism honestly. Both her parents were austere, driven, and highly critical. No matter how hard she worked or what she achieved, it never seemed like enough. She began being a maid in her own house at the age of 5 and began to do chores for others by the age of 9 so she could begin to save money ("a penny saved is a penny earned"). Nothing but As in school were acceptable to her parents. If she made a 95 on a test, her mother would ask her, "Where are the other 5 points?" Even though Ms. C can admit that she often found her parents' attitude painful and frustrating, she finds herself reacting to her own children in much the same way. Although she tries to praise them for their accomplishments, she always finds herself demanding that they work harder and perform better, even when they have done very well.

DSM-IV-TR Diagnosis

Axis I: V71.09   No diagnosis
Axis II: 301.4   Obsessive-Compulsive Personality Disorder
Axis III: None
Axis IV: About to be fired from her job, marital dissatisfaction
Axis V: GAF = 55

DSM-IV-TR diagnostic criteria for
301.4 Obsessive-Compulsive Personality Disorder

A pervasive pattern of preoccupation with orderliness, perfectionism, and mental and interpersonal control, at the expense of flexibility, openness, and efficiency, beginning by early adulthood and present in a variety of contexts, as indicated by four (or more) of the following:

(1) is preoccupied with details, rules, lists, order, organization, or schedules to the extent that the major point of the activity is lost

(2) shows perfectionism that interferes with task completion (e.g., is unable to complete a project because his or her own overly strict standards are not met)

(3) is excessively devoted to work and productivity to the exclusion of leisure activities and friendships (not accounted for by obvious economic necessity)

(4) is overconscientious, scrupulous, and inflexible about matters of morality, ethics, or values (not accounted for by cultural or religious identification)

(5) is unable to discard worn-out or worthless objects even when they have no sentimental value

(6) is reluctant to delegate tasks or to work with others unless they submit to exactly his or her way of doing things

(7) adopts a miserly spending style toward both self and others; money is viewed as something to be hoarded for future catastrophes

(8) shows rigidity and stubbornness

Guidelines for Differential Diagnosis of
Obsessive-Compulsive Personality Disorder

In diagnosing Obsessive-Compulsive Personality Disorder, the first differential is with individuals who are merely extremely well organized, hardworking, and conscientious. Up to a point, obsessive-compulsive traits are very adaptive and correlate with success. However, a characteristic feature of individuals with Obsessive-Compulsive Personality Disorder and one that helps to distinguish them is that they are often not very productive despite their hard work. They find it impossible to complete projects because of their perfectionism and are unable to work constructively with others because no one can live up to their "standards." In these individuals, the "excellent" is indeed the enemy of the "good."

Under certain circumstances, such as when a Mood Disorder or a general medical illness is present or the individual is under a lot of stress, obsessive-compulsive traits that are normally adaptive or that do not usually cause any impairment may be exacerbated and cause problems for the individual. This would not, however, warrant a diagnosis of Obsessive-Compulsive Personality Disorder. This distinction is somewhat complicated because individuals with Obsessive-Compulsive Personality Disorder are likely to develop Mood or Anxiety Disorders, especially when they are faced with their lack of success in living up to their own impossibly high standards. This is one of those situations in which it may not be clear whether there was a preexisting Personality Disorder that is being complicated by the development of an Axis I disorder or whether preexisting personality traits that would not have warranted a Personality Disorder diagnosis are being temporarily exacerbated by an Axis I condition. The clinician should obtain a careful history and information from other informants whenever possible; it may also be necessary to treat the symptoms of the Axis I condition first and then see whether the obsessive-compulsive traits remit or improve with the remission of the Axis I condition.

Despite the similarity in names and the apparent association between the two, Obsessive-Compulsive Personality Disorder can be distinguished from Obsessive-Compulsive Disorder by the lack of true obsessions and compulsions.

For example, even though Ms. C is driven to work extremely hard and to be superconscientious, she does not appear to have any specific obsessions or to perform any compulsive rituals.

Although individuals with Narcissistic Personality Disorder are also perfectionists, they tend to believe that they are already perfect, whereas those with Obsessive-Compulsive Personality Disorder are constantly driving themselves and others to do better. Although those with Obsessive-Compulsive Personality Disorder seem emotionally cold and stilted, they are able to form close and intimate relationships (often with those they can dominate). Their lack of emotional expression is the result of their almost exclusive focus on being in control and their discomfort with excessive emotionalism. This should be distinguished from the lack of interest in social intercourse that characterizes Schizoid and Schizotypal Personality Disorders.

Treatment Planning for
Obsessive-Compulsive Personality Disorder

These are often the most satisfying patients to work with in psychotherapy. They work hard in treatment and often make substantial gains. Psychodynamic treatment focuses on their scrupulosity in an attempt to deal with the superego triad of "blaming yourself, blaming others, and expecting others to blame you" that characterizes them. Another focus may be on the forbidden wishes, particularly aggressive ones, that these individuals are warding off with reaction formation. Because these individuals have such difficulty with emotional expression and relaxation and usually appear formal, stilted, and hypervigilant, the therapist should try to find areas of emotional expression, to take advantage of humor, and to encourage them to relax and become comfortable expressing emotions. The cognitive approach focuses on the unrealistic expectations associated with this disorder and tries to desensitize the person to the need to be perfect. It is also often helpful for the clinician to have the patient find opportunities in which to practice not being perfect. Family and group treatments can also be useful.

The supportive treatment of Obsessive-Compulsive Personality Disorder respects and recognizes an individual's need to be in control. For example, an individual with Obsessive-Compulsive Personality Disorder who has recently had a heart attack should be given a lot of information about alternative treatments, dosages, and rehabilitation schedules and, whenever possible, be encouraged to design his or her own regimen. In contrast, the individual with Dependent Personality Disorder would find this array of choices overwhelming and anxiety provoking. The supportive treatment for such an individual would be to prescribe from above and to offer little choice.

Summary

Personality Disorders are not easy to distinguish from normal personality functioning, Axis I conditions, and the difficulty in adjusting to particular role expectations. They also lack clear boundaries with one another; if one Personality Disorder is present, it is likely that others may also be diagnosed. The diagnosis of a Personality Disorder requires an evaluation of an individual's long-term functioning and may often be enhanced by data received from other informants and from a patient's previous records. Finally, it is important to evaluate for possible biases in diagnosis created by the clinician's own personality, cultural background, and gender biases.

Chapter 16

Medication-Induced Movement Disorders

A new section on Medication-Induced Movement Disorders is included in DSM-IV-TR as part of the section on "Other Conditions That May Be a Focus of Clinical Attention." Proposed criteria for each of these disorders are included in Appendix B of DSM-IV-TR for further study.

The following Medication-Induced Movement Disorders are listed in DSM-IV-TR:

332.1 Neuroleptic-Induced Parkinsonism

Parkinsonian tremor, muscular rigidity, or akinesia developing within a few weeks of starting or raising the dose of a neuroleptic medication (or after reducing a medication used to treat extrapyramidal symptoms).

333.92 Neuroleptic Malignant Syndrome

Severe muscle rigidity, elevated temperature, and other related findings (e.g., diaphoresis, dysphagia, incontinence, changes in level of consciousness ranging from confusion to coma, mutism, elevated or labile blood pressure, elevated creatine phosphokinase [CPK]) developing in association with the use of neuroleptic medication.

333.7   Neuroleptic-Induced Acute Dystonia

Abnormal positioning or spasm of the muscles of the head, neck, limbs, or trunk developing within a few days of starting or raising the dose of a neuroleptic medication (or after reducing a medication used to treat extrapyramidal symptoms).

333.99   Neuroleptic-Induced Acute Akathisia

Subjective complaints of restlessness accompanied by observed movements (e.g., fidgety movements of the legs, rocking from foot to foot, pacing, or inability to sit or stand still) developing within a few weeks of starting or raising the dose of a neuroleptic medication (or after reducing a medication used to treat extrapyramidal symptoms).

333.82   Neuroleptic-Induced Tardive Dyskinesia

Involuntary choreiform, athetoid, or rhythmic movements (lasting at least a few weeks) of the tongue, jaw, or extremities developing in association with the use of neuroleptic medication for at least a few months (may be for a shorter period of time in elderly persons).

333.1   Medication-Induced Postural Tremor

Fine tremor occurring during attempts to maintain a posture that develops in association with the use of medication (e.g., lithium, antidepressants, valproate).

333.90   Medication-Induced Movement Disorder
Not Otherwise Specified

This category is for Medication-Induced Movement Disorders not classified by any of the specific disorders listed above. Examples include 1) parkinsonism, acute akathisia, acute dystonia, or dyskinetic movement that is associated with a medication other than a neuroleptic; 2) a presentation that resembles neuroleptic malignant syndrome that is associated with a medication other than a neuroleptic; or 3) tardive dystonia.

Neuroleptic Malignant Syndrome/Bipolar I

❖ Case Study: A Very Bad Reaction to Medicine

Ms. C is a 17-year-old girl with a 2-year history of recurrent Manic Episodes. She is now admitted with an acute Manic Episode and accompanying psychotic features. Ms. C's mother has Bipolar Disorder, and the patient has mild cerebral palsy in addition to Bipolar Disorder. Ms. C's Manic Episodes have necessitated two previous hospitalizations.

During Ms. C's first admission, a "sensitivity" to neuroleptic antipsychotics was noted. The summaries from that admission stated that "catatonia, incoherence, and incontinence" developed when she was treated with chlorpromazine and thiothixene.

During Ms. C's second hospitalization for another Manic Episode, she was treated daily with 250 mg of chlorpromazine and 200 mg of amantadine. Within a few days she developed a fever, tachypnea, labile blood pressure, profound cogwheel rigidity with hyperreflexia and dystonias, dysphagia, grunting, mutism, and incontinence. Laboratory tests demonstrated elevated creatine phosphokinase (350 U/L) and white blood count (14,100/mm^3).

Chlorpromazine was discontinued, and diphenhydramine was used for symptomatic treatment of the preexisting extrapyramidal side effects. The presumed Neuroleptic Malignant Syndrome cleared within 8 days. Thirty-five days after that episode, lithium was begun with no adverse effects, and Ms. C's psychosis gradually resolved.

During the past 20 months, Ms. C has been functioning fairly well in a residential school. She made frequent visits home that were somewhat stressful because of constant parental fighting. As summer vacation approached, she developed another Manic Episode With Psychotic Features that necessitated this hospitalization.

During this admission, Ms. C's maintenance lithium is continued, but despite serum lithium levels in the 1–1.25 mEq/L range, her condition has continued to worsen. The treatment team, believing that antipsychotics are necessary but also making the retrospective diagnosis of Neuroleptic Malignant Syndrome, elects to add a low dose of 100 mg of chlorpromazine daily.

Ms. C does not develop Neuroleptic Malignant Syndrome, but her orthostatic hypotension and continuing mania prompt a cautious switch to a low dose of 8 mg of trifluoperazine daily. Ms. C becomes somewhat less agitated, but rigidity and mildly elevated creatine phosphokinase (476 U/L) and white blood count (12,200/mm^3) lead to a dosage reduction to 6 mg/day. Ms. C is continued on that dose for 11 days, with little change in either her mania or in the parameters monitored for Neuroleptic Malignant Syndrome.

Persistent rigidity and the onset of confusion prompt another lowering of trifluoperazine to 4 mg/day. However, within 1 week, Neuroleptic Malignant Syndrome recurs. Ms. C's temperature rises to 101.6°F, pulse to 134 beats per minute, creatine phosphokinase to 659 U/L, and white blood count to 17,500/mm^3.

The trifluoperazine is immediately stopped, lithium is discontinued 5 days later, and electroconvulsive therapy (ECT) is begun on the eighth day after this episode of Neuroleptic Malignant Syndrome began.

Ms. C receives a course of 12 unilateral ECT treatments during which both the mania and the Neuroleptic Malignant Syndrome resolved. Six weeks later she is discharged on lithium alone.

DSM-IV-TR Diagnosis

Axis I:	333.92	Neuroleptic Malignant Syndrome
	296.44	Bipolar I Disorder, Most Recent Episode Manic, Severe With Psychotic Features
Axis II:	V71.09	No diagnosis
Axis III:	343.9	Cerebral palsy
Axis IV:	Family discord, end of school year approaching, mother with Bipolar Disorder	
Axis V:	GAF = 35 (during this admission); 70 (highest level in past year)	

DSM-IV-TR research criteria for
333.92 Neuroleptic Malignant Syndrome

A. The development of severe muscle rigidity and elevated temperature associated with the use of neuroleptic medication.

B. Two (or more) of the following:

(1) diaphoresis
(2) dysphagia
(3) tremor
(4) incontinence
(5) changes in level of consciousness ranging from confusion to coma
(6) mutism
(7) tachycardia
(8) elevated or labile blood pressure
(9) leucocytosis
(10) laboratory evidence of muscle injury (e.g., elevated CPK)

C. The symptoms in Criteria A and B are not due to another substance (e.g., phencyclidine) or a neurological or other general medical condition (e.g., viral encephalitis).

D. The symptoms in Criteria A and B are not better accounted for by a mental disorder (e.g., Mood Disorder With Catatonic Features).

Guidelines for Differential Diagnosis of Neuroleptic Malignant Syndrome/Bipolar I

Medication-Induced Movement Disorders are frequently encountered by those who treat individuals with mental disorders. Although these conditions are not in themselves considered to be mental disorders, they are included in the manual because it is important that all clinicians be skillful in recognizing and treating them. If missed, they can lead to serious morbidity and even mortality—especially in the case of Neuroleptic Malignant Syndrome. Less dramatically, they are a major cause of the frequent noncompliance with treatment that occurs in patients taking antipsychotic medications.

Because the symptoms associated with Medication-Induced Movement Disorders can mimic the symptoms of certain primary mental disorders, including those that these medications are supposed to treat, it is very important to take them into account in the differential diagnosis. Certain patterns of symptoms, such as akathisia or dystonia, may be misinterpreted by the patient and the clinician as a worsening of primary symptoms, which in turn can lead to an increase in medication dose causing the side effects to worsen, thus setting up a vicious cycle. Medication-Induced Movement Disorders can also be confused with catatonia presenting as part of a Mood Disorder or Schizophrenia.

Treatment Planning for Neuroleptic Malignant Syndrome/Bipolar I

It is important that clinicians educate patients and their families about the possibility of developing Medication-Induced Movement Disorders. The patients and their families should be taught how to identify these symptoms, that they are caused by medications and do not represent a worsening of the disease process, that they are usually reversible, and that it is important to discuss these symptoms with the clinician as soon as they occur and not to stop medication on their own. Medication management of Movement Disorders depends on the situation but usually includes some combination of lowering the dose, changing the medication, adding adjunctive medications specifically targeted to the Movement Disorders (e.g., anticholinergics or diphenhydramine), and providing general supportive medical management. Fortunately, the newer atypical antipsychotics are much less likely to cause Medication-Induced Movement Disorders.

Summary

An ounce of prevention is worth a pound of cure in dealing with Medication-Induced Movement Disorders. It is also crucial to recognize that these conditions are often missed altogether or misinterpreted as evidence of the primary illness. All mental health professionals should be familiar with the appearance of abnormal movements in order to undertake appropriate medical and neurological diagnoses. Every patient and family member should be informed about these symptoms and instructed to report them immediately to the treating clinician.

Chapter 17

Test Yourself

W e now invite the reader to puzzle with us over some presentations that are much less clear-cut than the more straightforward cases presented in the earlier chapters of this book. It is important to realize that many, perhaps most, patients presenting in clinical practice do not fall neatly and obviously into one or another DSM-IV-TR category. Their symptoms often lie at the boundary between descriptive definitions of disorders, or they present with more than one disorder. We cannot emphasize enough the crucial role of clinical judgment and the danger of artificially forcing people into categories that are not good fits. A boundary patient is a boundary patient and will often require observation over time to gather more information and sequential systematic treatment trials before a definitive diagnosis can be made.

It will be useful for you to form your own conclusions about each of the following case presentations before reviewing our diagnostic choices and supporting discussion. Certainly, do not accept our suggested diagnoses as the last word. The more complicated the clinical situation, the less likely that any suggested diagnosis is definitive.

❖ Case Study: A Changed Boy

Eric is a 4½-year-old boy who is referred to a psychiatry clinic from a pediatrics service because of hyperactivity that developed after he was involved in a car accident 14 months earlier. He sustained basilar and parietal skull fractures, facial lacerations, and right parietal cerebral contusions and was in a coma for about 3 weeks. Over the following 6–8 weeks, he gradually regained language comprehension, speech, and the full use of his limbs.

However, Eric's mother said that for several weeks after he regained consciousness he refused to speak to her, avoided her gaze, and acknowledged only his father and three older siblings. Eric and his mother had been especially close before the accident.

The neurosurgeon who treated his head trauma had advised the parents to be prepared for some personality changes and hyperactivity as a result of the extensive injury. Over the ensuing 7–8 months, Eric manifested increasing motor restlessness, distractibility, and difficulties falling asleep. Interestingly, when Eric had climbed in his parents' bed before the accident, he got in on his mother's side; after the accident, he climbed in next to his father. Because his mother had difficulties controlling Eric, she felt progressively more helpless and resentful; on several occasions she threatened to "give him away."

Seven months after the accident, Eric was evaluated by a child psychiatrist, who described him as a "typical hyperactive"; he treated Eric with methylphenidate 5 mg tid, with apparent good initial response.

Ten months after the accident, Eric's mother was hospitalized for 6 weeks for treatment of a major depression. During the next 3 months, before Eric's psychiatric referral to the clinic, his behavior became increasingly difficult and was characterized by extreme motor restlessness, severe tantrums, fights with siblings, distractibility, and physical attacks on his mother, despite increases in methylphenidate to 30 mg q.d. Several days before the referral, his mother stopped the medication because she felt it was not helping.

Eric is the product of a full-term, uncomplicated pregnancy and delivery. Before the accident, his developmental and medical history were unremarkable, except that he was especially attached to his mother. Nonetheless, he rapidly adjusted to daily separations from her when she began working several months before the accident. Psychological testing approximately 8 months after the accident indicated normal intelligence despite the significant head trauma. Eric was rehospitalized for corrective surgery on his eye 4 months after the accident, and his father stayed with him. Plastic surgery to repair his eyebrow is scheduled for 4 months after this referral to the psychiatric clinic.

Eric is the youngest of four children (two brothers and a sister, ages 8 to 15). His 10-year-old brother was diagnosed as being hyperactive several years earlier. Despite stimulant treatment, his brother continues to manifest problems in school. Eric's great-grandmother suffered a "nervous breakdown" and committed suicide at age 62.

Eric's father is a sergeant in the army, with a successful military career. Although the parents' marriage was satisfactory up until the accident, both parents tended to "do their own thing." After the accident, Eric's mother noted that she resented her husband because he had "gotten off easy," whereas she was left with the burden of taking Eric back and forth from the hospital for repeated medical visits. During this time, Eric's father became very involved in his job. As problems mounted and family members became increasingly depressed, the father observed that he did not believe in depression. Despite Eric's mother's difficulties with Eric, his father says that Eric is no problem for him. The oldest son blames himself and his father for the accident and has begun to experience significant school and peer-relationship problems. Eric's 8-year-old sister has been having headaches.

When seen in the clinic for evaluation, Eric appears to be an energetic, handsome boy with a slight ptosis of the right eye and a scar through his eyebrow. He sits fairly still during the initial interview. Both parents have accompanied Eric to the evaluation, and he remains with his father, across the room from his mother. When questioned, he responds with good eye contact and a friendly smile.

Eric separates easily from his parents to come to the playroom for evaluation. Although his affect is slightly constricted and superficially bright, he cautiously reveals some anxiety about the accident. He nonetheless keeps up a generally talkative, cheerful, and active veneer, and his speech rate is slightly increased. His thought content and play themes concern his fears about bad things happening unexpectedly and people being killed in cars. His thought processes are clear, logical, and sequential; however, themes of death or violence result in abrupt shifts to different play material. When asked about three wishes he would make, he says he would ask for a boat, a motorcycle, and a car.

DSM-IV-TR Diagnosis

Axis I:	314.01	Attention-Deficit/Hyperactivity Disorder, Predominantly Hyperactive-Impulsive Type
	310.1	Personality Change Due to Head Trauma, Other Type
Axis II:	V71.09	No diagnosis
Axis III:	851.80	Status post-head trauma with right cerebral contusions
Axis IV:		Auto accident with head trauma, prolonged hospitalization, parents' marital conflict, major depression of mother, and upcoming plastic surgery
Axis V:		GAF = 60

DSM-IV-TR diagnostic criteria for 310.1 Personality Change Due to . . . *[Indicate the General Medical Condition]*

A. A persistent personality disturbance that represents a change from the individual's previous characteristic personality pattern. (In children, the disturbance involves a marked deviation from normal development or a significant change in the child's usual behavior patterns lasting at least 1 year).

B. There is evidence from the history, physical examination, or laboratory findings that the disturbance is the direct physiological consequence of a general medical condition.

C. The disturbance is not better accounted for by another mental disorder (including other Mental Disorders Due to a General Medical Condition).

D. The disturbance does not occur exclusively during the course of a delirium.

E. The disturbance causes clinically significant distress or impairment in social, occupational, or other important areas of functioning.

Specify type:

Labile Type: if the predominant feature is affective lability

Disinhibited Type: if the predominant feature is poor impulse control as evidenced by sexual indiscretions, etc.

Aggressive Type: if the predominant feature is aggressive behavior

Apathetic Type: if the predominant feature is marked apathy and indifference

Paranoid Type: if the predominant feature is suspiciousness or paranoid ideation

Other Type: if the presentation is not characterized by any of the above subtypes

Combined Type: if more than one feature predominates in the clinical picture

Unspecified Type

Coding note: Include the name of the general medical condition on Axis I, e.g., 310.1 Personality Change Due to Temporal Lobe Epilepsy; also code the general medical condition on Axis III.

Discussion

DSM-IV (and DSM-IV-TR) Personality Change Due to a General Medical Condition replaces the DSM-III-R category, Organic Personality Disorder. To make a diagnosis of Personality Change Due to a General Medical Condition, the clinician must establish that 1) a personality change has taken place, 2) an identifiable general medical condition is present, and 3) the change in personality is related to the direct physiological effects of the general medical condition. Each part of this connection can be difficult to establish. It is not always clear what represents a change in functioning or, in children, whether they have failed to achieve developmental steps they might otherwise have been expected to make. The clinician must rule out other possible causes of personality change (e.g., exposure to extreme psychosocial stressors resulting in Acute Stress or Posttraumatic Stress Disorder); the presence of another mental disorder such as Major Depressive Disorder or Panic Disorder, which may increase dependency and avoidant behavior; or Substance Abuse or Dependence.

There has clearly been a personality change in Eric that appears to have been a response to the severe head trauma. The more interesting, and perhaps unanswerable, question is whether the development of the Attention-Deficit/Hyperactivity Disorder is also related to the trauma or would have occurred anyway. One factor that may help to make this determination is family history (e.g., Eric's elder brother was diagnosed as being hyperactive several years earlier). However, Eric's behavioral problems and changes in attitude toward his mother started almost immediately after he recovered from the very severe head trauma he suffered in the car accident, which would seem to indicate that the development of the Attention-Deficit/Hyperactivity Disorder was related to the head trauma. Therefore, although it is impossible to be absolutely certain, it seems appropriate to diagnose both Personality Change Due to a Head Trauma and Attention-Deficit/Hyperactivity Disorder. This will help to direct attention to the etiological general medical condition, which can be crucial when there are reversible or untreated aspects of it that require attention.

The following different types of personality change are described in DSM-IV-TR: labile, disinhibited, aggressive, apathetic, paranoid, other, combined, and unspecified. These different presentations may require different kinds of management and treatment. Appropriate treatment may involve psychotherapy, medication, or environmental manipulation.

One caution: the clinician should recognize that there is a tendency to attribute all problems to traumatic events whenever such events are present in the history of the patient. It is possible that Eric would have developed Attention-Deficit/Hyperactivity Disorder even if he had never suffered the head trauma.

❖   Case Study: Trouble Doing Tax Shelters

Mr. B, a 62-year-old married tax attorney, is referred for inpatient evaluation of what the referring psychiatrist labeled a "treatment-resistant depression." Mr. B complains of poor appetite, with a 30-pound weight loss over a period of a year, difficulty falling asleep and early morning awakenings, pervasive feelings of sadness and hopelessness, and recurrent thoughts of death and suicide. Both the patient and his wife trace the onset of his illness to 14 months before this admission, when he first experienced work-related difficulties, including decreased motivation, diminished self-confidence, and fatigue while performing his high-pressure job in a New York City law firm.

On focused inquiry, however, Mr. B recalls that he had experienced conceptual and cognitive problems before the problems of diminished interest and self-esteem occurred. He says, "I found myself unable to design and negotiate the intricate tax shelters that are my specialty. I couldn't keep track of all the facts and factors that for years had been second nature to me. Even the mathematics of my job—which is relatively simple and straightforward—have become impossible for me to handle." Further questioning also reveals that Mr. B has been having increasing difficulty accomplishing the minor household repairs and the mechanical work on his car that he previously managed without difficulty. On numerous occasions, he has also missed appointments, misplaced documents, and lost his keys and eye glasses. He seems unable to keep order in what was previously a very well-ordered life.

Mr. B's wife was at first angered and frustrated by what she felt was her husband's "pure indolence and disinterest." Later, however, when Mr. B became increasingly tearful, unwilling to go to work and, finally, reluctant to get out of bed, she insisted that he seek psychiatric help. Mr. B's outpatient psychiatrist felt that he was depressed and initiated twice-a-week psychotherapy and low initial doses of amitriptyline. When the patient and his wife both associated a marked increase in his lethargy and confusion with the antidepressant, the amitriptyline was replaced with imipramine, also in low doses.

Despite Mr. B's increasing confusion and incoherence, the psychiatrist increased the daily dosage to 300 mg, reasoning that the patient's cognitive changes and clouding of sensorium were more likely related to depressive symptomatology than to the side effects of the tricyclic medication. In addition, the patient developed difficulty in starting urination and emptying his bladder. Eight months after the onset of symptoms, Mr. B is referred for this inpatient evaluation, with a recommendation that electroconvulsive therapy might be considered.

The most significant new information gleaned from the psychiatric history taken from inpatient admission is that Mr. B's cognitive impairments antedated the emergence of his affective symptoms. He began having difficulty remembering details of the contracts he was working on, missing appointments, and misplacing important papers more than a year before the affective symptoms developed. His partners noted an increased distractibility and reduced capacity for strategic planning. As a result of his numerous mistakes, a number of important clients had left his firm. Mr. B's physical and neurological history and examination are negative. However, magnetic resonance imaging (MRI) shows diffuse loss of cortical tissue in the patient.

Mr. B is switched from imipramine to a selective serotonin reuptake inhibitor. He receives intensive psychotherapy related to his poor job performance and family problems that is focused on decreasing his burden of responsibility. His wife also begins family counseling. Mr. B's mood begins to improve progressively after 1 week of hospitalization. He becomes more alert; his mood, sleep, and appetite improve; and family relationships become more positive and amicable.

Mr. B is released after a 3-week inpatient stay. Because he is unable to regain his conceptual capacity for formulating intricate tax shelters and shows a persistently impaired capacity to recall mathematical data, he is reassigned to less complex and demanding tasks within his law firm.

DSM-IV-TR Diagnosis

Axis I:	294.10	Dementia of the Alzheimer's Type, With Early Onset, With Depressed Mood
	293.83	Mood Disorder Due to Alzheimer's Disease, With Depressive Features
Axis II:	V71.09	No diagnosis
Axis III:	331.0	Alzheimer's disease
Axis IV:	Onset of a serious disabling illness in the context of high-pressure work responsibilities	
Axis V:	GAF = 45 (past year); GAF = 60 (current)	

Discussion

Mr. B's situation presents one of the most common and complex differential diagnostic distinctions: Is the individual's depression causing symptoms of "pseudodementia" or is the depression an early symptom of the dementia? Part of the confusion arises from the terms used to describe the major categories of disorders—they are necessarily simplified and do not do justice to the full range of psychopathology that is characteristic of each. Thus the Mood Disorders, although characterized by mood symptoms as the predominant complaint, are also frequently accompanied by cognitive impairment resembling that seen in dementia or psychotic symptoms such as those seen in Schizophrenia. At the same time, dementia, although most prominently a cognitive disorder, is also frequently accompanied by mood and psychotic symptoms. In any given clinical situation, particularly with late-onset depressions, it is crucial to thoroughly evaluate the possible contribution of both

Mood Disorder and dementia. Not infrequently, late-onset depression may be accompanied by brain changes that may be visible on sophisticated MRI. Because Mr. B's cognitive deficits preceded the onset of the depressive symptoms and persisted even after the depression improved, Dementia With Depressed Mood seems to be the appropriate diagnosis. Although Mr. B is obviously experiencing a clear-cut and significant impairment in memory and executive functioning, he is still able to function in his demanding job because of his previous high level of performance.

❖ Case Study: Hard to Call

Mr. M is 26 years old, single, and unemployed. He has a 6-year history of psychotic illness and is being treated in the aftercare program of a university hospital. He lives in a supervised apartment and is supported by Supplemental Security Income and Medicaid. The staff, frustrated by Mr. M's limited gains despite their active psychopharmacological and rehabilitative interventions, have prompted his presentation at a grand rounds for review and reassessment. Mr. M remains partly symptomatic and cannot function either vocationally or in peer relationships. Nevertheless, he and his parents continue to expect that he will become "normal" and be able to work.

As a child, Mr. M manifested a peculiar detached manner and consequently had trouble forming friendships. When he was 12, psychiatric consultation revealed a "personality problem." When he was 13, Mr. M's mother was diagnosed with cancer, and she died after 3 years of debilitating illness. During this period, Mr. M began weekly psychiatric treatment that continued for 5 years.

Despite declining school performance, Mr. M graduated from high school at age 18 and started college. He failed all his first-semester courses and returned home where he was socially isolated and unemployed. When he was 19 years old, a new psychiatrist diagnosed Mr. M with "borderline schizophrenia." Psychological testing suggested "incipient psychosis" in a "passive-aggressive individual with high anxiety and marked passive-dependency needs."

Mr. M's first psychotic episode and hospitalization occurred when he was 20, within a week of his father's remarriage. He had delusions of grandeur, insisting he could fly, and became sexually preoccupied and aggressive. Mental status examination revealed a suspicious, agitated man with inappropriate and blunted affect and thought processes characterized by derailment and racing. He felt that he could read minds and that sometimes his thoughts were not his own. He had vague suicidal and homicidal ideation without suicidal intent. Chlorpromazine 400 mg/day was prescribed. Mr. M's symptoms improved somewhat, and he was discharged after $3\frac{1}{2}$ weeks. The diagnostic impression at that time was Paranoid Schizophrenia.

Mr. M returned home to his family, began treatment with a new private psychiatrist, and entered a rehabilitative day hospital program and family therapy. At home, Mr. M had a very sheltered, undemanding role characterized by parental overinvolvement, protectiveness, and infantilization. For the next 2 years in the day program, he was socially isolated, had poor concentration, and frequently displayed provocative and intrusive behavior and depressive symptoms. Although Mr. M's parents were critical of his poor performance, they also showed strong denial about his degree of dysfunction.

When he was 22, his stepmother gave birth to a son. Mr. M's symptoms grew worse, and his parents decided to place him in an out-of-state residential program. Soon after, he had a second florid psychotic decompensation and was hospitalized in a condition similar to his first episode.

Mr. M was treated with an average of 40 mg/day of haloperidol and improved slightly. Because of the manic features in his presentation, his diagnosis was changed to Schizoaffective Disorder. He was started on lithium and soon grew more subdued and better able to focus. He had a more appropriate affect and was less hypersexual and delusional, although decreased concentration and intermittent childish impulsivity persisted.

After 2 months, Mr. M was discharged on haloperidol (10 mg/day) and lithium (900 mg/day). His lithium level was stable at 1 mEq/L. He was placed in a supervised apartment program and continued in the day program. He also continued outpatient treatment with his inpatient resident physician and over the next 2 years was maintained on low doses of haloperidol (5–10 mg/day) and lithium (900 mg/day). Although periodically symptomatic, he was never overtly psychotic.

Despite extensive work rehabilitation programs, Mr. M's prevocational and social functioning remained marginal. At age 23, he was referred to a new day program for ongoing social and vocational rehabilitation while continuing in the hospital's outpatient clinic, an "alumni group," and a family group with his parents.

Several months later, Mr. M was reassigned to a new female resident psychiatrist. The patient showed a resurgence of paranoid symptoms and would often call home for reassurance. Because mood symptoms were not prominent, the new resident reformulated the diagnosis from Schizoaffective Disorder to chronic Paranoid Schizophrenia. Haloperidol was increased from 5–20 mg/day, and lithium was discontinued without any evident change in symptoms.

Five months later, Mr. M's paranoid symptoms increased again despite the additional haloperidol. This development convinced another new resident to try a higher dose of antipsychotics, and the haloperidol was pushed to 50 mg/day. After 2 months, Mr. M showed minimal symptom improvement. Medications were switched from haloperidol to fluphenazine hydrochloride with moderate improvement.

Still another resident was assigned to Mr. M's case 4 months later. Mr. M continued to have "paranoid episodes" every 2 or 3 days, accompanied by intense anxiety. His stepmother noted that for the past 6 months his calls home had increased in frequency. He complained of being afraid to leave his apartment and showed suicidal ideation, which he denied. During these episodes, he usually responded to neuroleptic medication, support, and reassurance.

DSM-IV-TR Diagnosis

Axis I: 295.30   Schizophrenia, Paranoid Type, Episodic With
                        Interepisode Residual Symptoms (provisional,
                        rule out Schizoaffective Disorder)
Axis II: Passive-aggressive and dependent personality traits
             (premorbid)
Axis III: Childhood asthma, in remission
Axis IV: Unclear at present; in past, death of mother,
             father's remarriage, frequent changes in treatment
Axis V: GAF = 35

Discussion

The DSM-IV (and DSM-IV-TR) category Schizoaffective Disorder was included to describe individuals at the border between Schizophrenia and Mood Disorders, but it does not do this job well. It is hard to decide just how prominent mood symptoms must be before a diagnosis of Schizoaffective Disorder is justified. DSM-IV is fairly silent on this question, and there is a great deal of unreliability as a result. Although Mr. M's history has been characterized by partial remissions and exacerbations, it appears that this episode of illness has been more or less continuous since its initial onset 6 years earlier. He has periods in which his most prominent symptoms are delusions and hallucinations, some periods in which manic symptoms predominate, and some periods that are mainly characterized by the negative symptoms of Schizophrenia or by depression. This fairly common presentation at the border between Schizophrenia and Schizoaffective Disorder causes a great deal of both diagnostic and treatment confusion.

❖   Case Study: Nothing Ever Works Out Right

Ms. W is a 34-year-old woman, twice divorced, who comes to the outpatient clinic at the insistence of her boyfriend. She acknowledges being depressed but says that she was reluctant to seek help because she doubted it would do any good. For as long as she can remember, Ms. W has suffered from what she describes as a continuous depression. She feels that life is a series of hopeless struggles and disappointments, but she has never seriously contemplated suicide. She occasionally experiences hypersomnia and is modestly obese due to an excessive and uncontrollable appetite.

Ms. W has been dating her current boyfriend for more than 2 years and knows she wants to marry him but is nevertheless often stricken by doubts and worries. Her boyfriend broke up with his previous girlfriend the year before, but Ms. W continually suspects that they are still involved. She often drives by their houses to see whether she can catch them together and continues to do so even though the former girlfriend moved to another state. Once, after discovering an old love note in the closet of her boyfriend's bedroom, Ms. W was depressed to the point that she was unable to get out of bed for a week. She refused to discuss the note with him and remained very despondent for sometime thereafter.

Ms. W cannot understand why her boyfriend loves her because she considers herself unattractive and dull. She is often unable to enjoy their time together, even when they do things that she has been looking forward to. She gets the most depressed or anxious at these times, asks to go home, and then feels terribly guilty. She knows that if her boyfriend were not persistent, the relationship would have ended long ago.

Ms. W describes her relationship with her father as ambivalent. He punished both his children severely with a belt until they reached puberty, and, when he was drunk, he sometimes insulted and degraded her (e.g., calling her a "stupid slut" or "a waste of sperm"). Between drinking episodes, he could be very loving, affectionate, and remorseful. Ms. W was never quite sure whether what her father said when he was drunk was the alcohol talking or whether he was displaying his true feelings. It was apparent to her, however, that he preferred her older brother and regretted that he had a second child. Her father died of a heart attack when she was 17.

From ages 12 to 14, Ms. W had a sexual relationship with an uncle. The episodes occurred once or twice a week and progressed from her sitting on his lap through cuddling and fondling to masturbation and oral sex. It ended when he attempted intercourse, and she screamed in pain and fright. She always protested against these experiences but would eventually give in to his pleas, rationalizations, arguments, or threats of exposure. She was particularly fearful of what her father might do or say if he knew. However, she also felt ashamed and guilty ("I could have said no, but I never did"). She never told her parents.

Ms. W was an average student with no history of disciplinary or drug problems at school. Her school counselor suggested that her academic performance was considerably below her potential, but the patient felt that she was "at best a C student" and "got the grades I deserved." She had a few close friends and numerous interests. She was attractive, but shy and insecure, and had no serious boyfriend until she became engaged to be married at the age of 17. The marriage was called off 2 months before the wedding when she discovered that her fiancé was having an affair. She was willing to forgive him, but he wanted to end the engagement anyway.

The patient met her first husband soon after graduating from high school. She knew at the time that he was not the best choice. He was much older and had a history of poor employment and arrests, but she felt that a wife and family "would straighten him out." They were married for 8 years and had two children. The first 2 years were satisfying, but he became increasingly bored and began to feel trapped and eventually became physically and sexually abusive.

Friends and agencies attempted to intervene, but Ms. W continually rebuffed them. She acknowledges now that she should have left her husband, but at the time she did not find the situation to be as bad as others were suggesting, and she resented their efforts to end a relationship that she wanted to succeed. The marriage did end when her husband was sentenced to prison.

Ms. W then got her first job, as a waitress in a small bar, which provided little income. A friend offered her a better job, but she turned it down "because I don't like to accept charity." She enrolled in courses at a technical school to develop secretarial skills but failed to seek employment after completing the training because "I could never do it; I'm not the type of person they would hire."

She met her second husband at the bar, and he eventually got her a new job as a topless dancer. She found it demeaning, but "we did make more money, and I don't see how I could have refused him." He was not physically abusive or threatening, but he was verbally abusive and was an alcoholic. He divorced her after 2 years.

Ms. W met her current boyfriend, Mr. S, at a therapy group for relatives of alcoholics; she had entered the group at the request of her second husband during one of the times he was trying to abstain, and she continued attending after the divorce. Mr. S had no history of drug use or criminal or aggressive behavior. Ms. W found him to be the most supportive, reliable, attractive, and empathic of the men she had dated. Although she had wanted to marry her previous boyfriends after only about 2 months of dating, she continues to feel ambivalent and pessimistic about Mr. S after 2 years and more depressed than ever before, which led Mr. S to insist that she come to the outpatient clinic for psychiatric evaluation.

DSM-IV-TR Diagnosis

Axis I: 300.4   Dysthymic Disorder
Axis II: 301.9   Personality Disorder Not Otherwise Specified
                        (depressive or self-defeating personality disorder)
Axis III: None
Axis IV: Doubts about boyfriend
Axis V: GAF = 55 (current); 55 (highest level in past year)

Discussion

This type of presentation is commonly encountered in clinical practice and illustrates that it is often difficult to distinguish between personality and mood functioning. This was a source of considerable controversy in the DSM-IV deliberations. A criteria set for depressive personality disorder was developed and then tested in the DSM-IV Personality Disorder Field Trials. Somewhat surprisingly, this criteria set did not overlap completely with Dysthymic Disorder, but there was insufficient empirical evidence to include it as a separate category in DSM-IV. Instead, it is included as an example of a Personality Disorder Not Otherwise Specified, and a research criteria set is included in an appendix to DSM-IV (and DSM-IV-TR).

There was also considerable debate about the value of the construct of self-defeating personality disorder, which had been included in an appendix for future study in DSM-III-R. This proposed diagnosis was eliminated from DSM-IV because of concerns that it overlapped too much with the other Personality Disorders and the Mood Disorders and that it was very difficult or impossible to distinguish unconsciously motivated patterns of self-defeating behaviors from self-defeating behaviors that occur in response to an abusive environment or are associated with other mental disorders. Nevertheless, the construct of self-defeating personality disorder may be useful in specific cases, particularly when planning a psychodynamic treatment. The diagnosis may be coded as an example of Personality Disorder Not Otherwise Specified.

❖ Case Study: A Late Onset of Symptoms

Mrs. S is a 71-year-old widow who comes for psychiatric consultation at her daughter's request. The patient's symptoms began 10 months before this evaluation with episodes of difficult breathing, fear of having a heart attack, dizziness, palpitations, and trembling. Three months before this evaluation, she was seen by an otolaryngologist for an evaluation of the dizziness after her family practitioner made a presumptive diagnosis of Meniere's syndrome. The otolaryngologist found no inner ear damage, however, and diagnosed an Anxiety Disorder for which he prescribed a low dose of diazepam.

Mrs. S reports that the first episode occurred when she was getting ready to baby-sit with her grandchildren. She does not attribute the episodes to any life circumstances and feels that if she were the type to develop "nervousness," it should have occurred much earlier in her life when she had a young family to care for and a lot of financial worries. The panic episodes have occurred one to three times a month and on one occasion resulted in an emergency room evaluation for a possible myocardial infarction. The emergency room physician noted that the patient had a normal sinus arrhythmia with four or five premature atrial contractions per minute. Mrs. S was advised to reduce her caffeine and nicotine intake and to continue with the diazepam.

Since the onset of symptoms, the patient has reduced her social involvement, stays home most of the time, and is hesitant to drive by herself. During the evaluation, Mrs. S reluctantly admits that she feels discouraged and somewhat demoralized by her problem and the way it has restricted her activities. She feels unhappy because she can no longer function as the "rock" of the family, a position she has held since adolescence. She says that she has sometimes begun to wonder lately "what the point of it all is."

Mrs. S was the oldest of six children raised in a large immigrant family. When she was 13, her mother became seriously ill after a heart attack, leaving Mrs. S to care for the younger children and take over many of the household duties as well as care for her bedridden mother. She was 17 years old when her mother died.

Soon afterward, Mrs. S married a young man who was then drafted into the military, leaving Mrs. S to handle a move to a new house and the birth of their first child largely on her own. She says that her marriage was a happy one and describes her husband as a thoughtful but quiet provider. She enjoyed his "steadiness," reliability, old-fashioned manners, and the fact that he needed her. Throughout the marriage Mrs. S managed the finances of the family and made the major decisions. She worked throughout her adult life as a waitress and a secretary to supplement the family's income so that they could afford a college education for their two daughters. Mr. S died 2 years ago.

Mrs. S says that although she missed him very much, she thought she had done extremely well during the first 2 years after her husband's death. She feels that she has been a support and help to her daughters, who are now 43 and 40 years old and have two children each. Her youngest daughter has multiple sclerosis and is able to carry out only minimum household duties. A year ago, this daughter's husband had an affair with another woman, which led to an immediate separation and subsequent divorce. Because this son-in-law had been a great favorite of Mrs. S and had always been particularly helpful in doing household maintenance and handling other chores for her, the separation and divorce came as a great shock and "really hurt," although she claims her feelings were generated primarily by concern for her daughter's happiness.

An interview with Mrs. S's daughters indicates that they are both supportive of their mother. They wish that she would allow them to help her through her current emotional problems; instead, she portrays herself as totally independent, strong, and healthy.

DSM-IV-TR Diagnosis

Axis I:	300.21	Panic Disorder With Agoraphobia
	311	Depressive Disorder Not Otherwise Specified
Axis II:	V71.09	No diagnosis
Axis III:	401.9	Hypertension
Axis IV:	Death of husband 2 years previously, daughter's illness and divorce	
Axis V:	GAF = 50 (current); 60 (highest level in past year)	

Discussion

The most unusual aspect of this presentation is the late onset of symptoms. Most individuals with Panic Disorder have their first panic attack between their teens and mid-30s. An atypically late onset of any disorder should always alert the clinician to undertake a thorough workup to rule out the possible role of a general medical condition or a substance (in this case, caffeine and nicotine) or medication side effect. Elderly individuals are especially likely to have an underlying general medical condition; to be taking multiple medications; and to have difficulty clearing medications so that blood levels may become unduly elevated, resulting in psychopathology.

The relationship between Panic Disorder and depression is an interesting and variable one. Although Anxiety and Mood Disorders may develop in any temporal sequence, the picture described above, in which the anxiety symptoms precede the development of depressive symptoms, is most common. Depressive symptoms may often represent a kind of demoralization consequent to the sense of loss of control and inadequacy resulting from the panic symptoms and the avoidance that results from them.

❖ Case Study: A Panoply of Symptoms

> Mr. E is a 40-year-old recently married man who comes for psychiatric evaluation. He says, "I am nervous and worried about my health and afraid that this is affecting my marriage." He has had lifelong concerns about his health, but these became worse during his courtship and honeymoon. Mr. E's symptoms are legion. He has trouble falling asleep if the room is too dark or too light, if the sheets are cold or wrinkled, if he forgets his nose spray, or if there is any noise. He fears nightmares, nocturnal asthma attacks, or dying in his sleep. He often awakes from nightmares, typically of being chased or suffocated, in a panicky sweat. He worries that his lost sleep is shortening his life and ruining his work efficiency.
>
> Mr. E has always been anxious and worried. He expects the worst, dreads each time the phone rings lest it be bad news, and suspects that he

has a serious illness. He experiences frequent palpitations, shortness of breath, dizziness, and numb fingers and has had numerous physical exams and electrocardiograms. The negative findings of these exams do not reassure him. Mr. E is convinced that his doctors are withholding information, and he is determined to have additional checkups until his condition is diagnosed. He also has gastrointestinal flutters, frequent diarrhea or constipation, and occasional nausea and vomiting. His father died of heart disease and his mother of cancer, and he feels confident that he already has, or soon will have, one or both conditions.

Mr. E is also extremely anxious about his work. He is a stockbroker responsible for large financial transactions and cannot ever relax his concentration, even on vacations. He has also felt considerable performance anxiety about his recently more active sex life and has suffered from consistent premature ejaculation. There are many specific situations that make him intolerably nervous, such as waiting in line, sitting in the middle row of a movie, wearing a pair of pants a second time without having them cleaned, having dirty dollar bills, and so forth, but he manages to avoid most of these situations without great inconvenience. Mr. E has panic attacks at least every few weeks. They tend to occur whenever something new is expected of him, when he is forced to do one of the things he fears, when he has to give a talk, and sometimes for no apparent reason.

Mr. E is a very precise and demanding person who is difficult to live or work with (and to treat). He is controlling, self-absorbed, and maddeningly fastidious and meticulous. He did not marry when he was younger because of his very high expectations about the sort of woman he wanted to marry and because his constant worries and irritating habits are intolerable to many women. His wife has already begun to complain about some of his behavior, and he is afraid that she may leave him unless he is able to change quickly.

DSM-IV-TR Diagnosis

Axis I:	300.01	Panic Disorder Without Agoraphobia
	300.02	Generalized Anxiety Disorder
	300.7	Hypochondriasis
	302.75	Premature ejaculation, probable
Axis II:	301.4	Obsessive-Compulsive Personality Disorder
Axis III:	Physical disorders: not apparent; rule out hyperthyroidism and sympathomimetic abuse	
Axis IV:	Recent marriage and marital stress	
Axis V:	GAF = 60	

Discussion

This situation illustrates both the joys and the perils of the "splitter's" approach to classification that has informed the development of DSM-IV. That the patient's symptoms meet criteria for a number of different disorders should by no means be construed as evidence that these are independent disease entities, each with a separate pathogenesis. It must be recognized that the DSM-IV (and DSM-IV-TR) criteria sets are for the most part no more than descriptions of syndromes, without any presumption that separate disorders represent different disease processes. Mr. E's presentation would have been diagnosed as anxiety neurosis by Freud (who made as significant a contribution to the nosology of Anxiety Disorders as Kraepelin did to the nosology of the Psychotic and Mood Disorders). The DSM-IV splitter's approach of giving multiple diagnoses has the advantage of providing more specific and reliable information about the patient but the disadvantage of reifying what may be unimportant distinctions. The DSM-II (American Psychiatric Association 1968) "lumper's" approach, which provided a single category of anxiety neurosis, had the advantage of including under one rubric a variety of anxiety and somatic symptoms that often co-occur and seem likely to have a shared pathogenesis but had the disadvantage of losing information and presuming a greater relationship among symptoms than may be present. The DSM-IV splitter's system is very useful if the divisions are not reified and if clinicians realize that disorders may represent no more than descriptive building blocks for a diagnostic formulation. We would certainly assume that all Mr. E's anxiety, somatic, and compulsive symptoms are only different surface manifestations of a single underlying pathogenesis.

❖ Case Study: Out of Control

Sergeant D is a 35-year-old army cook who is brought to the psychiatrist by the military police because he threw a large butcher knife across the kitchen and narrowly missed killing his superior officer. He begins the interview tearfully and apologetically and says he must be going crazy.

The incident began in a seemingly trivial way when Sergeant D's superior mildly reprimanded him for burning the previous night's dessert. Although Sergeant D accurately remembers what happened next, he cannot explain it. He says that the criticism from his captain made him feel furious and misunderstood and that it was always this way and would never change: "It just wasn't fair and I deserved better." Sergeant D says that when he threw the knife he felt a sense of detachment, as if it was happening in a dream and to someone else.

Sergeant D has a long history of impulsive and violent behavior. As a child, he had great difficulty concentrating in school and was constantly playing truant, starting fights, and setting fires. He was unmanageable at home and finally was sent to a tightly structured military school, which settled him down considerably. However, the patient still had trouble with reading and arithmetic, and at age 17 he ran away from school to join the army.

The patient's military record has been blemished by many disciplinary actions. He has been fined eight times and reduced in rank three times. His offenses have included going AWOL three times, driving while drinking twice, hitting a superior officer, and instigating barroom fights. Sergeant D is ashamed of his record and of his behavior but feels he can't control his "short fuse." He recognizes that his behavior is aggravated by drinking, but he says he is unable to avoid alcohol. It is his long-standing practice to stay almost completely sober from Monday to Friday and almost completely drunk on weekends.

Since his tour in Vietnam, Sergeant D has felt even less in control of himself. During the Tet Offensive, he manned a machine gun while defending an encampment and killed dozens of the enemy during one 12-hour period. He acted in a mechanical and depersonalized way, but during the body count he began crying as he noticed how young the soldiers looked. There was no other immediate effect, but 3 weeks later he saw other dead bodies and began having battle nightmares, panic attacks, and intrusive guilty thoughts. He was given 3 days of evaluation and rest and was treated with benzodiazepines, and the symptoms disappeared. However, similar nightmares and intrusive thoughts continue to occur at irregular intervals, and he believes that he is now more nervous and violence prone than ever.

A warm, likable man, Sergeant D has many friends and is highly successful in attracting women. He has been married twice and has five children, but both wives divorced him because of his unreliability and unfaithfulness. He is an extremely able, energetic, and productive worker when he is not getting into trouble and was cited on several occasions for bravery in combat. Sergeant D's workup includes an electroencephalogram (EEG) and thorough neurological and psychological testing, which reveals no central nervous system pathology.

DSM-IV-TR Diagnosis

Axis I:	312.34	Intermittent Explosive Disorder
	309.81	Posttraumatic Stress Disorder, Chronic
	305.00	Alcohol Abuse
	312.81	Conduct Disorder (prior history)
	314.01	Attention-Deficit/Hyperactivity Disorder in partial remission

Axis II: 301.9   Personality Disorder Not Otherwise
                      Specified (impulsive personality)
Axis III: None
Axis IV: Reprimand from superior officer
Axis V: GAF = 40

Discussion

One of the weaknesses of the diagnostic system is its failure to adequately de-velop a nosology of impulsive and aggressive behaviors. This deficiency has probably occurred because aggressive individuals are more often incarcerated than hospitalized or treated as psychiatric outpatients and, consequently, the psychiatric research on such disorders is remarkably limited. Intermittent Ex-plosive Disorder is meant to be a residual diagnosis to be used only when there is not a better understood and more specific diagnosis that applies. It is unclear whether Sergeant D's current episode of violence is related to the delayed ef-fects of his wartime experience and Posttraumatic Stress Disorder or whether it would have occurred independently. The fact that these symptoms go back to his childhood is strong evidence that his impulsive behavior is not just a function of his adult experiences, although they may have exacerbated his aggressive ten-dencies. It must also be recognized, however, that claims about having Posttraumatic Stress Disorder symptoms are sometimes used in an effort to es-cape legal or other responsibility for actions. Sergeant D's description of his bat-tlefield experience and its consequences were compellingly vivid, however, and hard not to take seriously. Studies also suggest that individuals who abuse sub-stances have 10 times the risk of committing violent acts than those who do not. Sergeant D's Alcohol Abuse should certainly be a diagnostic and treatment tar-get.

The next two cases will be discussed together.

❖   Case Study: A Rocky Therapy

Ms. T is a 28-year-old operating room nurse who is seen in the emergency room after ingesting 15 tablets of meprobamate. Shortly after swallowing the pills, she induced vomiting. Now, after gastric lavage, she feels "terrific" and wants to go home.

Since age 12, Ms. T has been intermittently preoccupied with suicidal thoughts and has made three previous suicide attempts. Her state of mind preceding the event was characterized by intense anger and despair, pre-cipitated by her boyfriend's storming out of the apartment because he was fed up with her constant demands. Ms. T then called her psychiatrist and spoke to him for 10 minutes but found him perfunctory and not concerned enough about the extent of her suffering. As she took the pills, her thoughts were, "those bastards will be sorry when they realize what they made me do." Ms. T has a history of impulsive and self-destructive behaviors that go back to her early teens.

Ms. T had begun psychodynamically oriented, twice-a-week psychotherapy 9 months ago, following the breakup of one of her many stormy love affairs. For the first few months, her therapy seemed to be the solution to all her problems. She and her therapist discussed the meaning of her intensely pleasurable but ultimately disappointing relationships with men and were able to trace a clear line back to a similarly labile relationship with her father.

Ms. T is psychologically skilled and made rapid discoveries that clarified the roots of her feelings, thoughts, and behaviors. She was delighted that her therapist seemed so pleased with her progress and assumed that he regarded her with fondness as his best patient. It seemed like a promising treatment induction.

Then the roof fell in. Ms. T discovered, through a mutual friend, that her therapist was married, apparently happy, and had two children. She became increasingly jealous of his wife and preoccupied with wondering who the therapist would really prefer as a mate if he were given a choice. She discussed with him her many fantasies that they might marry or at least have an affair.

The patient's associations, dreams, and behavior were clear and focused enough to allow the therapist to make frequent pithy interpretations and to allow Ms. T to gain seemingly useful and affectively charged insights. Unfortunately, however, her desire to marry the therapist grew progressively stronger and was accompanied by a growing sense that he didn't like or prefer her after all. She accused him of treating her only for the money or the chance to play "mind games" with her. The treatment had been stuck in this bitter stalemate in the months preceding her suicide attempt.

Ms. T is now taking her suicide attempt lightly and treats the emergency room psychiatrist (a male) with a combination of contempt and seductiveness. She refuses to speak to anyone but "my own psychiatrist" and insists that he come to the emergency room to see her or that she be allowed to go home immediately.

DSM-IV-TR Diagnosis

Axis I:	309.0	Adjustment Disorder With Depressed Mood
Axis II:	301.83	Borderline Personality Disorder
	301.50	Histrionic Personality Disorder
Axis III:	None	
Axis IV:	Fights with boyfriend	
Axis V:	GAF = 25	

❖   Case Study: A Tempestuous Life

Ms. C is a 24-year-old woman who looks as if she is only 16 and sometimes acts as if she were 3. She can be tempestuous, fickle, manipulative, impossible to please, and is convinced that others are never doing enough for her. She becomes easily frustrated, especially in romantic relationships, and has already made half a dozen casual suicide attempts (so far with no harm done).

Although she is highly intelligent, makes a good first impression, and can be a very efficient worker, Ms. C's performance in school, work, and therapy has been characterized by fits and starts. She went through three prep schools and is a college dropout. She is working what she calls "below my station" as an office temporary because she has been fired from several jobs for insubordination. She doesn't feel that she can work at any one place and at any one thing for very long without becoming bored. She has been in and out of all sorts of psychotherapies since she was 17 years old, so far without showing any benefit.

Ms. C's course is characterized by periods of relative steadiness punctuated by stormy periods that are occasioned by her overreaction to the frustrations of everyday life, particularly romantic ones. Between these periods, she can be reasonable and responsible, but when she loses her calm "all hell breaks loose." Her strong, negative emotions, particularly anger, crowd rational thoughts out of her mind, and she becomes desperate and impulsive.

Ms. C comes in for the current consultation because she is disappointed with her current therapist, never wants to see him again, and is contemplating suicide. She began treatment with him several months ago, was initially very impressed with his manner and appearance, and seemed to be settling down and doing very well in the sessions. Two weeks ago, she learned through a friend that the therapist was married. In the next session, Ms. C felt that her therapist was being much less attentive to her and didn't smile at the end of the session. She felt rejected and angry and became convinced that he was "just like the others—an uncaring S.O.B." She went home and told her boyfriend that she was going to kill herself because "there is no love in the world."

Ms. C has never experienced mania, hypomania, or depression that lasted long enough to qualify for a diagnosis of Major Depressive or Bipolar Disorder. Her "downs" generally last only a few days and disappear "after I've blown off steam" or "when someone interesting asks me out."

DSM-IV-TR *Diagnosis*

Axis I:	311	Depressive Disorder Not Otherwise Specified
Axis II:	301.83	Borderline Personality Disorder
	301.50	Histrionic Personality Disorder

Axis III: None
Axis IV: Problems with her boyfriend, no permanent job
Axis V: GAF = 60

Discussion

The introduction of Axis II in DSM-III was useful because it called attention
to the Personality Disorders that were too often previously ignored. However,
the most common problem these days is the overdiagnosis of Personality
Disorders in patients whose symptoms are better attributable to Substance
Use, a Mood Disorder, or adjustment to a difficult situation. We cannot emphasize enough that, before making a diagnosis of Personality Disorder, the
clinician must evaluate the individual's long-term functioning to ensure that
symptoms had an early onset and a continuous and pervasive course. A diagnosis of Borderline Personality Disorder makes sense for Ms. T because of
the early onset of her symptoms and their continuous course. Nevertheless,
the presence of a Personality Disorder does not preclude, and may in fact predispose to, the development of Mood, Adjustment, or Substance Use Disorders that may exacerbate the patient's personality problems. For example,
Ms. T developed depressive symptoms in response to her disillusionment
with her therapist; however, they were not sufficiently severe to meet full
criteria for a Major Depressive Episode.

Some clinicians would emphasize the Axis II personality features in
Ms. C's presentation and would see the dysphoric symptoms as secondary results of the Personality Disorders. Others would regard the patient's personality symptoms as being secondary to a Mood Disorder, which has been
characterized as "hysteroid dysphoria" or "atypical depression" in the literature. DSM-IV (and DSM-IV-TR) includes the term "atypical depression" as
a specifier but requires that this be applied only when the patient's symptoms
meet criteria for Major Depressive or Dysthymic Disorder, neither of which
applies to Ms. C's depressive symptoms. ICD-10 has included a diagnosis
called "brief recurrent depression," which consists of frequent depressive
episodes, each lasting for only a few days. DSM-IV (and DSM-IV-TR) does
not include this as a separate category but does mention recurrent brief
depressive disorder as an example of Depressive Disorder Not Otherwise
Specified and includes a research criteria set for this proposed disorder in an
appendix for further study.

Although the distinction between Axis I and Axis II often serves a useful
purpose, these cases illustrates how, in some instances, it can be more confusing
than helpful. The distinction between Mood and Personality Disorders should
not be reified, particularly when considering cases that lie at the boundary be-

tween them and have features of each. Mood Disorders that have an early on-set and a pervasive impact on an individual's functioning are indistinguishable from Personality Disorders. The most useful diagnostic approach is to include all the Axis I and Axis II disorders that apply without any assumption about their underlying etiology or relationship to one another. Treatment should be based on whichever target symptoms are most distressing to the patient and most amenable to treatment.

❖   Case Study: Impossible to Tell

Mr. W is a 42-year-old man whom the police bring to the county hospital's psychiatric emergency service from a local hotel that serves as a publicly funded shelter for the homeless mentally ill. Mr. W is agitated but cooperative. He begins the interview by saying, "I just want to go out and find work today. Do you think I'll be able to do that? I don't want to go back to that hospital."

According to the director, Mr. W has been living at the shelter hotel for the past 18 months. Five days before this evaluation, he attempted to contact his mother, with whom he has been out of touch for 8 years. He could not reach her and began to threaten and assault people at the shelter. The police were called, and they took Mr. W to a nearby crisis clinic where he was put on legal hold because of his grave disability and the danger he posed to others. The clinic was full, and he was involuntarily hospitalized in a neighboring county.

After a few days, he managed to leave the hospital, hitchhike to San Francisco, and return to the hotel that had been his home. Although the shelter staff did not find him threatening or violent, they were concerned about his reappearance and called the police to take him to the county emergency service.

Little is known of Mr. W's psychiatric history. His only formal contact with the community mental health system was the episode 5 days ago. The shelter workers, extended over too many clients, have obtained no formal psychiatric history on Mr. W. They do note that he has been "decompensated and belligerent" for some time and that he has been setting small fires at the shelter for several months.

Mr. W gives a rather vague history but does say that he has been in psychiatric hospitals in the past, that he served in the Navy, and that he has worked. He claims to have lived at the hotel for 6 years rather than 18 months.

On mental status examination, Mr. W is cooperative and oriented in all spheres. He denies having hallucinations but appears preoccupied. At times he seems hypervigilant but denies feeling threatened in any way. His associations are not loose. His speech is slightly pressured but of normal tone, and he has a slight tremor in his legs. His short-term memory is grossly intact, but confabulations and wishes seem to be clouding his long-term memory.

DSM-IV-TR Diagnosis

Axis I: 799.9   Diagnosis deferred
Axis II: 799.9   Diagnosis deferred
Axis III: Deferred
Axis IV: Homelessness, unsuccessful attempt to contact mother,
            minimal social support structure
Axis V: GAF = 35

Discussion

Not infrequently, particularly in an emergency room setting, a patient may be a confused and confusing informant. There may be insufficient collateral information on which to base a presumptive diagnosis. All that we know about Mr. W is that he is functioning very poorly and has been behaving in a threatening and assaultive manner. We do not know whether he has been using drugs or medications; whether he is suffering from a general medical condition; or whether he has delusions or hallucinations, mood symptoms, delirium, or dementia. We know nothing about his earlier course or history, and no informants are available. It is better to acknowledge our ignorance in these types of situations than to go out on a diagnostic limb and perhaps do more harm than good. DSM-IV-TR provides a number of ways of dealing with diagnostic uncertainty, listed below from least specific to most specific:

799.9   Diagnosis or Condition Deferred on Axis I
799.9   Diagnosis Deferred on Axis II
300.9   Unspecified Mental Disorder (nonpsychotic)
298.9   Psychotic Disorder Not Otherwise Specified
[Class of disorder] Not Otherwise Specified (e.g., Depressive
          Disorder Not Otherwise Specified)
[Specific diagnosis] (provisional) (e.g., Schizophreniform
          Disorder [provisional])

Working on DSM-IV over the past many years was always interesting but sometimes somewhat dry and technical. In contrast, working on this book has been rather like having dessert, giving us the opportunity to see how the system works in real life. Although there is something very special about patient contact that can never be reduced to the written page, discussing actual cases was a welcome relief after dealing with diagnoses and diagnostic criteria in isolation. We hope that your study of the examples in this book has been as valuable to you as it was for us in learning how to translate DSM-IV (and DSM-IV-TR) into the reality of clinical practice.

Index